Esophageal Cancer

Nabil F. Saba • Bassel F. El-Rayes
Editors

Esophageal Cancer

Prevention, Diagnosis and Therapy

Second Edition

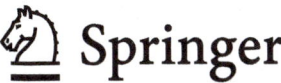 Springer

Editors
Nabil F. Saba
Hematology and Medical Oncology
Emory University Winship Cancer Institute
Atlanta, GA
USA

Bassel F. El-Rayes
Hematology and Medical Oncology
Emory University Winship Cancer Institute
Atlanta, GA
USA

ISBN 978-3-030-29834-0   ISBN 978-3-030-29832-6   (eBook)
https://doi.org/10.1007/978-3-030-29832-6

This Springer imprint is published by the registered company Springer Nature Switzerland AG
The registered company address is: Gewerbestrasse 11, 6330 Cham, Switzerland

In memory of Dr. Hanna Jean Khoury

To patients affected by esophageal cancer and their loved ones

Preface

Esophageal cancer is a major cause of cancer-related mortality worldwide. In the Western world, there has been a change in esophageal cancer presentation due to the rapidly rising incidence of distal esophageal adenocarcinoma. The heterogeneity of the disease and its aggressive clinical course has rendered the task of the development of an optimal multimodal management approach a challenging one. On the brighter side, there has been a noted surge in exploring novel therapeutic approaches in medical, surgical, and radiation therapy, including immune-based and targeted approaches, as well as palliative and nutritional supportive care.

Esophageal Cancer: Prevention, Diagnosis and Therapy, second edition, provides a unique and updated comprehensive review of the current epidemiology, molecular biology, staging, and treatment of cervical, thoracic, and junctional tumors. In addition, it highlights the differences in etiology, prognosis, and management of squamous cell and adenocarcinomas of the esophagus.

Promising novel diagnostic approaches and an in-depth review of cellular and molecular biology of premalignant lesions, the role of immunotherapy, as well as palliative and nutritional aspects are discussed in depth. We hope this second edition will further incite the interest of specialists from various diagnostic and therapeutic disciplines and will promote further research in the field of esophageal cancer.

Atlanta, GA, USA   Nabil F. Saba
                                                                      Bassel F. El-Rayes

Acknowledgments

The editors acknowledge

Anthea Hammond for editorial contribution

Nefertiti Hawthorne for communication

Contents

1   **Epidemiology and Risk Factors for Esophageal Cancer**............   1
Keshini Vijayan and Guy D. Eslick

2   **Cellular and Molecular Biology of Esophageal Cancer** 33
Alfred K. Lam

3   **Pathology of Premalignant and Malignant Disease
of the Esophagus**... 61
Jessica Tracht, Brian S. Robinson, and Alyssa M. Krasinskas

4   **Barrett's Esophagus: Diagnosis and Management** 83
Adam Templeton, Andrew Kaz, Erik Snider, and William M. Grady

5   **Chemoprevention of Esophageal Cancer** 113
Elizabeth G. Ratcliffe, Mohamed Shibeika, Andrew D. Higham,
and Janusz A. Jankowski

6   **Staging of Cancer of the Esophagus and
Esophagogastric Junction** 127
Thomas W. Rice and Eugene H. Blackstone

7   **Radiologic Assessment of Esophageal Cancer** 139
Valeria M. Moncayo, A. Tuba Kendi, and David M. Schuster

8   **Role of Endoscopy in the Diagnosis, Staging,
and Management of Esophageal Cancer** 159
Michelle P. Clermont and Field F. Willingham

9   **Principles and Approaches in Surgical Resection
of Esophageal Cancer**....................................... 185
Nassrene Elmadhun and Daniela Molena

10   **Principles of Radiation Therapy** 199
Neil Bryan Newman and A. Bapsi Chakravarthy

11   **The Multidisciplinary Management of Early-Stage
Cervical Esophageal Cancer** 221
Jarred P. Tanksley, Jordan A. Torok, Joseph K. Salama,
and Manisha Palta

**12   The Multidisciplinary Management of Early-Stage
       Thoracic Esophageal Cancer** 237
       Brandon Mahal and Theodore S. Hong

**13   The Multidisciplinary Management of Early Distal Esophageal
       and Gastroesophageal Junction Cancer** 251
       Megan Greally and David H. Ilson

14   Systemic Treatment for Metastatic or Recurrent Disease 275
       Daniel H. Ahn and Tanios Bekaii-Saab

15   Immunotherapy in Esophageal Cancer 289
       Megan Greally and Geoffrey Y. Ku

16   Palliative Approaches in Esophageal Cancer 311
       Baiwen Li, Shanshan Shen, Cicily T. Vachaparambil,
       Vladimir Lamm, Qunye Guan, Jie Tao, Hui Luo, Huimin Chen,
       and Qiang Cai

17   Nutritional Support in Esophageal Cancer 323
       Tiffany Barrett

Epidemiology and Risk Factors for Esophageal Cancer

Keshini Vijayan and Guy D. Eslick

Introduction

Esophageal cancer has a long and fascinating history and the epidemiology is geographically dynamic with wide variation from region to region [1]. There have been several recent publications reporting the global epidemiology of esophageal cancer. The majority of these published papers have used the International Agency for Research on Cancer (IARC) databases (e.g., GLOBOCAN 2012) data as the basis for any data analysis conducted. Esophageal cancer remains the eighth most common cancer worldwide, with 455,784 new cases in 2012, and it is the sixth most common cause of death from a cancer with approximately 400,156 deaths annually [2]. Figures 1.1 and 1.2 show the breakdown of new cases and deaths associated with esophageal cancer by gender and also comparing developed and developing countries. Future predictive models estimate that by the year 2035, the number of new cases of esophageal cancer will almost double to 808,508 and the number who will die from the disease will reach 728,945 individuals in that year, making it an enormous cancer burden globally [3]. In fact, it is one of a handful of cancers for which the number of new cases in some regions of the world is actually increasing [4], with average annual increase ranging from 3.5% in Scotland to 8.1% in Hawaii [5]. It is disappointing, given the increases in rates of esophageal cancer and the continued poor prognosis for this cancer, that it receives very little attention relative to other cancers; however, there has recently been a call for a greater research focus and funding for male-dominated cancers like esophageal cancer [6]. There is an urgent need for cancer research organizations to provide increased and dedicated funding to gain a greater understanding of the dynamic epidemiology of esophageal cancer. This will be crucial to determine the causes and risk factors associated with

K. Vijayan · G. D. Eslick (✉)
The Whiteley-Martin Research Centre, The Discipline of Surgery, The University of Sydney, Sydney Medical School, Nepean Hospital, Penrith, NSW, Australia
e-mail: guy.eslick@sydney.edu.au

© Springer Nature Switzerland AG 2020
N. F. Saba, B. F. El-Rayes (eds.), *Esophageal Cancer*,
https://doi.org/10.1007/978-3-030-29832-6_1

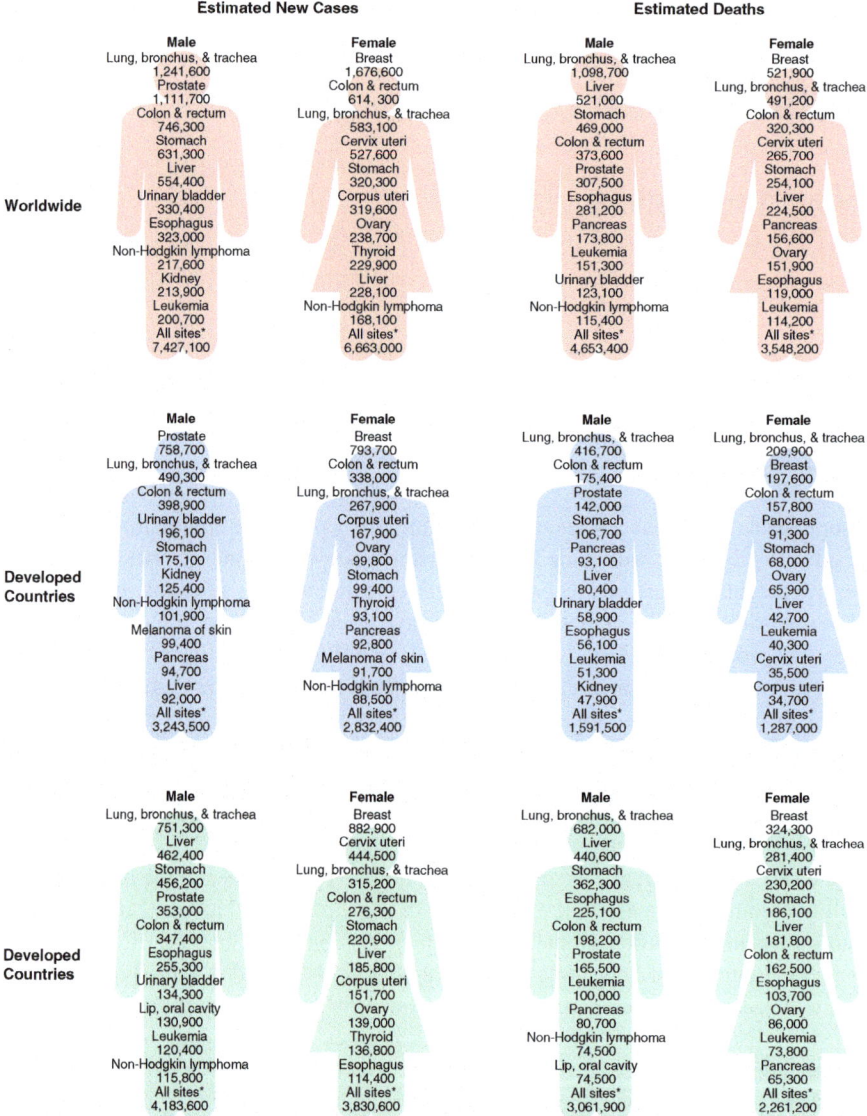

Fig. 1.1 The incidence and mortality for all cancers, note esophageal cancer

developing this lethal cancer and, more importantly, form the cornerstone of developing any prevention strategies.

There are two main histological types of esophageal cancer: adenocarcinoma and squamous cell carcinoma [7]. The epidemiology and risk factors for esophageal cancer vary substantially by these two different histological cell types. Published studies usually categorize esophageal cancer studies into either "adenocarcinoma" or "squamous cell carcinoma" histological types or a combined "esophageal cancer" grouping which contains both histological types.

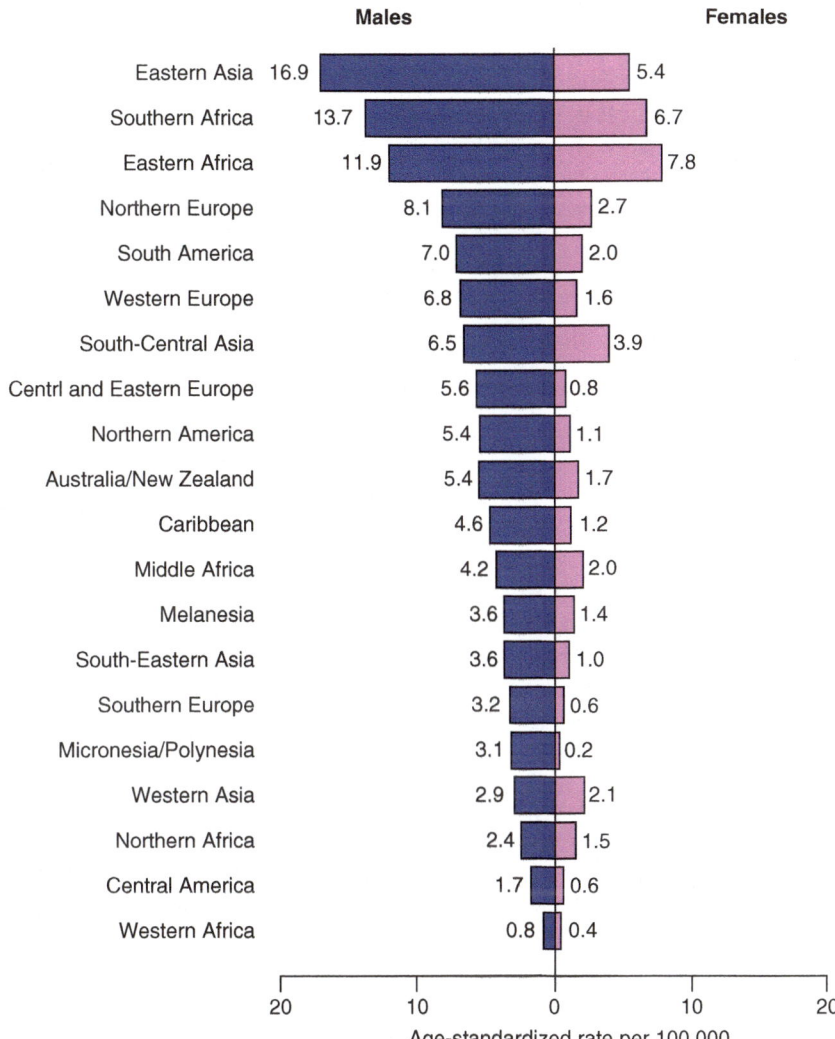

Fig. 1.2 Age-standardized incidence rates of esophageal cancer among males and females globally (GLOBOCAN 2012)

Epidemiology

Incidence

Esophageal Adenocarcinoma

The global age-standardized incidence rate of esophageal adenocarcinoma (EAC) was estimated at 0.7 per 100,000 (1.1 in men and 0.3 in women) in 2012, with 52,000 estimated cases occurring during the year [8]. The highest incidence rates were observed in Northern and Western Europe (3.4 in men and 0.6 in women), Northern America (3.5 in men and 0.4 in women), and Oceania (3.4 in men and 0.6 in women)—contributed to mainly by Australia and New Zealand—while the lowest rates were found in Eastern/Southeastern and Central Asia (0.6 in men and 0.2 in women) and sub-Saharan Africa (0.4 in men and 0.2 in women) [8]. The highest national rates were observed in the UK (7.2 in men and 2.5 in women), the Netherlands (7.1 in men and 2.8 in women), Ireland (5.4 in men and 2.9 in women), Iceland (3.9 in men and 2.7 in women), and New Zealand (4.0 in men and 1.5 in women), while the highest absolute incidence occurred in the United States, with 10,000 cases occurring in 2012, of which 88% were in men [8].

In the United States, there has been a disturbing trend in which the number of new cases of EAC has been increasing faster than that of any other cancer, and incidence data suggests that this increase commenced sometime in the mid-1970s. The reasons for this dramatic increase in EAC are multifactorial and complex and are not explained by known risk factors. Data from the National Cancer Institute (NCI) Surveillance, Epidemiology, and End Results (SEER) database have shown an increase in the incidence of EAC from 0.40 cases per 100,000 in 1975 to 2.58 cases per 100,000 in 2009, with an average annual percentage increase in incidence of 6.1% in men and 5.9% in women during the period from 1975 to 2009 [9]. Interestingly, geographic variability was observed in the incidence of EAC across the United States, with the highest age-standardized incidence rates observed in the Northeast and Midwest and the lowest observed in the South and West [10]. Likewise, the annual percentage change over the 10-year period from 1999 to 2008 varied widely, a 3.19% annual increase for men in the Northeast, in contrast to the 0.80% annual increase observed in the West [10]. The increase in EAC incidence is predicted to continue until 2030 with a plateauing trend, reaching 8.4–10.1 cases per 100,000 person-years for males and 1.3–1.8 per 100,000 person-years for females [11].

In Europe, increasing EAC incidence trends were observed in most countries during the period from 1980 to 2002, with the steepest increases observed in the male population in Denmark, the Netherlands, England, and Scotland, where the incidence of EAC has overtaken that of esophageal squamous cell carcinoma [12]. Overall, the age-standardized incidence rate in Northern and Western Europe was 3.4 per 100,000 for men and 0.6 per 100,000 for women in 2012 [8].

Esophageal Squamous Cell Carcinoma

Globally, esophageal squamous cell carcinoma (ESCC) is the more commonly occurring of the two histological subtypes, with 398,000 estimated incident cases in 2012 and a global age-standardized incidence rate of 5.2 per 100,000 (7.7 in men and 2.8 in women). The highest incidence rates occurred in Eastern/Southeastern Asia (13.6 in men and 4.3 in women), sub-Saharan Africa (6.4 in men and 4.0 in women), and Central Asia (5.9 in men and 3.6 in women) [8]. The highest estimated national rates were calculated for Malawi, Turkmenistan, Kenya, Mongolia, and Uganda [8]. The lowest incidence regions were North America (1.7 in men and 0.7 in women), Oceania (2.0 in men and 1.2 in women), and Southern Europe (2.4 in men and 0.4 in women) [8].

Approximately 80% of ESCC cases in 2012, or 315,000 cases, occurred within what is termed the "esophageal cancer belt," an area stretching across Central to Eastern Asia from the Caspian littoral region through Iran, Iraq, and Kazakhstan to the northern provinces of China [8]. Additionally, 210,000, more than half of all ESCC cases, occurred in China in 2012 [8]. This dramatic concentration of ESCC cases to this particular geographical area is likely to reflect local risk factors.

In China, 2015 data reported that esophageal cancer (predominantly squamous cell carcinoma) was the fourth most commonly diagnosed and the leading cancer cause of death for both males and females [13]. Data analyzed between 2000 and 2011 revealed that the incidence of cancer of the esophagus had decreased for both males (annual percentage change −3.2) and females (annual percentage change −5.5). Mortality rates also decreased for both males (annual percentage change −6.1) and females (annual percentage change −6.4) during this period.

In the United States, the national age-standardized incidence rate for ESCC is 4.93 per 100,000 in men and 2.30 per 100,000 in women [10]. In contrast with the trends observed in EAC, incidence rates of ESCC in the United States have been decreasing at a rate of around 3% per year in both genders and across regions, which has generally been attributed to a decrease in the practice of smoking [10, 14]. Figure 1.3 shows that ethnic variation exists within the United States for esophageal cancer rates. An excellent graph highlights the differences between States in North America in terms of both EAC and ESCC by gender (Fig. 1.4).

This trend has been mirrored in Europe, where ESCC incidence has been decreasing or stabilizing over the last several decades in most countries [10]. The incidence

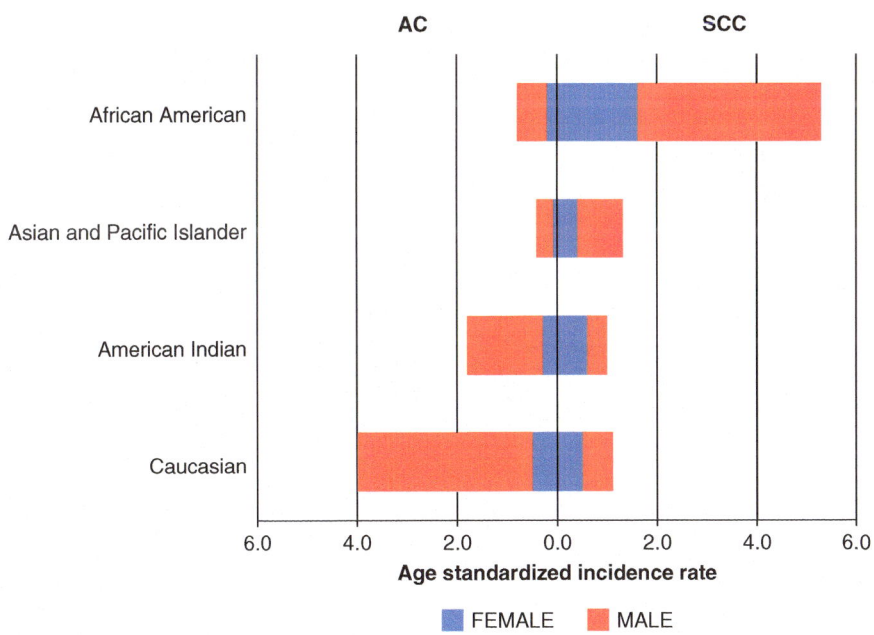

Fig. 1.3 Incidence rates of esophageal cancer in the United States by ethnic group

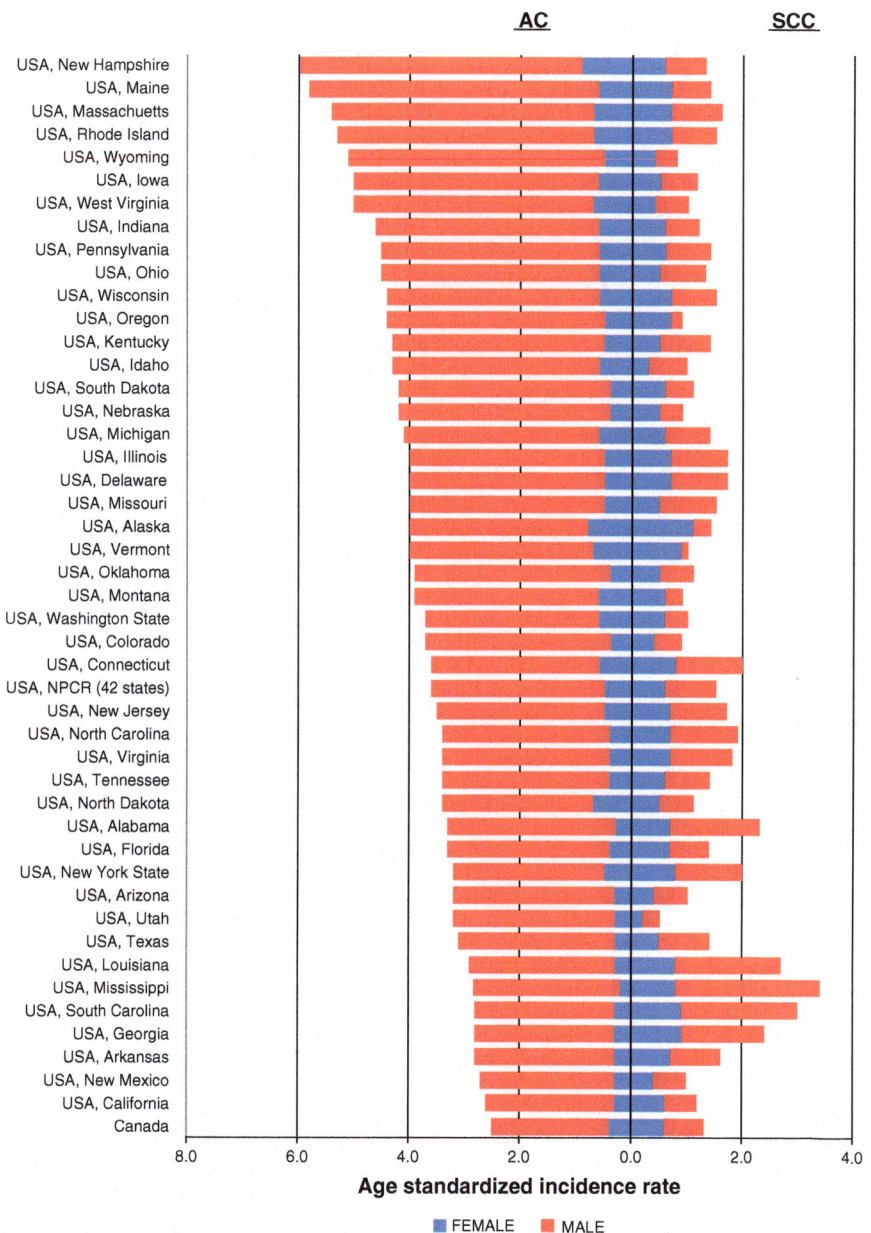

Fig. 1.4 Age-standardized incidence rates in the United States and Canada

rates in most European countries were between 2 and 4 per 100,000 in 2002, with the exceptions of France, which although experiencing a steep decrease in incidence over the last couple of decades still had an incidence rate of above 5 per 100,000, and Slovenia, which has not followed the trend and has actually seen an increase in ESCC incidence rates from just below 2 per 100,000 in 1980 to around 5 per 100,000 in 2002.

Mortality

In the United States, the estimated number of deaths from esophageal cancer in 2018 was 15,850, with a large male predominance (12,850 male deaths versus 3000 female deaths) [15]. The mortality rate from esophageal cancer increased from 4.67 to 5.44 cases per 100,000 during the period from 1993 to 2007 for white males and experienced only a minor increase from 0.76 to 0.77 in white females during the same period [16]. Esophageal cancer mortality rates are predicted to increase in the United States, with most of the deaths contributed to by EAC [11]. Cause-specific EAC deaths for years 2011–2030 are estimated to range between 142,300 and 186,298, almost double the number of deaths in the past 20 years, and EAC mortality rates are estimated to reach 5.4–7.4 cases per 100,000 person-years for males and 0.9–1.2 cases per 100,000 person-years for females by 2030 [11].

In EU, decreasing trends were observed for esophageal cancer mortality in males in a number of several southern and western European countries, and in central Europe mortality has also stabilized or declined since the mid-1990s [12]. In some northern European countries, mortality rates from esophageal cancer are still increasing, likely due to the continued increase in EAC observed in that region. Similar to the situation in the United States, the female mortality rate from esophageal cancer in Europe was comparatively low and remained stable or decreased [12]. Overall, deaths from esophageal cancer have declined in European men, from 5.34 to 4.99 per 100,000 during the period from 2000 to 2009. European women also experienced a modest decrease in mortality during this period, from 1.12 to 1.09 per 100,000 [12]. European mortality rates from esophageal cancer are predicted to decline to 4.46 per 100,000 men (resulting in approximately 22,300 deaths) and 1.07 per 100,000 women (resulting in approximately 7400 deaths) by 2015 [12]. Significantly, the predicted mortality rate for UK men is 8.51 per 100,000 by 2015, above the European average [12], which again is likely due to the expected continued increase in EAC incidence.

A recent analysis of esophageal cancer mortality data shows that Bulgaria and the Philippines have escalating rates of cancer death among females [17]. These results can be seen in Fig. 1.5, which also shows changes in incidence and mortality rates for other countries.

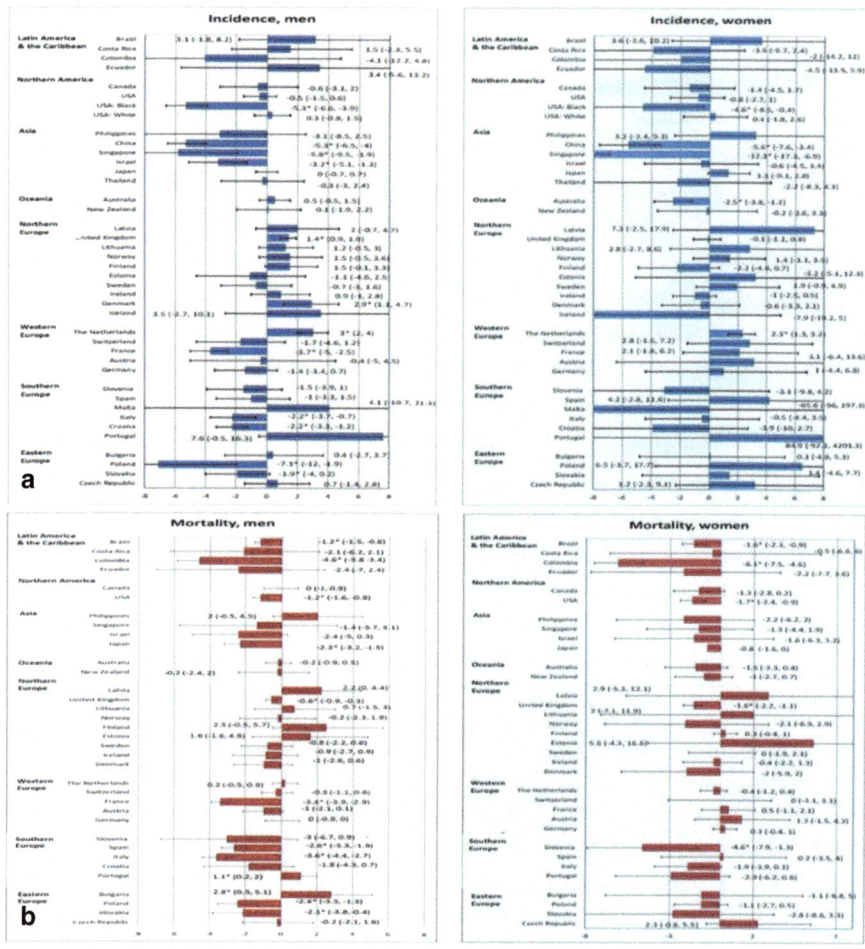

Fig. 1.5 (A) Incidence trend of esophageal cancer in males (left panel) and females (right panel). (B) Mortality trend of esophageal cancer in males (left panel) and females (right panel)

Survival

Esophageal cancer remains a rapidly fatal disease. The current 5-year survival rates are 19% in the United States [15] and 12% in Europe, with the highest European rate observed in Belgium (21.8%) and the lowest occurring in Lithuania (5.7%) [18]. There is generally no difference reported in survival between the two histological types, EAC and ESCC [18].

One study which did investigate EAC separately reported improved 5-year relative age-adjusted EAC survival rates in the United States since 1975, with the greatest improvement observed in cases with localized disease [9]. The 5-year survival rate in this group has increased from only 2.1% in 1975 to just over 50% in 2009 [9]. The 5-year survival for all stages of EAC in the United States has increased from just under 5% in 1975 to just over 20% in 2009 [9].

Risk Factors

An evidence-based approach has been taken with this section of the chapter. Where possible, meta-analyses or systematic reviews of the literature were used to summarize the current level of evidence for each risk factor.

Esophageal Adenocarcinoma

The risk factors for EAC are presented diagrammatically in Fig. 1.6 and are discussed individually below.

Age and Gender

The majority of individuals with EAC are aged 50–60 years [19]. The incidence of EAC has a strong male preponderance. Globally, the incidence of EAC was

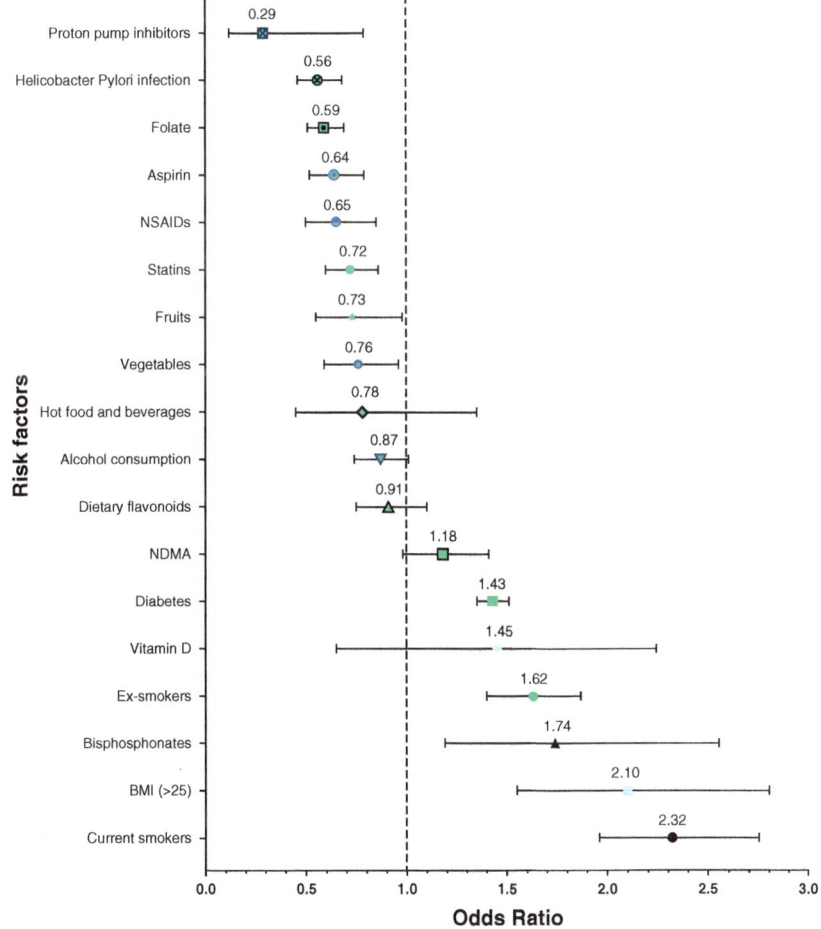

Fig. 1.6 Risk factors associated with esophageal adenocarcinoma

estimated to be 1.1 per 100,000 in men and 0.3 per 100,000 in women in 2012, a difference in incidence of over threefold [8]. The difference was most obvious in the highest incidence areas of Northern and Western Europe (3.4 in men and 0.6 in women), Northern America (3.5 in men and 0.4 in women), and Oceania (3.4 in men and 0.6 in women). Also striking are the predicted incidence rates in 2030, which are estimated at 8.4–10.1 cases per 100,000 person-years for males and 1.3–1.8 per 100,000 person-years for females [11].

Ethnicity

Several studies have found that Caucasians are more likely to develop EAC compared to ESCC. Most recently, two studies conducted in 2017 afforded further evidence that Caucasians had a higher risk of developing EAC. The first study compared Caucasian individuals to Africans, non-white Hispanics, Asians, Pacific Islanders, and Native Americans, concluding that Caucasians were more likely to develop EAC ($p < 0.002$) [20]. The second study confirmed this finding, reaffirming that the incidence rate of EAC was higher in Caucasians than in Asian and African ethnic groups upon analysis of the SEER database ($p < 0.05$) [21]. This study also suggested that molecular patterns associated with the relevant genes for EAC are similar between Asians and Caucasians (however, small differences do preside) and that these differences may be crucial in tumorigenesis and personalized treatment.

Eating Disorders

Obesity

A 2015 review found a consistent relationship in which patients with higher-than-normal BMIs had a higher risk of developing EAC compared to patients with normal BMI. Patients with BMI ≥ 40 kg/m^2 had a higher risk of developing this cancer (OR, 4.76, 95% CI, 2.96–7.66), compared to patients with BMI 35–39.9 kg/m^2 (OR, 2.79, 95% CI, 1.89–4.12), BMI 30–34.9 kg/m^2 (OR, 2.39, 95% CI, 1.86–3.06), and BMI 25–29.9 kg/m^2 (OR, 1.54, 95% CI, 1.26–1.88) [22].

As discussed above, there has been a dramatic increase in the incidence of EAC over the last several decades in many Western countries such as the United States, the UK, and the Netherlands. One of the contributing factors to this increase is thought to be the obesity epidemic, which has risen to prominence during a similar time period. Obesity is linked with gastroesophageal reflux disease (GERD) and Barrett's esophagus, a precursor lesion to EAC. A meta-analysis conducted in 2012 found a positive association between a body mass index (BMI) between 25 and 30 and EAC (relative risk (RR), 1.71, 95% confidence interval (CI), 1.50–1.96) [23]. The risk increased even further for BMI ≥ 30 (RR, 2.34, 95% CI, 1.95–2.81) [23]. The continuous RR for a 5-point increase in BMI was RR 1.11 and 95% CI 1.09–1.14 [23].

This is a consistent finding, with an earlier meta-analysis likewise finding an increased risk of EAC associated with a BMI of over 25 (males, OR, 2.2, 95% CI, 1.7–2.7; females, OR, 2.0, 95% CI, 1.4–2.9) [24]. A population-based study from Australia which included 367 EAC patients also reported an increased risk for BMIs of 30–35 (OR, 2.1, 95% CI, 1.4–3.1) which increased almost threefold (OR, 6.1, 95% CI, 2.7–13.6) for BMIs over 40, after adjusting for reflux [25].

Bulimia Nervosa

Historically, it has been proposed that the risk of EAC may be elevated in individuals who suffer from eating disorders like bulimia, caused by the acidic damage to esophageal mucosa in the process of self-induced vomiting [26]. A retrospective 2015 study reported seven cases that were hospitalized for anorexia nervosa, later developing ESCC (SIR, 6.1, 95% CI, 2.5–12.6), with a mean interval period of 22 years. However, this did not support the authors' hypothesis that patients with bulimia would experience higher risks of developing EAC, but the authors emphasize that it is premature to rule out an increased risk entirely due to the small sample size in their analysis [27].

Gastroesophageal Reflux Disease

Gastroesophageal reflux disease (GERD) is an important risk factor for EAC. A review from 2002 reported an increased risk of EAC associated with GERD, with the risk estimates ranging from OR 2.50 and 95% CI 1.50–4.50 to OR 16.40 and 95% CI 8.30–28.40 for individuals who had experienced GERD symptoms for 5 years or more, compared with asymptomatic subjects [28]. There was a very apparent dose response, with EAC risk increasing with longer duration, as well as with increased frequency of symptoms. In one study included in the review, the risk was increased by almost eightfold (95% CI, 5.30–11.40) for those who reported at least weekly symptoms of GERD. Severity and duration of symptoms appeared to act synergistically, with individuals who had experienced severe symptoms for over 20 years being 43.5 times more likely (95% CI, 18.30–103.50) to have EAC than asymptomatic subjects. Recall bias does not seem to have influenced the results, because the study also included ESCC subjects, in whom an association was not found between reflux and the risk of cancer.

A more recent population-based case-control study from Australia published in 2008 also reported an increased risk of EAC associated with reflux (OR, 6.40, 95% CI, 4.50–9.0) [25]. There was also an apparent synergistic relationship with obesity, with the risk increasing threefold between nonobese subjects with reflux (OR, 5.60, 95% CI, 2.80–11.30) and obese patients with reflux (OR, 16.50, 95% CI, 8.9–30.6).

Barrett's Esophagus

Barrett's esophagus is defined as a change in the distal esophageal epithelium of any length that can be recognized as columnar-type mucosa at endoscopy and is confirmed to have intestinal metaplasia by biopsy [29]. It is recognized as the precursor lesion of EAC and patients with Barrett's esophagus are 30–125 times more likely to develop EAC compared with the general population [30]. However, despite the alarming appearance of these figures, investigators have repeatedly concluded that in relative terms, Barrett's esophagus patients remain at low risk of malignant progression and predominantly die due to causes other than EAC [30–32].

In a large meta-analysis from 2010 consisting of 51 studies, Sikkema et al. [30] reported a pooled estimate for EAC incidence of 6.3 per 1000 person-years of follow-up (95% CI, 4.7–8.4), corresponding to an annual risk of 0.6% and a pooled incidence of fatal EAC of 3.0 per 1000 person-years of follow-up (95% CI, 2.2–3.9). The mortality rate due to causes other than EAC was 12-fold higher with an estimate of 37 deaths per 1000 person-years, as compared with the mortality rate due to EAC. Put another way, only 7% of the total number of patients died from EAC, while 93% died due to other causes.

A more recent meta-analysis from 2014 analyzed the incidence of EAC and high-grade dysplasia in Barrett's esophagus patients with low-grade dysplasia [32]. The annual incidence of EAC was 0.54% (95% CI, 0.32–0.76). A subgroup analysis looking at mortality from EAC included four studies and 318 patients with Barrett's esophagus and low-grade dysplasia. 4.4% of the patients developed EAC and 1–2.2% died due to the cancer, while 28.3% died due to causes other than esophageal disease.

Socioeconomic Status

There is very little information on the role of socioeconomic status in relation to EAC and the data is conflicting. A Swedish case-control study with 189 EAC cases and 820 control subjects aimed to determine the role of various socioeconomic factors in relation to EAC [33]. The data suggested that skilled manual workers were at an increased risk of developing EAC (OR, 3.70, 95% CI, 1.70–7.7); however after adjustment for tobacco smoking, BMI, and reflux symptoms, the result became nonsignificant (OR, 2.00, 95% CI, 0.90–4.50). There was also an increased adjusted risk for those who lived alone (OR, 2.30, 95% CI, 1.20–4.50). An earlier case-control study of 554 patients with EAC and 695 controls from the United States reported that there was an increased risk of developing EAC including junctional tumors among those with a lower level of education (<12 years); however, these findings were not statistically significant (OR, 1.3, 95% CI, 0.90–2.10; OR, 1.3, 95% CI, 0.80–2.00, respectively) [34]. The findings adjusted for age, sex, geographic center, BMI, smoking status, and alcohol consumption. A recent study which assessed sociodemographic and geographical factors in relation to esophageal cancer mortality in Sweden found that individuals with a lower education were at an increased risk (HR, 1.64, 95% CI, 1.11–2.38), as were those living in densely populated areas (HR, 1.31, 95% CI, 1.14–1.50) [35].

Occupation

A recent large cohort study found that men had higher risks of developing EAC if they were waiters (SIR, 2.58, 95% CI, 1.41–4.32), cooks and stewards (SIR, 1.72, 95% CI, 1.04–2.69), seamen (SIR, 1.52, 95% CI, 1.16–1.95), food workers (SIR, 1.51, 95% CI, 1.18–1.90), miscellaneous construction workers (SIR, 1.24, 95% CI, 1.04–1.48), and drivers (SIR, 1.16, 95% CI, 1.01–1.33). The same study found lower risks of developing EAC in men who were technical workers (SIR, 0.81, 95% CI, 0.72–0.92), physicians (SIR, 0.40, 95% CI, 0.16–0.81), teachers (SIR, 0.72, 95% CI, 0.57–0.90), religious workers (SIR, 0.75, 95% CI, 0.56–0.98), and gardeners (SIR, 0.77, 95% CI, 0.61–0.95). Among women, elevated risks for EAC were observed in food workers (SIR, 0.76, 95% CI, 0.31–1.57) and wait staff (SIR, 0.84, 95% CI, 0.40–1.55), while decreased risks were seen in teachers (SIR, 0.88, 95%

CI, 0.56–1.33), nurses (SIR, 0.79, 95% CI, 0.38–1.45), and assistant nurses (SIR, 1.02, 95% CI, 0.60–1.61). This study exemplifies that the risk for esophageal cancer varies with occupation; however the authors assert that the risk posed by most occupational categories do not differ according to histological type [36]. As such, a 1995 Swedish study found higher incidences of esophageal cancer in men that were employed in specific industries, including the food (SIR, 1.3, $p < 0.05$) and beverage and tobacco (SIR, 1.8, $p < 0.05$) industries, vulcanizing shops within the rubber industry (SIR, 4.7, $p < 0.01$), breweries (SIR, 4.2, $p < 0.01$), and butchery (SIR, 2.1, $p < 0.01$), as well as waiters, particularly employed in hotels and restaurants (SIR, 3.1, $p < 0.01$) [37]. It is important to note that some of these observations could be attributable to lifestyle factors like alcohol consumption and smoking, which are known risk factors for esophageal cancer. Occupational exposure to other risk factors of EAC could also render individuals of a certain occupation more susceptible to the development of EAC. Examining occupational exposure to smoke, an American study reported that firefighters are more likely to develop cancers of the esophagus, after adjusting for race (OR, 1.6, 95% CI, 1.2–2.1) [38].

Helicobacter pylori Infection
There has been conflicting data regarding the role of *Helicobacter pylori* infection in the development of ESCC and EAC. A meta-analysis of case-control studies reported that EAC ($n = 9$) risk was significantly reduced in patients with *H. pylori* infection (OR, 0.58, 95% CI, 0.48–0.70), which was similar for studies of *H. pylori* cagA-positive strains ($n = 6$) (OR, 0.54, 95% CI, 0.40–0.73) [39]. Another meta-analysis of case-control or nested case-control studies published in the same year assessed the relationship between *H. pylori* infection and EAC and ESCC [40]. The link between *H. pylori* infection and EAC ($n = 13$) was consistent with the previous meta-analyses (OR, 0.56, 95% CI, 0.46–0.68), as was the relationship with *H. pylori* cagA-positive studies ($n = 5$) (OR, 0.41, 95% CI, 0.28–0.62).

Diet

Hot Food and Beverage
A meta-analysis reported that hot food and beverage increases the odds of developing esophageal adenocarcinoma; however, the relationship observed was not significant (OR, 0.78, 95% CI, 0.45–1.35) [41]. A recent IARC report into the potential carcinogenic properties of very hot beverages found that there was limited evidence in humans for the carcinogenicity of drinking very hot beverages. However, there were a number of positive associations reported linking drinking very hot beverages and esophageal squamous cell carcinoma. The overall finding was that drinking very hot beverages at temperatures above 65 °C is probably carcinogenic to humans (Group 2A) [42].

Meat Consumption
Meat consumption and in particular red meat consumption is a known risk factor for colorectal cancer. A meta-analysis to determine the association between meat

consumption and risk of esophageal cancer analyzed 29 studies involving 1,208,768 individuals [43]. Any meat consumption was associated with an increased risk of developing EAC (OR, 1.53, 95% CI, 1.16–2.03), as was red meat (OR, 1.19, 95% CI, 1.08–1.33) and barbecued meat (OR, 1.23, 95% CI, 1.07–1.42). There was an increased risk associated with processed meat consumption, but it was not statistically significant (OR, 1.11, 95% CI, 1.00–1.23). Consumption of white meat (chicken) decreased the risk of EAC (OR, 0.87, 95% CI, 0.75–0.99), along with fish (OR, 0.79, 95% CI, 0.54–1.15) which was not statistically significant.

Fruit and Vegetables
Another meta-analysis of observational studies aimed to determine the association between fruit and vegetable intake and risk of EAC [44]. The analysis included 12 studies with 1572 cases of EAC and found that intake of both fruit (OR, 0.73, 95% CI, 0.55–0.98) and vegetables (OR, 0.76, 95% CI, 0.59–0.96) was associated with a decreased risk of developing EAC.

Minerals and Vitamins

Flavonoids
Flavonoids are a class of plant pigments, often responsible for the vivid colors of fruits and vegetables. Common dietary sources of flavonoid include black tea, orange and grapefruit juice, and wines. Historically, little or no consistent association was found for a possible relationship between flavonoids and esophageal adenocarcinoma. However, a 2015 study found that the intake of anthocyanidins, present in wine and fruit juice, reduced the risk of developing EAC (OR = 0.43, 95% CI, 0.29–0.66) [45]. A 2016 meta-analysis confirmed this finding, reporting that intake of dietary flavonoids reduces the risk of developing esophageal cancer, regardless of histological type (OR, 0.91, 95% CI, 0.75–1.10; $I(2)$, 0.0%) [46]. This was also reflected in another meta-analysis conducted in 2016, which compared patients of highest intake and lowest intake for total flavonoids and for each flavonoid subclass. It reported lower risks for developing esophageal cancers, regardless of histological type, in the intake of anthocyanidins (OR, 0.60, 95% CI, 0.49–0.74), flavanones (OR, 0.65, 95% CI, 0.49–0.86), flavones (OR, 0.78, 95% CI, 0.64–0.95), and total flavonoids (OR, 0.78, 95% CI, 0.59–1.04) [47].

Vitamin D
Most recently, a 2016 meta-analysis found a nonsignificant elevated risk for developing adenocarcinoma and vitamin D intake (OR, 1.45, 95% CI, 0.65–2.24). This meta-analysis also discussed the results obtained from one study that reported a decreased risk (OR, 0.49, 95% CI, 0.31–0.79) of esophageal adenocarcinoma in individuals who had a higher lifetime mean daily UV radiation exposure [48].

N-Nitrosodimethylamine (NDMA)
NDMA is a semi-volatile organic compound found in industrial waste and sometimes in very low concentrations in food, such as meats. A 2016

meta-analysis reported no significant relationship with EAC (RR, 1.18, 95% CI, 0.98–1.41) [49].

Folate

There is conflicting evidence regarding the role of folate in the development of upper gastrointestinal cancers. Evidence exists both implicating folate in carcinogenesis and suggesting that folate may reduce cancer risk. A recent meta-analysis of 9 studies and including 2574 esophageal cancer cases found high dietary folate intake to be associated with a decreased risk of any histological type of esophageal cancer (OR, 0.59, 95% CI, 0.51–0.69) [50]. The study also found a risk reduction for EAC (OR, 0.57, 95% CI, 0.43–0.76) associated with a high dietary folate intake [50]. These results are supported by findings that polymorphisms in genes involved in folate metabolism that result in lower circulating folate levels are associated with an increased risk of esophageal cancer.

Drugs

Sex Steroids

A recent study reported that higher levels of sex steroids may be linked with a decreased risk of developing EAC. As such, higher levels of dehydroepiandrosterone (DHEA) were associated with a 72% decreased risk (OR, 0.28, 95% CI, 0.13–0.64; $p = 0.001$). Similarly, estradiol was also associated with a 48% reduced risk (OR, 0.52, 95% CI, 0.29–0.93; $p = 0.03$) [51].

Proton Pump Inhibitors

Acid-suppressive medications such as proton pump inhibitors (PPIs) are commonly used in the management of GERD. It has been suggested that PPI use may decrease the risk of progression from Barrett's esophagus to EAC. A meta-analysis from 2014 based on seven observational studies investigated this possibility and found a decreased risk of EAC or high-grade dysplasia in patients with Barrett's esophagus taking PPIs (OR, 0.29, 95% CI, 0.12–0.79) [52]. There is no clinical evidence indicating that PPI therapy may increase the risk of neoplastic progression to EAC, and therefore if this finding is supported by further studies, it could warrant the use of PPI therapy in patients with Barrett's esophagus for its chemopreventive effects.

Bisphosphonates

Following a report by the US Food and Drug Administration of 23 cases of esophageal cancer between 1995 and 2008, which implicated the bisphosphonate alendronate as a possible causative agent, there has been an increase in interest and investigation into the potential for an increased carcinogenic risk associated with bisphosphonate use, particularly for esophageal cancer. However, several studies have subsequently reported conflicting results. A meta-analysis from 2012 of seven studies with 19,700 esophageal cancer cases did find an increased risk of esophageal cancer associated with any bisphosphonate use (OR, 1.74, 95% CI, 1.19–2.55) [53]. In addition, the study found the risk to be increased with longer duration of use compared with shorter duration (OR, 2.32, 95% CI, 1.57–3.43, versus OR, 1.35, 95% CI, 0.77–2.39) [53].

Nonsteroidal Anti-inflammatory Agents and Aspirin

A number of studies have reported conflicting results on the relationship between aspirin and nonsteroidal anti-inflammatory agents (NSAIDs) and esophageal cancer, especially EAC. A prospective cohort study and meta-analysis failed to find a statistically significant association between either aspirin (OR, 1.00, 95% CI, 0.73–1.37) or NSAID (OR, 0.90, 95% CI, 0.69–1.17) use and EAC risk in the results from the cohort study [54]. The meta-analysis conducted by the same investigators did however find a decreased risk of EAC associated with both aspirin (OR, 0.64, 95% CI, 0.52–0.79) and NSAID (OR, 0.65, 95% CI, 0.50–0.85) use. A more recent meta-analysis from 2011 likewise found a decreased risk of EAC associated with both aspirin (OR, 0.73, 95% CI, 0.65–0.83) and NSAID (OR, 0.84, 95% CI, 0.72–0.98) use [55]. The meta-analysis also found a reduced risk of EAC among patients with Barrett's esophagus associated with either aspirin or NSAID use (RR, 0.64, 95% CI, 0.42–0.96) [55].

Statins

Recently, a chemopreventive role for statins in esophageal cancer has been suggested. An early meta-analysis that included seven studies (n = 6895 esophageal cancer cases) found a reduced risk of esophageal cancer associated with statin use (OR, 0.75, 95% CI, 0.67–0.84) [56]. Moreover, a greater reduction was observed for a longer duration of use (OR, 0.45, 95% CI, 0.31–0.67), with no heterogeneity (I^2 = 0%, p = 0.79). There was also a reduction in the risk of progression to EAC in BE patients (OR, 0.56, 95% CI, 0.41–0.76), with no heterogeneity (I^2 = 0%, p = 0.93). Only atorvastatin and simvastatin showed a statistically significant reduction in risk, with OR 0.68, 95% CI 0.55–0.86, and OR 0.76, 95% CI, 0.66–0.89, respectively; no heterogeneity was present. Subgroup analyses for prospective and retrospective studies both showed a reduced risk, with OR 0.75, 95% CI 0.67–0.86, and OR 0.68, 95% CI 0.54–0.86, respectively; heterogeneity was not present [56]. A recent meta-analysis of 20 studies included 372,206 cancer cases and 6,086,906 controls [57]. Statin use was not associated with an increased risk of esophageal cancer among patients with Barrett's esophagus (OR, 0.59, 95% CI, 0.50–0.68). In addition, statin use was associated with a lower incidence of both EAC (OR, 0.57, 95% CI, 0.43–0.76) and all esophageal cancers (OR, 0.82, 95% CI, 0.70–0.88) [57].

Alcohol Consumption and Tobacco Smoking

The lack of a relationship between alcohol consumption and EAC is consistent across studies. No relationship between alcohol consumption and EAC was found in a recent large prospective cohort study from the Netherlands [58]. In fact, the lack of relationship between alcohol consumption and EAC was confirmed by a meta-analysis which included 20 case-control and 4 cohort studies (RR, 0.87, 95% CI, 0.74–1.01) [59].

Smoking, however, has been linked with EAC. A meta-analysis of 33 studies published found that compared to never smokers, there was an increased risk of EAC among current smokers (RR, 2.32, 95% CI, 1.96–2.75), ever smokers (RR, 1.76, 95% CI, 1.54–2.01), and ex-smokers, (RR, 1.62, 95% CI, 1.40–1.87) [60]. Similarly, in a large prospective follow-up study of 474,606 participants, current smokers were at increased risk for EAC (HR, 3.70, 95% CI, 2.20–6.22), as were former smokers (HR, 2.82, 95% CI, 1.83–4.34), when compared with never smokers [61].

Another meta-analysis found that the risk of EAC increased with greater BMI. However, after adjusting for other confounding factors, it was noted that there was a significant inverse relationship with drinking-years in those drinkers that consumed <5 drinks per day, who had particularly reported no acid reflux. Conversely, no such association was found for heavier drinkers [62]. In 2017, a meta-analysis examined the effect of water pipe smoking and esophageal cancer, without classifying the histological type of the cancer [63]. Water pipe smoking is a method of tobacco smoking originating from the Middle East that involves smoking a variety of flavored tobacco using a water pipe. Some modern terms that describe this type of smoking are shisha, hookah, hubble-bubble, narghile, and qalyan. The paper collected data from five case-control studies, reporting that water pipe smoking confers a significant positive association (OR, 3.63, 95% CI, 1.39–9.44) [63].

Metabolic Disorders

A recent population-based study reported that EAC is mildly associated with metabolic syndrome in elderly patients (OR, 1.16, 95% CI, 1.06–1.26) [63]. The association in males is linked to individuals without prior diagnosis of GERD; however, it was noted that in females, the occurrence of EAC was not related to GERD status [64]. Over the last 30 years, the incidence of EAC and diabetes mellitus has been increasing steadily in the United States. Investigating a possible association to explain this trend, a recent study found that diabetes mellitus is significantly associated with EAC independent of obesity, another known risk factor for EAC (OR, 2.20, 95% CI, 1.70–2.80) [65]. This was confirmed in a meta-analysis, reporting that diabetes mellitus conferred an increased risk for EAC (RR, 1.43, 95% CI, 1.35–1.51) [66].

Esophageal Squamous Cell Carcinoma

The risk factors for ESCC are presented diagrammatically in Fig. 1.7 and are discussed individually below.

Age and Gender

The incidence of esophageal cancer increases with age. The majority of individuals with ESCC are aged between 60 and 70 years, an older age group than for EAC; however, there are some specific groups that are at much higher risk very early in life (in their 20s) [19]. As with EAC, ESCC is more common in men than in women. The global incidence was estimated at 7.7 per 100,000 in men and 2.8 per 100,000 in

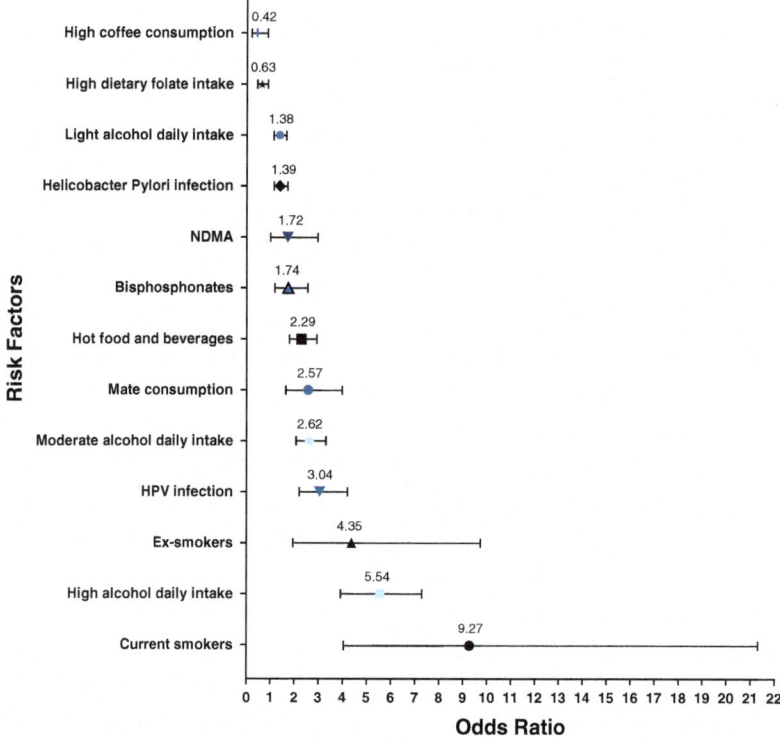

Fig. 1.7 Risk factors associated with esophageal squamous cell carcinoma

women. Again, as with EAC, the difference in incidence between the genders is most evident in the high-incidence region of Eastern and Southeastern Asia (13.6 in men and 4.3 in women) [8]. In the United States, the national age-standardized incidence rate for ESCC is 4.93 per 100,000 in men and 2.30 per 100,000 in women [10]. This difference is thought to be due to risk factors such as smoking and alcohol consumption which historically have had a larger male participation rate.

Ethnicity

A recent finding reported a higher incidence of ESCC in individuals of African descent compared to Caucasians. However, it also highlights that the racial disparities in this cancer have declined over time in the United States [67]. This observation was supported by another study that found the incidence of ESCC to be the highest among African-Americans compared with white non-Hispanics, Hispanics, or Asians, according to the SEER database. Additional analysis determined that the estimated incidence of ESCC in African-American men (at age 60) who consumed alcohol and tobacco (30/100,000) was relatively similar to the incidence of EAC in white non-Hispanic men (at age 60) with GERD (40/100,000) [68]. In another study, it was reported that ESCC rates varied in different Asian ethnic groups, but it was far more prevalent in both foreign-born and US-born Asian-Americans. This study reported that rates of ESCC were higher in US-born Asian men (4.0 cases per 100,000) compared with foreign-born Asian men (3.2 cases per 100,000) and Caucasian men (2.2 cases per 100,000) ($p = 0.03$). This suggests that there are genetic and environmental factors that come to play in the incidence of ESCC [69].

Alcohol Consumption and Tobacco Smoking

The distinct risk outcomes of alcohol consumption observed in EAC and ESCC are plausibly attributable to the varying pathogeneses between the two histological types [70]. The association between alcohol consumption, smoking, and ESCC is well established, as is the synergistic increase in risk that heavy alcohol consumption and smoking have on this cancer. A large prospective cohort study from the Netherlands consisting of 120,852 participants and published in 2010 found a greatly increased risk of ESCC in consumers of >30 g of ethanol per day compared with nondrinkers (RR, 4.61, 95% CI, 2.24–9.50) [58]. The RR for current smokers who consumed between 5 and 15 g of ethanol per day was 4.48 (95% CI, 1.97–10.20), and this increased in daily drinkers of 15 g of ethanol to 8.05 (95% CI, 3.89–16.60), when compared with never smokers who consumed <5 g/day of ethanol.

A recent meta-analysis specifically analyzed the effects of alcohol consumption and tobacco use on ESCC, both alone and in combination [71]. This study found an increased risk in nonsmoking drinkers (OR, 1.21, 95% CI, 0.81–1.81), though this was statistically nonsignificant, and in nondrinking smokers (OR, 1.36, 95% CI, 1.14–1.61). This increased to OR 3.28 (95% CI, 2.11–5.08) in concurrent smokers and drinkers. Studies have reported ORs as high as 50.1 for the increased risk of ESCC in the highest smoking and highest alcohol consumption group, compared with nonsmokers and nondrinkers [72].

Recently, meta-analyses have been conducted analyzing the dose-response risk of alcohol consumption on esophageal cancer, with particular emphasis on light and moderate alcohol drinkers, nonsmokers, and, in recognition of genetic polymorphisms involved in alcohol metabolism, different racial groups. A meta-analysis which included 40 case-control and 13 cohort studies found that after adjusting for age, sex, and tobacco smoking, there was an increased risk of ESCC associated with light alcohol drinking (≤12.5 g/day) (RR, 1.38, 95% CI, 1.14–1.67), which increased for moderate drinkers (12.5–50 g/day) (RR, 2.62, 95% CI, 2.07–3.31) and for high alcohol intake (>50 g/day) (RR, 5.54, 95% CI, 3.92–7.28) [73]. The association was slightly stronger in Asian studies for light drinkers (RR, 1.52, 95% CI, 1.06–2.19), but was weaker for moderate (RR, 2.52, 95% CI, 1.69–3.74) and heavy (RR, 4.31, 95% CI, 2.46–7.55) consumption. Among never-smokers, the risk estimates were RR 0.74, 95% CI, 0.47–1.16, for light; RR 1.54, 95% CI, 1.09–2.17, for moderate; and RR 3.09, 95% CI, 1.75–5.46, for heavy drinkers.

Another meta-analysis which also examined racial effects on risks of ESCC found that compared to nondrinkers, weekly consumption of more than 200 g of alcohol was associated with an increased risk of ESCC, and the risk was greater in Asian never drinkers (OR, 5.05, 95% CI, 3.40–7.49) than for Europeans (OR, 3.42, 95% CI, 2.29–5.09) [74]. This observation could be due to the effect of polymorphisms of genes involved in alcohol metabolism occurring more commonly in those populations.

Another meta-analysis examined the relationship between light alcohol drinking and various cancers by comparing light drinkers (defined as consuming $\leq$12.5 g of ethanol or $\leq$1 drink per day) to nondrinkers [75]. The study found a positive relationship even for light drinkers (RR, 1.30, 95% CI, 1.09–1.56) and estimated that 24,000 deaths from esophageal ESCC were attributable to light drinking in 2004 worldwide.

Tobacco smoking is also independently associated with an increased risk of ESCC. A large prospective follow-up study of 474,606 participants found that current smokers were at increased risk for ESCC (HR, 9.27, 95% CI, 4.04–21.29), as were former smokers (HR, 4.35, 95% CI, 1.95–9.72), when compared with never smokers [61]. The association was much stronger for ESCC in current smokers than the same study found for EAC.

Further evidence analyzing race-specific effects of alcohol and tobacco on the risk of ESCC also found an increased risk of ESCC, with the effect of current smoking versus never smoking being weaker among Asians (OR, 2.31, 95% CI, 1.78–2.99) than among Europeans (OR, 4.21, 95% CI, 3.13–5.66) [74].

Socioeconomic Status

The evidence for a relationship between socioeconomic status and ESCC appears to be much clearer than for EAC. In a case-control study, 347 male cases and 1354 male controls consisting of both African-Americans and Caucasians from the United States were compared in terms of social class [76]. Income was an important factor and those individuals with a low income (<$10,000 per year compared with those earning $25,000 or more annually) had a substantially increased risk of developing ESCC (African-American OR, 8.00, 95% CI, 4.30–15.00; Caucasian OR, 4.30, 95% CI, 2.10–8.70). Another case-control study from India compared 703 cases of ESCC with 1664 controls matched by age, sex, and geographic area [77]. After adjusting for ethnicity, place of residence, religion, education, fruit intake, vegetable intake, smoking status, hookah, nass, ever-use of bidi and gutka, and alcohol consumption, there was a strong relationship between occupations requiring physical activity and ESCC (OR, 5.65, 95% CI, 3.49–9.12).

Occupation

As noted previously, the risk of developing esophageal cancer based on occupational categories does not generally vary with the histological type of tumor. However, a study reported that among men, increased risks of ESCC were seen in waiters (SIR, 3.22, 95% CI, 2.30–4.38), cooks and stewards (SIR, 2.53, 95% CI, 1.94–3.25), seamen (SIR, 1.77, 95% CI, 1.53–2.05), food workers (SIR, 1.21, 95% CI, 1.03–1.42), miscellaneous construction workers (SIR, 1.39, 95% CI, 1.25–1.54), and drivers (SIR, 1.23, 95% CI, 1.13–1.34) [36]. As seen with EAC, lower risks for ESCC were observed among technical workers (SIR, 0.72, 95% CI, 0.66–0.79), physicians (SIR, 0.46, 95% CI, 0.27–0.74), teachers (SIR, 0.49, 95% CI, 0.40–0.60), religious workers (SIR, 0.59, 95% CI, 0.47–0.74), and gardeners (SIR, 0.72, 95% CI, 0.63–0.82).

Opium

This potential link was first reported in 1977 based on a 2-year clinical study undertaken in Northern Iran [78]. One potential mechanism by which opium may assist in esophageal cancer formation relates to papaverine (1% in crude opium) affecting esophageal peristalsis and causing esophageal relaxation and stasis [79]. This combined with micronutrient deficiency makes the esophageal mucosa vulnerable to carcinogenic attack. A case-control study was conducted in the Golestan Province in Northeastern Iran with 300 ESCC cases and 571 controls whose age, gender, and neighborhood of residence matched [80]. An adjusted analysis found that opium use was associated with a twofold increased risk of developing ESCC (OR, 2.12, 95% CI, 1.21–3.74).

Diet

Hot Food and Beverages

A comprehensive meta-analysis found an increased risk associated with the consumption of hot food and beverages and the development of ESCC (OR, 2.29, 95% CI, 1.79–2.93), which remained even after adjusting for the confounding variables like smoking and alcohol consumption (OR, 2.39, 95% CI, 1.71–3.33) [41].

There have been numerous studies assessing the level of risk associated with diet and nutrition in the development of esophageal cancer. Several recent evidence-based meta-analyses have determined the risk associated with various food groups and vitamins in relation to esophageal cancer.

Eggs

A risk assessment of egg consumption and esophageal cancer reported that among seven studies ($n = 2223$ cases), there was an increased risk (OR, 1.25, 95% CI, 0.98–1.61); however, this was not statistically significant [81].

Meat Consumption

A recent meta-analysis to determine the association between meat consumption and risk of esophageal cancer analyzed 29 studies involving 1,208,768 individuals [43]. The study found an increased risk of ESCC associated with the consumption of red meat (OR, 1.41, 95% CI, 1.24–1.61), processed meat (OR, 1.54, 95% CI, 1.06–2.23), and barbequed meat (OR, 1.33, 95% CI, 1.15–1.45). The consumption of white meat (chicken) (OR, 0.73, 95% CI, 0.65–0.83) and fish (OR, 0.66, 95% CI, 0.58–0.76) both conferred a protective effect on the development of ESCC.

Pickles

A relationship between Asian pickled vegetable consumption and ESCC has been suggested by experimental studies; however, the results of epidemiological studies have been inconsistent. A meta-analysis from 2009 sought to investigate the relationship and included 34 studies, of which 3 were prospective studies [82]. They found an increased risk of ESCC associated with the consumption of pickled vegetables (OR, 2.08, 95% CI, 1.66–2.60). The adjusted studies retained the positive relationship (OR, 2.15, 95% CI, 1.64–2.81). However, the subgroup analysis of the three prospective studies revealed a nonstatistically significant relationship (OR, 1.52, 95% CI, 0.82–1.63), illustrating the need for more prospective studies to confirm the potential relationship.

Tea and Coffee Consumption

A number of studies have investigated whether a relationship exists between the consumption of tea and coffee and esophageal cancer. The most recent is a large European study which included 442,143 participants from nine European countries [83]. The results showed a decreased risk of esophageal cancer of any type among current smokers who consumed high levels of coffee (HR, 0.48, 95% CI, 0.28–0.83), as well as a decreased risk of ESCC among current smokers who consumed high levels of tea (HR, 0.46, 95% CI, 0.23–0.93) and coffee (HR, 0.37, 95% CI, 0.19–0.73). There was also a decreased risk of ESCC in men who consumed high levels of coffee (HR, 0.42, 95% CI, 0.20–0.88). There were no statistically significant associations with EAC.

Another large study from Norway examined the relationship between coffee intake and oral and ESCC in a follow-up of 389,624 Norwegian men and women aged 40–45 years [84]. Using 1–4 cups per day as the reference level of consumption, the study did not find a statistically significant relationship, neither protective nor harmful, linking different levels of coffee consumption and ESCC.

A large follow-up study from the United States with 481,563 subjects, including 123 ESCC and 305 EAC cases, also investigated the relationship between hot tea, iced tea, and coffee consumption and risk of upper gastrointestinal tract cancers [85]. The only statistically significant relationship observed was an inverse association between high levels of coffee drinking and EAC for the cases occurring in the last 3 years of follow-up—the risk estimate for drinking >3 cups/day compared to <1 cup/day was HR 0.54 (95% CI, 0.31–0.92).

A Cochrane review conducted in 2009 investigated the consumption of green tea (from the *Camellia sinensis* plant) for the prevention of cancer and found no evidence that green tea consumption reduces the risk of gastrointestinal cancers, including esophageal cancer [86].

In addition, a recent IARC report into the potential carcinogenic properties of very hot beverages found that there was limited evidence in humans for the carcinogenicity of drinking very hot beverages. However, there were a number of positive associations reported linking drinking very hot beverages and esophageal squamous cell carcinoma. The overall finding was that drinking very hot beverages at temperatures above 65 °C is probably carcinogenic to humans (Group 2A) [42].

Minerals and Vitamins

Toenail Mineral Concentration

A recent study examined the concentration of selenium (OR, 0.78, 95% CI, 0.41–1.49), zinc (OR, 0.80, 95% CI, 0.42–1.53), chromium (OR, 0.9, 95% CI, 0.46–1.80), and mercury (OR, 0.61, 95% CI, 0.27–1.38) in a population based study and found no significant evidence asserting a correlation between toenail mineral concentration and SCC [87].

NDMA

Though NDMAs have not been proven to be significantly associated with EAC, evidence has been published suggesting that there is a significant positive relationship with ESCC (RR, 1.72, 95% CI, 1.01–2.96) [88].

Folate

A recent meta-analysis of 9 studies including 2574 esophageal cancer cases found high dietary folate intake to be associated with a decreased risk of any histological type of esophageal cancer (OR, 0.59, 95% CI, 0.51–0.69) [50]. The study also found a risk reduction for ESCC (OR, 0.63, 95% CI, 0.44–0.89) associated with a high dietary folate intake [50]. These results are supported by findings that polymorphisms in genes involved in folate metabolism that result in lower circulating folate levels are associated with an increased risk of esophageal cancer.

Diet-Related Inflammation

Chronic diet-related inflammation has been linked to increased risk of developing diabetes [89], heart disease [90], and obesity [91]. Several studies have detected a positive association between diet-related inflammation and ESCC. A 2015 study investigated participants with varying dietary inflammatory indices (DII), uncovering that higher DII scores (i.e., more pro-inflammatory diets) were associated with a higher risk of ESCC with the DII being used as a categorical variable (OR quintile 5 versus 1, 2.46, 95% CI, 1.40–4.36) [92]. This result was further supported by a study conducted a year later that presented significant associations for ESCC (OR quartile 4 versus 1, 4.35, 95% CI, 2.24–8.43) and EAC (OR quartile 4 versus 1, 3.59, 95% CI, 1.87–6.89) for individuals with higher recorded DIIs [93].

Maté Consumption

Maté is a tealike infusion made from the leaves of the perennial tree *Ilex paraguariensis*, which is native to Argentina, Brazil, Paraguay, and Uruguay. It is a popular drink in some parts of South America, where it is also variously also referred to as yerba maté, erva maté, chimarraõ, and cimarrón. The consumption of maté is suspected to be a risk factor for cancers of the upper aerodigestive tract, including ESCC. In a recent meta-analysis of nine studies, 1565 ESCC cases were analyzed to determine the relationship [94]. ESCC was associated with exposure to maté drink (OR, 2.57, 95% CI, 1.66–3.98). There was an increased risk of ESCC associated with a higher consumption of maté, versus low consumption (OR, 2.76, 95% CI, 1.33–5.73, versus OR, 1.84, 95% CI, 1.12–3.00).

Tooth Loss and Oral Hygiene

There is a dearth of data on the relationship between oral hygiene/tooth loss and esophageal cancer. A recent case-control study conducted in Kashmir on ESCC patients ($n = 703$) and matched controls ($n = 1664$) reported an inverse association between never cleaning teeth and developing ESCC (OR, 0.41, 95% CI, 0.28–0.62) [95]. There was also an association made with the combined number of decayed, missing, or filled teeth (3–4) (OR, 2.44, 95% CI, 1.47–4.03). The adjusted data suggest that the greatest risk is associated with an increased number of decayed, missing, or filled teeth.

There have been a couple of other studies which have focused on tooth loss in relation to risk of developing esophageal cancer. A study from China found an increased risk of esophageal cancer associated with tooth loss (RR, 1.30, 95% CI, 1.10–1.60) [96]. An increased risk of ESCC was also found in subjects in Iran who had 32 decayed, missing, or filled teeth compared with those who had 15 or less decayed, missing, or filled teeth (OR, 2.10, 95% CI, 1.19–3.70) [97]. In addition, compared with daily toothbrushing, practicing no regular oral hygiene resulted in more than a twofold increase of ESCC risk (OR, 2.37, 95% CI, 1.42–3.97). These results were not significantly changed when the analysis was restricted to never smokers. Another study also confirmed the increased risk of ESCC associated with tooth loss in two other regions, namely, Central Europe and Latin America [98]. The study found missing 6–15 teeth was an independent risk factor for esophageal cancer in Central Europe (OR, 2.84, 95% CI, 1.26–6.41) and Latin America (OR, 2.18, 95% CI, 1.04–4.59). An increased risk of esophageal cancer associated with missing teeth was also reported in Japan (OR, 2.36, 95% CI, 1.17–4.75) [99].

By contrast, a study from Finland found no statistically significant relationship between tooth loss and ESCC [100]. Likewise, a Swedish study from 2011 which included 6156 ESCC cases found no association between oral disease and ESCC after adjustment for diseases related to alcohol consumption (OR, 1.3, 95% CI, 0.9–1.9) or tobacco smoking (OR, 1.1, 95% CI, 0.8–1.7) [101].

Oral Cancer

Oral cancer and ESCC share similar risk factors, namely, smoking and alcohol consumption. The occurrence of primary oral cancer has been reported to increase the risk of developing secondary ESCC, based on a population-based study conducted in Taiwan over 28 years [102]. The study suggested that there was a bidirectional relationship between oral cancer leading to esophageal cancer and vice versa. Primary oral cancers were ten times more likely to develop a secondary cancer of the esophagus (SIR, 10.40, 95% CI, 9.35–11.53), and those individuals with primary esophageal cancer were seven times more likely to develop a secondary oral cancer (SIR, 7.31, 95% CI, 6.11–8.67). An Iranian study found that in its analysis of a possible relationship between these two cancers, a relatively high rate of opium abuse (9%) was observed in the patients affected by oral cancer [103]. There is some correlation between opium addiction and oral and ESCC, as opium is also a proposed risk factor (OR, 1.77, 95% CI, 1.17–2.68) for ESCC [104].

Infectious Disease

Viral Disease

A 2015 study found that HIV infection was correlated with the incidence of SCC (OR, 2.30, 95% CI, 1.00–5.10); however, it also noted that there is a more prominent risk in individuals under 60 years of age (OR, 4.30, 95% CI, 1.50–13.20) [105].

Another study that investigated 51 mucosotropic HPV types detected no such association between SC and mucosal alpha-papillomaviruses [106]. A meta-analysis reported that a prior HPV infection increases the risk of ESCC by threefold (OR, 3.04, 95% CI, 2.20–4.20). The authors also indicated that studies that were conducted in countries with low to medium ESCC incidence presented a stronger relationship with HPV (OR, 4.65, 95% CI, 2.47–8.76) than that in areas of high OSCC incidence (OR, 2.65, 95% CI, 1.80–3.91) [107].

Helicobacter pylori Infection

There has been conflicting data regarding the role of *Helicobacter pylori* infection in the development of ESCC and EAC. An early meta-analysis of 18 studies reported a decreased risk for ESCC in patients with *H. pylori* infection (OR, 0.85, 95% CI, 0.55–1.33) and a nonsignificant increased risk associated with *H. pylori cagA*-positive strains (OR, 1.22, 95% CI, 0.70–2.13) [108]. In addition, there was an inverse statistically significant association with *H. pylori* infection and EAC (OR, 0.52, 95% CI, 0.37–0.73) and for *H. pylori cagA*-positive strains (OR, 0.51, 95% CI, 0.31–0.82).

A meta-analysis of case-control studies reported that the level of risk for ESCC ($n = 5$) was decreased but not statistically significant (OR, 0.80, 95% CI, 0.45–1.43), but studies of *cagA*-positive strains ($n = 2$) showed an increased nonsignificant risk (OR, 1.20, 95% CI, 0.45–3.18) [39].

Moreover, in the same year there was another meta-analysis of case-control or nested case-control studies assessing the relationship between *H. pylori* infection and esophageal adenocarcinoma and squamous cell carcinoma [40]. When assessing ESCC ($n = 9$), the risk was increased but not statistically significant (OR, 1.10, 95% CI, 0.78–1.55), and the link with *cagA* studies ($n = 4$) was null (OR, 1.01, 95% CI, 0.80–1.27).

A more recent systematic review and quantitative meta-analysis aimed to determine the relationship between *H. pylori* infection and ESCC [109]. There were 40 studies that were included in the final analysis which included 3806 cases and 15,897 controls. The relationship between *H. pylori* infection and ESCC ($n = 17$) appeared protective but not statistically significant (OR, 0.82, 95% CI, 0.63–1.06). There was no evidence of publication bias ($p = 0.53$), but there was significant heterogeneity ($I^2 = 74.00$; $p < 0.001$). However, among those with *H. pylori cagA*-positive strains ($n = 12$), there was an increased risk of developing ESCC (OR, 1.39, 95% CI, 1.14–1.71; $I^2 = 0.00$, $p = 0.88$). There was no heterogeneity among these studies ($I^2 = 0.00$). This finding was further enforced by the strong relationship demonstrated in developing countries (OR, 1.70, 95% CI, 1.25–2.32). This meta-analysis identified a statistically significant relationship between *H. pylori cagA* positivity and ESCC, which had not previously been identified.

Medications

Bisphosphonates

Following a report by the US Food and Drug Administration of 23 cases of esophageal cancer between 1995 and 2008 which implicated the bisphosphonate alendronate as a possible causative agent, there has been an increase in interest and investigation into the potential for an increased carcinogenic risk associated with bisphosphonate use, particularly for esophageal cancer. A meta-analysis from 2012 of seven studies with 19,700 esophageal cancer cases did find an increased risk of esophageal cancer associated with any bisphosphonate use (OR, 1.74, 95% CI, 1.19–2.55) [53]. In addition, the study found the risk to be increased with longer duration of use compared with shorter duration (OR, 2.32, 95% CI, 1.57–3.43, versus OR, 1.35, 95% CI, 0.77–2.39) [53].

Conclusions

Esophageal cancer, while not a common cancer, continues to increase in incidence, with predictive models estimating cases of esophageal cancer to almost double to 808,508 by the year 2035, resulting in 728,920 deaths in that year from the disease. The two histological subtypes, esophageal adenocarcinoma and esophageal squamous cell carcinoma, differ in their epidemiology and risk factors by geographic region.

EAC has experienced a surge in incidence rates during the past few decades, most strikingly in Western countries, where incidence rates have increased up to six- to sevenfold during the period from 1975 to 2009. In Northern and Western Europe, North America, and Australia, its incidence continues to increase and is expected to plateau by 2030. ESCC is still the more common of the two histological subtypes, and in certain countries its incidence has stabilized or decreased recently. Approximately 80% of ESCC cases in 2012, or 315,000 cases, occurred within what is termed the "esophageal cancer belt," which stretches across Central and Eastern Asia, with more than half of all ESCC cases occurring in China.

Risk factors for the two subtypes vary widely. While both are more common in men, EAC is associated with GERD, Barrett's esophagus, and obesity, whereas ESCC seems to result from exposure to carcinogens and is associated with tobacco smoking, the consumption of alcohol and certain foods and beverages, poor oral hygiene, and a low socioeconomic status. Recent developments have included investigations into the effects, both protective and harmful, of different commonly used medications such as PPIs, bisphosphonates, and NSAIDs on esophageal cancer; studies looking into the impact of food and beverage subgroups such as meat, pickles, folate, and maté drink on esophageal cancer; as well as studies evaluating the effects of light to moderate alcohol drinking on esophageal cancer and how alcohol consumption affects the risk of esophageal cancer among different racial groups.

Esophageal cancer remains a rapidly fatal disease, with 5-year survival rates of 19% in the United States and 12% in Europe. Given its poor prognosis and that it is one of the few cancers which continue to increase in incidence, greater research focus and funding into this disease is urgently required.

References

1. Eslick GD. Esophageal cancer: a historical perspective. Gastroenterol Clin N Am. 2009;38:1–15.
2. Torre LA, Bray F, Siegel RL, Ferlay J, Lortet-Tieulent J, Jemal A. Global cancer statistics, 2012. CA Cancer J Clin. 2015;65:87–108.
3. Ferlay J, Soerjomataram I, Ervik M, Dikshit R, Eser S, Mathers C, Rebelo M, Parkin DM, Forman D, Bray F. GLOBOCAN 2012 v1.0, cancer incidence and mortality worldwide: IARC CancerBase no. 11 [internet]. Lyon, France: International Agency for Research on Cancer; 2013. Available from: http://globocan.iarc.fr, accessed on 12/06/2018
4. Simard EP, Ward EM, Siegel R, et al. Cancers with increasing incidence trends in the United States: 1999 through 2008. CA Cancer J Clin. 2012;62(2):118–28.
5. Edgren G, Adami HO, Weiderpass E, et al. A global assessment of the oesophageal adenocarcinoma epidemic. Gut. 2013;62(10):1406–14.
6. Cook MB. Optimization and expansion of predictive models for Barrett's esophagus and esophageal adenocarcinoma: could a life-course exposure history be beneficial? Am J Gastroenterol. 2013;108(6):923–5.
7. Scudiere JR, Montgomery EA. New treatments, new challenges: pathology's perspective on esophageal carcinoma. Gastroenterol Clin N Am. 2009;38:121–33.
8. Arnold M, Soerjomataram I, Ferlay J, et al. Global incidence of oesophageal cancer by histological subtype in 2012. Gut. 2014;64:381–7.
9. Hur C, Miller M, Kong CY, et al. Trends in esophageal adenocarcinoma incidence and mortality. Cancer. 2013;119(6):1149–58.
10. Drahos J, Wu M, Anderson WF, et al. Regional variations in esophageal cancer rates by census region in the United States, 1999–2008. PLoS One. 2013;8(7):e67913.
11. Kong CY, Kroep S, Curtius K, et al. Exploring the recent trend in esophageal adenocarcinoma incidence and mortality using comparative simulation modeling. Cancer Epidemiol Biomark Prev. 2014;23(6):997–1006.
12. Castro C, Bosetti C, Malvezzi M, et al. Patterns and trends in esophageal cancer mortality and incidence in Europe (1980-2011) and predictions to 2015. Ann Oncol. 2014;25(1):283–90.
13. Chen W, Zheng R, Baade PD, Zhang S, Zeng H, Bray F, Jemal A, Yu XQ, He J. Cancer statistics in China, 2015. CA Cancer J Clin. 2016;66:115–32.
14. Giri S, Pathak R, Aryal MR, et al. Incidence trend of esophageal squamous cell carcinoma: an analysis of surveillance epidemiology, and end results (SEER) database. Cancer Causes Control. 2015;26:159–61.
15. Siegel R, Miller KD, Jemal A. Cancer statistics, 2018. CA Cancer J Clin. 2018;68:7–30.
16. Jemal A, Simard EP, Xu J, et al. Selected cancers with increasing mortality rates by educational attainment in 26 states in the United States, 1993–2007. Cancer Causes Control. 2013;24(3):559–65.
17. Wong MCS, Hamilton W, Whiteman DC, Jiang JY, Qiao Y, Fung FDH, Wang HHX, Chiu PWY, Ng EKW, Wu JCY, Yu J, Chan FKL, Sung JJY. Global incidence and mortality of oesophageal cancer and their correlation with socioeconomic indicators temporal patterns and trends in 41 countries. Sci Rep. 2018;8:4522.
18. De Angelis R, Sant M, Coleman MP, et al. Cancer survival in Europe 1999–2007 by country and age: results of EUROCARE-5 – a population-based study. Lancet Oncol. 2014;15(1):23–34.
19. Dawsey SP, Tonui S, Parker RK, et al. Esophageal cancer in young people: a case series of 109 cases and review of the literature. PLoS One. 2010;5(11):e14080.
20. David YN, Vignesh S, Martinez M, Mcfarlane S, Kabrawala A. Eliminating racial disparities: esophageal cancer treatment and outcomes in a va healthcare system. Gastroenterology. 2017;152(5 Supplement 1):S880–1.
21. Chen Z, Ren Y, Du XL, Shen Y, Li S, Wu Y, Lv M, Dong D, Li E, Li W, Liu P, Yang J, Yi M. Incidence and survival differences in esophageal cancer among ethnic groups in the United States. Oncotarget. 2017;8:47037–51.

22. Elliott JA, Donohoe CL, Reynolds JV. Obesity and increased risk of esophageal adenocarcinoma. Expert Rev Endocrinol Metab. 2015;10:511–23.
23. Turati F, Tramacere I, La Vecchia C, et al. A meta-analysis of body mass index and esophageal and gastric cardia adenocarcinoma. Ann Oncol. 2013;24(3):609–17.
24. Kubo A, Corley DA. Body mass index and adenocarcinomas of the esophagus or gastric cardia: a systematic review and meta-analysis. Cancer Epidemiol Biomark Prev. 2006;15(5):872–8.
25. Whiteman DC, Sadeghi S, Pandeya N, et al. Combined effects of obesity, acid reflux and smoking on the risk of adenocarcinomas of the oesophagus. Gut. 2008;57(2):173–80.
26. Denholm M, Jankowski J. Gastroesophageal reflux disease and bulimia nervosa – a review of the literature. Dis Esophagus. 2011;24:79.
27. Brewster DH, Nowell SL, Clark DN. Risk of oesophageal cancer among patients previously hospitalised with eating disorder. Cancer Epidemiol. 2015;39(3):313–20.
28. Shaheen N, Ransohoff DF. Gastroesophageal reflux, Barrett esophagus, and esophageal cancer: scientific review. JAMA. 2002;287(15):1972–81.
29. Wang KK, Sampliner RE. Updated guidelines 2008 for the diagnosis, surveillance and therapy of Barrett's esophagus. Am J Gastroenterol. 2008;103(3):788–97.
30. Sikkema M, de Jonge PJ, Steyerberg EW, et al. Risk of esophageal adenocarcinoma and mortality in patients with Barrett's esophagus: a systematic review and meta-analysis. Clin Gastroenterol Hepatol. 2010;8(3):235–44.
31. Yousef F, Cardwell C, Cantwell MM, et al. The incidence of esophageal cancer and high-grade dysplasia in Barrett's esophagus: a systematic review and meta-analysis. Am J Epidemiol. 2008;168(3):237–49.
32. Singh S, Manickam P, Amin AV. Incidence of esophageal adenocarcinoma in Barrett's esophagus with low-grade dysplasia: a systematic review and meta-analysis. Gastrointest Endosc. 2014;79(6):897–909.
33. Jansson C, Johansson AL, Nyrén O, et al. Socioeconomic factors and risk of esophageal adenocarcinoma: a nationwide Swedish case-control study. Cancer Epidemiol Biomark Prev. 2005;14(7):1754–61.
34. Gammon MD, Schoenberg JB, Ahsan H, et al. Tobacco, alcohol, and socioeconomic status and adenocarcinomas of the esophagus and gastric cardia. J Natl Cancer Inst. 1997;89(17):1277–84.
35. Ljung R, Drefahl S, Andersson G, et al. Socio-demographic and geographical factors in esophageal and gastric cancer mortality in Sweden. PLoS One. 2013;8(4):e62067.
36. Jansson C, Oh JK, Martinsen JI, Lagergren J, Plato N, Kjaerheim K, Pukkala E, Sparen P, Tryggvadottir L, Weiderpass E. Occupation and risk of oesophageal adenocarcinoma and squamous-cell carcinoma: the Nordic occupational cancer study. Int J Cancer. 2015;137:590–7.
37. Chow WH, Mclaughlin JK, Malker HS, Linet MS, Weiner JA, Stone BJ. Esophageal cancer and occupation in a cohort of Swedish men. Am J Ind Med. 1995;27:749–57.
38. Tsai RJ, Luckhaupt SE, Schumacher P, Cress RD, Deapen DM, Calvert GM. Risk of cancer among firefighters in California, 1988–2007. Am J Ind Med. 2015;58:715–29.
39. Zhuo X, Zhang Y, Wang Y, et al. Helicobacter pylori infection and oesophageal cancer risk: association studies via evidence-based meta-analyses. Clin Oncol (R Coll Radiol). 2008;20(10):757–62.
40. Islami F, Kamangar F. Helicobacter pylori and esophageal cancer risk: a meta-analysis. Cancer Prev Res. 2008;1(5):329–38.
41. Andrici J, Eslick GD. Hot food and beverage consumption and the risk of esophageal cancer: a meta-analysis. Am J Prev Med. 2015;49:952–60.
42. IARC monographs on the evaluation of carcinogenic risks to humans. Volume 116. Drinking Coffee, Mate, and Very Hot Beverages/IARC Working Group on the Evaluation of Carcinogenic Risks to Humans. Lyon, France. 2016.
43. Narang B, Cox MR, Eslick GD. Meat consumption and risk of developing esophageal cancer: a meta-analysis. Am J Cancer Epidemiol Prev. 2013;1:36–54.
44. Li B, Jiang G, Zhang G, et al. Intake of vegetables and fruit and risk of esophageal adenocarcinoma: a meta-analysis of observational studies. Eur J Nutr. 2014;53(7):1511–21.

45. Petrick JL, Steck SE, Bradshaw PT, Trivers KF, Abrahamson PE, Engel LS, He K, Chow WH, Mayne ST, Risch HA, Vaughan TL, Gammon MD. Dietary intake of flavonoids and oesophageal and gastric cancer: incidence and survival in the United States of America (USA). Br J Cancer. 2015;112:1291–300.
46. Bo Y, Sun J, Wang M, Ding J, Lu Q, Yuan L. Dietary flavonoid intake and the risk of digestive tract cancers: a systematic review and meta-analysis. Sci Rep. 2016;6:24836.
47. Cui L, Liu X, Tian Y, Xie C, Li Q, Cui H, Sun C. Flavonoids, flavonoid subclasses, and esophageal cancer risk: a meta-analysis of epidemiologic studies. Nutrients. 2016;8:350.
48. Zgaga L, O'sullivan F, Cantwell MM, Murray LJ, Thota PN, Coleman HG. Markers of vitamin D exposure and esophageal cancer risk: a systematic review and meta-analysis. Cancer Epidemiol Biomark Prev. 2016;25:877–86.
49. Cui J, Guo XM, Bao HL, Tan JB. Relationship between N-nitrosodimethylamine and risk of digestive tract cancers: a meta analysis based on cohort studies. Zhonghua liu xing bing xue za zhi Zhonghua liuxingbingxue zazhi. 2016;37:725–9.
50. Tio M, Andrici J, Cox MR, et al. Folate intake and the risk of upper gastrointestinal cancers: a systematic review and meta-analysis. J Gastroenterol Hepatol. 2014;29:250–8.
51. Petrick J, Hyland PL, Carron P, Falk RT, Pfeiffer R, Dawsey SM, Abnet CC, Taylor PR, Weinstein SJ, Albanes D, Freedman ND, Guillemette C, Campbell PT, Cook MB. Association between circulating levels of sex steroid hormones and esophageal/gastric cardia adenocarcinoma. Gastroenterology. 2017;152(5 Supplement 1):S34–5.
52. Singh S, Garg SK, Singh PP, et al. Acid-suppressive medications and risk of oesophageal adenocarcinoma in patients with Barrett's oesophagus: a systematic review and meta-analysis. Gut. 2014;63(8):1229–37.
53. Andrici J, Tio M, Eslick GD. Meta-analysis: oral bisphosphonates and the risk of oesophageal cancer. Aliment Pharmacol Ther. 2012;36(8):708–16.
54. Abnet CC, Freedman ND, Kamangar F, et al. Non-steroidal anti-inflammatory drugs and risk of gastric and oesophageal adenocarcinomas: results from a cohort study and a meta-analysis. Br J Cancer. 2009;100(3):551–7.
55. Wang F, Lv ZS, Fu YK. Nonsteroidal anti-inflammatory drugs and esophageal inflammation – Barrett's esophagus – adenocarcinoma sequence: a meta-analysis. Dis Esophagus. 2011;24(5):318–24.
56. Andrici J, Tio M, Eslick GD. Statin use reduces the risk of esophageal cancer: a meta-analysis. Gastroenterology. 2013;144(Suppl 1):S675.
57. Thomas T, Loke Y, Beales ILP. Systematic review and meta-analysis: use of statins is associated with a reduced incidence of oesophageal adenocarcinoma. J Gastrointest Canc. 2018;49(4):442–54.
58. Steevens J, Schouten LJ, Goldbohm RA, et al. Alcohol consumption, cigarette smoking and risk of subtypes of oesophageal and gastric cancer: a prospective cohort study. Gut. 2010;59(1):39–48.
59. Tramacere I, La Vecchia C, Negri E. Tobacco smoking and esophageal and gastric cardia adenocarcinoma: a meta-analysis. Epidemiology. 2011;22(3):344–9.
60. Tramacere I, Pelucchi C, Bagnardi V, et al. A meta-analysis on alcohol drinking and esophageal and gastric cardia adenocarcinoma risk. Ann Oncol. 2012;23(2):287–97.
61. Freedman ND, Abnet CC, Leitzmann MF, et al. A prospective study of tobacco, alcohol, and the risk of esophageal and gastric cancer subtypes. Am J Epidemiol. 2007;165(12):1424–33.
62. Lubin JH, Cook MB, Pandeya N, Vaughan TL, Abnet CC, Giffen C, Webb PM, Murray LJ, Casson AG, Risch HA, Ye W, Kamangar F, Bernstein L, Sharp L, Nyrén O, Gammon MD, Corley DA, Wu AH, Brown LM, Chow W-H, Ward MH, Freedman ND, Whiteman DC. The importance of exposure rate on odds ratios by cigarette smoking and alcohol consumption for esophageal adenocarcinoma and squamous cell carcinoma in the Barrett's Esophagus and Esophageal adenocarcinoma consortium. Cancer Epidemiol. 2012;36:306–16.
63. Montazeri Z, Nyiraneza C, El-Katerji H, Little J. Waterpipe smoking and cancer: systematic review and meta-analysis. Tob Control. 2017;26(1):92–7.

64. Drahos J, Ricker W, Pfeiffer RM, Cook MB. Metabolic syndrome and risk of esophageal adenocarcinoma in elderly patients in the United States: an analysis of SEER-Medicare data. Cancer. 2017;123(4):657–65.

65. Dixon JL, Copeland LA, Zeber JE, Maccarthy AA, Reznik SI, Smythe WR, Rascoe PA. Association between diabetes and esophageal cancer, independent of obesity, in the United States veterans affairs population. Dis Esophagus. 2016;29(7):747–51.

66. Xu B, Zhou X, Li X, Liu C, Yang C. Diabetes mellitus carries a risk of esophageal cancer: a meta-analysis. Medicine. 2017;96(35):e7944.

67. Xie SH, Rabbani S, Petrick JL, Cook MB, Lagergren J. Racial and ethnic disparities in the incidence of esophageal cancer in the United States, 1992–2013. Am J Epidemiol. 2017;186(12):1341–51.

68. Prabhu A, Obi K, Lieberman D, Rubenstein JH. The race-specific incidence of esophageal squamous cell carcinoma in individuals with exposure to tobacco and alcohol. Am J Gastroenterol. 2016;111(12):1718–25.

69. Kim JY, Winters JK, Kim J, Bernstein L, Raz D, Gomez SL. Birthplace and esophageal cancer incidence patterns among Asian-Americans. Dis Esophagus. 2016;29(1):99–104.

70. Siewert JRMD, Ott KMD. Are squamous and adenocarcinomas of the esophagus the same disease? Semin Radiat Oncol. 2006;17(1):38–44.

71. Prabhu A, Obi KO, Rubenstein JH. The synergistic effects of alcohol and tobacco consumption on the risk of esophageal squamous cell carcinoma: a meta-analysis. Am J Gastroenterol. 2014;109(6):822–7.

72. Morita M, Kumashiro R, Kubo N, et al. Alcohol drinking, cigarette smoking, and the development of squamous cell carcinoma of the esophagus: epidemiology, clinical findings, and prevention. Int J Clin Oncol. 2010;15(2):126–34.

73. Islami F, Fedirko V, Tramacere I, et al. Alcohol drinking and esophageal squamous cell carcinoma with focus on light-drinkers and never-smokers: a systematic review and meta-analysis. Int J Cancer. 2011;129(10):2473–84.

74. Prabhu A, Obi KO, Rubenstein JH. Systematic review with meta-analysis: race-specific effects of alcohol and tobacco on the risk of oesophageal squamous cell carcinoma. Aliment Pharmacol Ther. 2013;38(10):1145–55.

75. Bagnardi V, Rota M, Botteri E, et al. Light alcohol drinking and cancer: a meta-analysis. Ann Oncol. 2013;24(2):301–8.

76. Brown LM, Hoover R, Silverman D, et al. Excess incidence of squamous cell esophageal cancer among US black men: role of social class and other risk factors. Am J Epidemiol. 2001;153(2):114–22.

77. Dar NA, Shah IA, Bhat GA, et al. Socioeconomic status and esophageal squamous cell carcinoma risk in Kashmir. India Cancer Sci. 2013;104(9):1231–6.

78. Joint Iran-IARC Study Group. Esophageal cancer studies in the Caspian littoral of Iran: results of population studies – a prodrome. Joint Iran-International Agency for Research on Cancer study group. J Natl Cancer Inst. 1977;59(4):1127–38.

79. Dowlatshahi K, Miller RJ. Role of opium in esophageal cancer: a hypothesis. Cancer Res. 1985;45(4):1906–7.

80. Nasrollahzadeh D, Kamangar F, Aghcheli K, et al. Opium, tobacco, and alcohol use in relation to oesophageal squamous cell carcinoma in a high-risk area of Iran. Br J Cancer. 2008;98(11):1857–63.

81. Tse G, Eslick GD. Egg consumption and risk of GI neoplasms: dose-response meta-analysis and systematic review. Eur J Nutr. 2014;53(7):1581–90.

82. Islami F, Ren JS, Taylor PR, et al. Pickled vegetables and the risk of oesophageal cancer: a meta-analysis. Br J Cancer. 2009;101(9):1641–7.

83. Zamora-Ros R, Luján-Barroso L, Bueno-de-Mesquita HB, et al. Tea and coffee consumption and risk of esophageal cancer: the European prospective investigation into cancer and nutrition study. Int J Cancer. 2014;135(6):1470–9.

84. Tverdal A, Hjellvik V, Selmer R. Coffee intake and oral-oesophageal cancer: follow-up of 389,624 Norwegian men and women 40–45 years. Br J Cancer. 2011;105(1):157–61.

85. Ren JS, Freedman ND, Kamangar F, et al. Tea, coffee, carbonated soft drinks and upper gastrointestinal tract cancer risk in a large United States prospective cohort study. Eur J Cancer. 2010;46(10):1873–81.
86. Boehm K, Borrelli F, Ernst E, et al. Green tea (Camellia sinensis) for the prevention of cancer. Cochrane Database Syst Rev. 2009;3(3):CD005004. https://doi.org/10.1002/14651858. CD005004.pub2.
87. Hashemian M, Murphy G, Etemadi A, Poustchi H, Brockman JD, Kamangar F, Pourshams A, Khoshnia M, Gharavi A, Dawsey SM, Brennan PJ, Boffetta P, Hekmatdoost A, Malekzadeh R, Abnet CC. Toenail mineral concentration and risk of esophageal squamous cell carcinoma, results from the Golestan cohort study. Cancer Med. 2017;6(12):3052–9.
88. Cui J, Guo XM, Bao HL, Tan JB. Relationship between N-nitrosodimethylamine and risk of digestive tract cancers: a meta analysis based on cohort studies. [Chinese]. Zhonghua liu xing bing xue za zhi = Zhonghua liuxingbingxue zazhi. 2016;37(5):725–9.
89. Kolb H, Mandrup-Poulsen T. The global diabetes epidemic as a consequence of lifestyle-induced low-grade inflammation. Diabetologia. 2010;53(1):10–20.
90. Pearson TA, Mensah GA, Alexander RW, Anderson JL, Cannon RRO, Criqui M, Fadl YY, Fortmann SP, Hong Y, Myers GL, Rifai N, Smith JSC, Taubert K, Tracy RP, Vinicor F, Centers for Disease, C, Prevention, American Heart, A. Markers of inflammation and cardiovascular disease: application to clinical and public health practice: a statement for healthcare professionals from the Centers for Disease Control and Prevention and the American Heart Association. Circulation. 2003;107(3):499–511.
91. Gregor MF, Hotamisligil GS. Inflammatory mechanisms in obesity. Annu Rev Immunol. 2011;29(1):415–45.
92. Shivappa N, Zucchetto A, Serraino D, Rossi M, La Vecchia C, Hebert JR. Dietary inflammatory index and risk of esophageal squamous cell cancer in a case-control study from Italy. Cancer Causes Control. 2015;26(10):1439–47.
93. Lu Y, Shivappa N, Lin Y, Lagergren J, Hebert JR. Diet-related inflammation and oesophageal cancer by histological type: a nationwide case-control study in Sweden. Eur J Nutr. 2016;55(4):1683–94.
94. Andrici J, Eslick GD. Maté consumption and the risk of esophageal squamous cell carcinoma: a meta-analysis. Dis Esophagus. 2013;26(8):807–16.
95. Dar NA, Islami F, Bhat GA, et al. Poor oral hygiene and risk of esophageal squamous cell carcinoma in Kashmir. Br J Cancer. 2013;109(5):1367–72.
96. Abnet CC, Qiao YL, Mark SD, et al. Prospective study of tooth loss and incident esophageal and gastric cancers in China. Cancer Causes Control. 2001;12(9):847–54.
97. Abnet CC, Kamangar F, Islami F, et al. Tooth loss and lack of regular oral hygiene are associated with higher risk of esophageal squamous cell carcinoma. Cancer Epidemiol Biomark Prev. 2008;17(11):3062–8.
98. Guha N, Boffetta P, Wünsch Filho V, et al. Oral health and risk of squamous cell carcinoma of the head and neck and esophagus: results of two multicentric case-control studies. Am J Epidemiol. 2007;166(10):1159–73.
99. Hiraki A, Matsuo K, Suzuki T, Kawase T, et al. Teeth loss and risk of cancer at 14 common sites in Japanese. Cancer Epidemiol Biomark Prev. 2008;17(5):1222–7.
100. Abnet CC, Kamangar F, Dawsey SM, et al. Tooth loss is associated with increased risk of gastric non-cardia adenocarcinoma in a cohort of Finnish smokers. Scand J Gastroenterol. 2005;40(6):681–7.
101. Ljung R, Martin L, Lagergren J. Oral disease and risk of oesophageal and gastric cancer in a nationwide nested case-control study in Sweden. Eur J Cancer. 2011;47(14):2128–32.
102. Lee KD, Wang TY, Lu CH, Huang CE, Chen MC. The bidirectional association between oral cancer and esophageal cancer: a population-based study in Taiwan over a 28-year period. Oncotarget. 2017;8(27):44567–78.
103. Saedi B, Razmpa E, Ghalandarabadi M, Ghadimi H, Saghafi F, Naseri M. Epidemiology of oral cavity cancers in a country located in the esophageal cancer belt: a case control study. Iran J Otorhinolaryngol. 2012;24(68):113–8.

104. Shakeri R, Kamangar F, Nasrollahzadeh D, Nouraie M, Khademi H, Etemadi A, Islami F, Marjani H, Fahimi S, Sepehr A, Rahmati A, Abnet CC, Dawsey SM, Brennan P, Boffetta P, Malekzadeh R, Majdzadeh R. Is opium a real risk factor for esophageal cancer or just a methodological artifact? Hospital and neighborhood controls in case-control studies. PLoS One. 2012;7(3):e32711.
105. Kayamba V, Bateman AC, Asombang AW, Shibemba A, Zyambo K, Banda T, Soko R, Kelly P. HIV infection and domestic smoke exposure, but not human papillomavirus, are risk factors for esophageal squamous cell carcinoma in Zambia: a case-control study. Cancer Med. 2015;4(4):588–95.
106. Halec G, Schmitt M, Egger S, Abnet CC, Babb C, Dawsey SM, Flechtenmacher C, Gheit T, Hale M, Holzinger D, Malekzadeh R, Taylor PR, Tommasino M, Urban MI, Waterboer T, Pawlita M, Sitas F. Mucosal alpha-papillomaviruses are not associated with esophageal squamous cell carcinomas: lack of mechanistic evidence from South Africa, China and Iran and from a world-wide meta-analysis. Int J Cancer. 2016;139(1):85–98.
107. Liyanage SS, Rahman B, Ridda I, Newall AT, Tabrizi SN, Garland SM, Segelov E, Seale H, Crowe PJ, Moa A, Macintyre CR. The aetiological role of human papillomavirus in oesophageal squamous cell carcinoma: a meta-analysis. PLoS One. 2013;8(7):e69238.
108. Rokkas T, Pistiolas D, Sechopoulos P, et al. Relationship between helicobacter pylori infection and esophageal neoplasia: a meta-analysis. Clin Gastroenterol Hepatol. 2007;5(12):1413–7.
109. Eitzen K, Eslick GD, Cox MR. Helicobacter pylori cag-a positivity – an important determinant for esophageal squamous cell carcinoma risk: a systemtic review and meta-analysis. J Gastroenterol Hepatol. 2011;26(Suppl 4):81–2.

Cellular and Molecular Biology of Esophageal Cancer

2

Alfred K. Lam

Introduction

Histological Differences

Esophageal cancers comprise cancers of different histological types of diverse cellular and molecular bases [1, 2]. The two major histological types of esophageal cancers are squamous cell carcinoma and adenocarcinoma. It is important to note that there are histological variants of both squamous cell carcinoma and adenocarcinoma, such as basaloid squamous cell carcinoma, spindle cell carcinoma, mucoepidermoid carcinoma, and adenosquamous carcinoma [3–6]. In addition, neuroendocrine neoplasms such as small cell carcinoma of the esophagus account for approximately 1% of primary esophageal carcinoma [7]. All these carcinomas have distinct clinicopathological features. Limited studies have revealed that the cellular and molecular biology of these uncommon types of esophageal carcinomas is different from those of esophageal squamous cell carcinoma or adenocarcinoma [4, 8, 9].

The current understanding of the cellular and molecular biology of esophageal cancers focuses on esophageal squamous cell carcinoma and esophageal adenocarcinoma. The difference in prevalence of these two major histological types in different geographic regions is likely due to the complex interactions of genetic and environmental factors. In general, esophageal squamous cell carcinoma predominates in areas with high incidence of esophageal cancer, whereas esophageal adenocarcinoma is more common in areas with low incidence of esophageal cancer. In addition, the genetic mechanisms of esophageal squamous cell carcinoma are complex with multiple genetic factors proposed [2]. On the other hand, most esophageal

A. K. Lam (✉)
School of Medicine, Griffith University and Pathology Queensland, Gold Coast University Hospital, Gold Coast, Australia
e-mail: a.lam@griffith.edu.au

© Springer Nature Switzerland AG 2020
N. F. Saba, B. F. El-Rayes (eds.), *Esophageal Cancer*,
https://doi.org/10.1007/978-3-030-29832-6_2

adenocarcinomas show genetic changes of the progression of lesions related to acid reflux. The histological progression from reflux esophagitis to Barrett's metaplasia to dysplasia to adenocarcinoma is well known.

Applications of Molecular and Cellular Biology

Esophageal cancer is one of the leading causes of cancer death worldwide despite recent improvements in surgical and adjuvant therapies. Better understanding of the cellular and molecular biology of these cancers will allow us to apply this knowledge to clinical management, thereby increasing the quality of life of patients with esophageal cancer. Thus, the study of cellular and molecular biology of esophageal cancer serves the following purposes: (1) to establish the presence or absence of an infectious cofactor, (2) to understand the genetic mechanisms of disease, (3) to provide prognostic information, and (4) to predict response to medical therapies and new modalities of treatment. In performing research and interpreting and applying knowledge in this area, it is important to bear in mind the histological differences between esophageal cancers.

Establishment of an Infectious Cofactor

For esophageal adenocarcinoma, gastroesophageal reflux and the resulting Barrett's esophagus (intestinal metaplasia) are the most important risk factors [1]. Obesity, tobacco use, drugs, and dietary factors also play roles as risk factors [10]. Besides these, the role of infection in the development of esophageal cancer has long been suspected, in particular the role of human papillomavirus (HPV).

Human Papillomavirus

In esophageal cancers, the main infectious cofactor under intensive study is HPV. HPV is a non-enveloped double-stranded DNA virus that can infect the basal cells of the skin or mucosa. The majority of patients with HPV infections are asymptomatic. After the infection, approximately 10% of patients may have persistent infection, which may lead to cancer [11]. In squamous cell carcinomas of the upper aerodigestive tract, in particular in the oropharynx, identification of the presence of HPV in the carcinomas is of important value [12]. In these sites, patients with HPV-positive cancers have better prognosis when compared to patients with HPV-negative cancers. The detection of HPV in oropharyngeal squamous cell carcinomas also predicts better response to radiotherapy. The detection of HPV in clinical settings is indirectly achieved by the identification of expression of p16 protein by immunohistochemistry (IHC) [13].

The esophagus is distal to the oropharynx and histologically lined by stratified squamous epithelium as in the oropharynx. Studies to investigate HPV in esophageal squamous cell carcinomas have been underway for 30 years [14, 15]. Thus, there is considerable data on the role of HPV infection in the development of esophageal cancer. The majority of studies were in esophageal squamous cell carcinoma.

Pooled analysis of five studies (in the years 2006–2013) from the literature revealed that HPV prevalence in esophageal adenocarcinoma was 35.0% (range, 1–90%) and HPV-16 prevalence was 11.4% [16]. Due to the limited number of studies on esophageal adenocarcinoma, no detailed analysis of the impact was available. Nevertheless, the hypothesis is that progressive acid damage to the esophagus increases the likelihood of mucosal breaks and allows the virus to enter the basal layer of the transformation zone. Recently, transcriptionally active HPV was noted to be strongly associated with Barrett's dysplasia and esophageal adenocarcinoma, suggesting a potential role of HPV in esophageal carcinogenesis. The involvement of HPV is reported to be via wild-type p53 and aberrations of the retinoblastoma protein pathway [17]. On the other hand, Antonsoon and colleagues in 2016 showed no evidence of HPV DNA in a large cohort ($n = 233$) of histologically confirmed archived esophageal adenocarcinomas [18]. Thus, HPV alone is unlikely to cause esophageal adenocarcinoma.

In esophageal squamous cell carcinoma, summarized HPV prevalence from both early and recent meta-analysis was 22% [16]. In general, HPV prevalence was higher in studies conducted in Asian countries and was much lower in studies conducted in Western countries such as in Europe and America [2]. Stratified analysis by localization of cancer showed that esophageal squamous cell carcinoma was only slightly higher in the cervical portion but not significantly higher than the middle or lower portion of the esophagus [19].

With respect to HPV DNA detection in meta-analysis, the prevalence of esophageal squamous cell carcinoma detected by type-specific primer PCR method (30.4%) was significantly higher than that by broad-spectrum primers (20.8%) [16]. Limited studies have employed the IHC method to detect p16 protein to study HPV infection in esophageal carcinoma. Nevertheless, the current data using p16 detection in esophageal squamous cell carcinoma did not reflect the HPV status in the cancer [20]. Detection of HPV DNA is thus the preferred means of studying HPV in esophageal carcinoma.

Human papillomaviruses are a group of more than 100 subtypes of viruses [11]. Slightly more than 30 subtypes are oncogenic in humans and are defined as high risk and low risk for cancers [21]. From pooled data, HPV-16 was the most frequently observed subtype with a summarized prevalence of 11.4% [2, 16]. The other six most frequent individual HPV subtypes identified in esophageal squamous cell carcinoma, in order of decreasing prevalence, were HPV-18 (2.9%), HPV-6 (2.1%), HPV-11(2.0%), HPV-52 (1.1%), HPV-33 (0.8%), and HPV-31 (0.6%). Apart from HPV-6 (low-risk type), all the detected types belong to high-risk carcinogenic HPV types. HPV-16 can induce cancer stem-like cell phenotypes in esophageal squamous cell carcinoma through the activation of the p13K/AKT signaling pathway [22].

Overall, HPV infection was associated with an increased risk of esophageal squamous cell carcinoma. However, the association was not as strong as that for oropharyngeal squamous cell carcinoma or cervical squamous cell carcinoma. The impact on survival of patients with esophageal squamous cell carcinoma has not been clearly determined. Patients with HPV-positive esophageal squamous cell carcinoma had better response to chemoradiation [23, 24]. Wang and colleagues also reported better 3-year survival in patients with HPV-positive cancers [24]. On the other hand, de Costa and colleagues showed no predictive values of HPV, p16, and p53 status on the survival of patients with esophageal squamous cell carcinoma in a recent multivariate analysis [25]. At this stage, routine evaluation of HPV or p16 status is not required in the management of esophageal cancer.

The importance of studying the pathogenesis of HPV in cancers also stems from the availability of effective vaccines against HPV in the market. Prophylactic HPV vaccine is now in its second generation [26]. The vaccine is useful to prevent premalignant genital and anal lesions arising from infection with HPV when given to young females. Australia was the first country to offer complimentary HPV vaccines to boys and girls. The clinical impact of the vaccination program is already visible in the population. Although there is no data from clinical trials regarding the efficacy of the vaccines for HPV-related cancers outside the genital tract, it is likely that universal vaccination could affect the prevalence of HPV-related esophageal cancers in the future.

Epstein-Barr Virus

The detection rates of Epstein-Barr virus (EBV) in esophageal cancer are variable and range from 0% to 35% [27–29]. This variability likely results from differences in racial, geographical, and detection methods used. It is worth noting that lymphocytes in the cancer stroma can harbor EBV, and thus detection of virus in esophageal cancer by PCR-based methods may show false-positive results [28]. On the other hand, in situ hybridization may provide false-negative results due to a higher rate of RNA degradation. Most studies have shown that EBV-associated esophageal cancer demonstrates similar morphologic findings to undifferentiated carcinoma of the nasopharynx, which is associated with EBV. At the current time, the identification of EBV in esophageal carcinoma has no clinical application.

Bacteria

Helicobacter pylori, previously known as *Campylobacter pylori*, is a Gram-negative microaerophilic spiral bacterium, which is the major cause of peptic ulcer disease and a recognized cause of gastric carcinoma. Some strains of *H. pylori* may protect patients from gastroesophageal reflux disease and esophageal adenocarcinoma [27, 29]. This effect may result from the bacterium decreasing acid production through the production of cytokines [29]. It is worth noting that the decreased prevalence of *H. pylori* worldwide because of antibiotics use parallels the increased prevalence of esophageal adenocarcinoma [29]. Overall, there is no consensus on the role of *H. pylori* in esophageal adenocarcinoma, with substantial differences between the results of Asian and Western studies. Metagenomics studies have identified many other types of bacteria in the esophagus [27, 30]. Metagenomics is the study of microbiota in their natural habitat using next-generation sequencing through a PCR-based analysis of bacterial 16S rRNA genes. Two distinct clusters, a predominantly Gram-positive cluster (type I) and a predominately Gram-negative cluster (type II), were noted. The type II cluster may stimulate expression of different proteins and genes leading to reflux and trigger the process of adenocarcinoma formation.

Understanding Genetic Mechanisms

Genetic Profiles

Esophageal carcinomas are biologically aggressive cancers and thus their genetic profiles are complex. Oncogenes, tumor-suppressor genes, metastatic genes, apoptosis genes, proliferation-related factors, epigenetic factors, and proteins related to metastases have roles in the pathogenesis of both esophageal squamous cell carcinoma and esophageal adenocarcinoma [2, 31]. In recent years, studies have suggested that many components of the *P13/AKT* (phosphatidylinositol 3-kinase/ protein kinase B) pathway may be important in the pathogenesis of esophageal squamous cell carcinoma. The expressions of different markers such as E-cadherin, N-cadherin, p120, DNAJB6 (DnaJ homolog subfamily B member 6), and phosphorylated AKT play roles in progression of the cancer as well as predicting the prognosis of patients with the cancer [32–34]. Oncogenic proteins such as receptors for vascular endothelial growth factor (VEGF) and calpain 10 (CAPN10), which is regulated by gene amplified in esophageal cancer 1 (GAEC1), are related to the clinical progression of esophageal squamous cell carcinoma [35, 36]. In addition, epigenetic changes such as promoter methylation of nidogen-2 (NID2, a key component of the basement membrane) could suppress the epidermal growth factor receptor (EGFR)/AKT metastasis-related pathway and control cancer metastases [37]. In general, for both esophageal squamous and adenocarcinoma, p53 mutation is an important genetic change [38, 39].

DNA copy number alterations and methylation analysis could detect many of the genetic and epigenetic changes in esophageal carcinomas [40–43]. Studies from about 2000 onwards have used comparative genomic hybridization (CGH) and expression array to identify the differences in genetic profiles between esophageal cancer and noncancerous esophageal tissue [44–47]. Chromosomal regions with amplification may harbor oncogenes, and chromosomal regions with deletion may harbor tumor-suppressor genes. CGH can identify the whole profile of cytogenetic changes in an individual cancer. Using this approach, researchers have identified many new cancer-related genes in both esophageal squamous cell carcinoma and esophageal adenocarcinomas [48–54]. These provide more information regarding the carcinogenesis of esophageal cancers as well as defining gene candidates as prognostic markers and molecular targets for therapy.

The traditional method of detecting genetic mutations is by Sanger sequencing [55]. The introduction of next-generation sequencing in research and clinical practice has led to the sequencing of many new genes and generated vast quantities of genetic data at a low cost [56, 57]. These recent technologies allow researchers to sequence DNA much more quickly and economically than the previously used Sanger sequencing and as such have revolutionized the study of genomics and molecular biology. The first commercially available next-generation sequencer was available in 2007, and many newer versions offer the ability to detect multiple genes in one experimental run using smaller size equipment (Fig. 2.1). Using these robust new sequencing platforms, whole exome sequencing and whole genome sequencing of patients with esophageal carcinoma are possible. In the literature, reports of whole exome sequencing have been noted mainly in esophageal squamous cell carcinoma and occasionally in esophageal adenocarcinoma [58–67]. Many novel mutations and genetic pathways have been detected which could help us to understand the pathogenesis of this group of cancers with complex genetic alterations (Table 2.1).

The International Cancer Genome Consortium (ICGC) coordinates a large number of research projects that have the common aim of comprehensively elucidating the genomic changes present in many cancers [68]. The preliminary meeting was in 2007 and the consortium launched a public notice in 2010. The primary goals of the ICGC are to generate comprehensive catalogues of genomic abnormalities (somatic mutations, abnormal expression of genes, epigenetic modifications). For esophageal cancer, the genomic study of esophageal squamous cell carcinoma was conducted by researchers in China, whereas the study of esophageal adenocarcinoma was performed by researchers in the United Kingdom.

Whole genome sequencing data for esophageal cancer began to appear in the literature in 2013 [69–83]. A large volume of information is available for the two major histological subtypes of esophageal cancer, which provides substantial resources for future research directions for the better management of patients with esophageal carcinoma (Table 2.1). The information includes (1) the first report of many novel driver gene mutations, (2) the relevant frequencies of key mutations in esophageal carcinomas, (3) the identification of predominant mutation pathways in esophageal cancers, (4) mutational signatures related to risk factors and (5) progression of the cancer as well as changes related to adjuvant chemotherapy. It is worth noting that as predicted from the biological aggressiveness of esophageal cancer, the genomic changes obtained are very complex. It will take time for research into

Fig. 2.1 Use of next-generation sequencer to study esophageal carcinoma. A chip (arrow) in which DNA to be sequenced is loaded. On the right side, the chip (arrow) is in the grounding plate on the benchtop sequencer

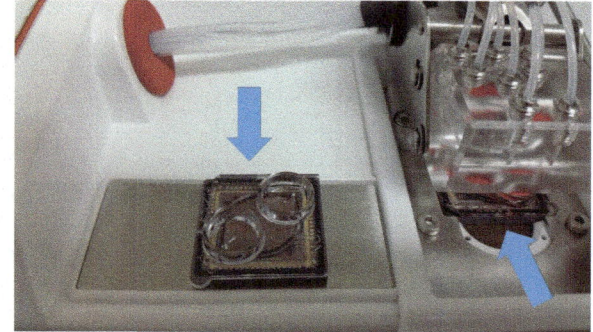

Table 2.1 Whole exome and whole genome sequencing results in esophageal carcinoma

Author/year/place	Samples	Findings
Whole exome sequencing in esophageal carcinoma		
Lin/2014/China	139 ESCC	Novel mutated genes, RTK-MAPK-PI3K pathways, cell cycle, and epigenetic regulation are frequently dysregulated
Wang/2015/China	9 ESCC and matched blood samples	Importance of deletion of 9p21.3 covering *CDKN2A/2B*, amplification of 11q13.3 covering *CCND1*, and *p53* mutation
Stachler/2015/ USA	30 EAC and Barrett's esophagus	Importance of p53 in the progression
Rajendra/2016/ Australia	EAC (4 HPV-positive and 78 HPV-negative)	Distinct genomic differences between HPV-positive and HPV-negative EAC
Findlay/2016/UK	30 EAC before and after neoadjuvant chemotherapy	Changes in driver mutations and acquire new mutations after chemotherapy
Liu/2016/Africa	59 ESCC	Mutational signature analysis revealed common signatures associated with aging, cytidine deaminase activity (APOBEC), and a third signature of unknown origin
Hao/2016/China	13 ESCC	Evidence of spatial intra-tumor heterogeneity with multiple mutations
Chen/2017/China	45 ESCC with matched dysplasia	Mutations in p53 and gains in 3q are early alterations in ESCC development
Forouzanfar/2017/ Iran	9 familial ESCC	Identify Notch signaling pathway in ESCC pathogenesis
Dai/2017/Hong Kong	41 ESCC with 15 matched lymph nodes with ESCC	Critical roles of ZNF750 mutations, TP53 putative GOF mutations, and nucleosome disorganization in ESCC metastasis
Whole genome sequencing in esophageal carcinoma		
Dulak/2013/UK	15 EAC	Novel genes (include chromatin-modifying factors and candidate contributors *SPG20, TLR4, ELMO1*, and *DOCK2*) identified as well as the potential activation of the *RAC1* pathway
Song/2014/China	17 ESCC	Frequent mutations in well-known tumor-associated genes (*p53, RB1, CDKN2A, PIK3CA, NOTCH1, NFE2L2*), and two novel genes (*ADAM29* and *FAM135B*) as well as in histone regulator genes
Nones/2014/ Australia	22 EAC	Oncogene amplification through chromothripsis-derived double-minute chromosome formation (*MYC* and *MDM2*) or breakage-fusion-bridge (*KRAS, MDM2*, and *RFC3*). Telomere shortening is more prominent in EACs bearing localized complex rearrangements. Mutational signature analysis also confirms that extreme genomic instability in EAC can be driven by somatic BRCA2 mutations
Weaver/2014/UK	12 EAC and Barrett' esophagus	The majority of recurrently mutated genes in EAC were mutated in non-dysplastic Barrett's esophagus. Only *p53* and *SMAD4* mutations occurred in a stage-specific manner, confined to high-grade dysplasia and EAC

(continued)

Table 2.1 (continued)

Author/year/place	Samples	Findings
Paterson/2015/ UK	22 EAC and matched normal tissue/ blood	Somatic mobile elements insertions are abundant in EAC
Ross-Innes/2015/ UK	23 pairs of EAC and Barrett's esophagus	(i) Barrett's esophagus is polyclonal and highly mutated even in the absence of dysplasia; (ii) when cancer develops, copy number increases and heterogeneity persists such that the spectrum of mutations often shows little overlap between EAC and adjacent Barrett's esophagus; and (iii) despite differences in specific coding mutations, the mutational context suggests a common causative insult underlying these two conditions
Zhang/2015/ China	104 ESC and previous reports	Cytidine deaminase activity (APOBEC)-mediated mutational signature, high activity of hedgehog signaling, and the PI3K pathway
Qin/2016/China	10 ESCC	Identify mutations in *VANGL1* as well as in three coding genes (*SHANK2, MYBL2, FADD*) and two noncoding genes (*miR-4707-5p, PCAT1*)
Sawada/2016/ Japan	144 ESCC	Patients were assigned to three groups, which are associated with environmental (drinking and smoking) and genetic (polymorphisms in *ALDH2* and *CYP2A6*) factors. Many tumors contained mutations in genes that regulate the cell cycle, epigenetic processes, and the *NOTCH, WNT,* and *receptor-tyrosine kinase-phosphoinositide 3-kinase* signaling pathways
Secrier/2016/UK	129 EAC	Mutational signatures showed three distinct molecular subtypes with potential therapeutic implication: (i) enrichment for BRCA signature with prevalent defects in the homologous recombination pathway, (ii) dominant T > G mutational pattern associated with a high mutational load and neoantigen burden, and (iii) C > A/T mutational pattern with evidence of an aging imprint
Cheng/2016/ China	31 ESCC	Molecular defects such as chromothripsis and breakage-fusion-bridge are important in malignant transformation of ESCCs and demonstrate diverse models of somatic variation-derived target genes in ESCCs
Cheng/2016/ China	A portion of 104 ESCC (stage I or II)	*FAM84B* and the *NOTCH* pathway are involved in the progression of ESCC
Fels Elliott/2017/ UK	171 EAC	Toll-like receptor pathway genes are recurrently mutated
Noorani/2017/ UK	10 EAC matched pre- and post-chemotherapy	The genomic landscape of pre- and post-chemotherapy is similar for EAC
Liu/2017/China	70 ESCC and squamous dysplasia	Squamous dysplasia and ESCCs each had similar mutations and markers of genomic instability, including apolipoprotein B messenger RNA editing enzyme, catalytic polypeptide-like

ESCC esophageal squamous cell carcinoma, EAC esophageal adenocarcinoma, HPV human papilloma virus the functional aspects of these genomic changes to be applied to the clinical management of patients with this group of cancers.

MicroRNAs (miRNAs)

MicroRNAs (miRNAs) are a class of small, well-conserved, non-coding RNAs that regulate the translation of RNAs. Many studies have shown that miRNAs have important biological and pathological functions in many cancer types [84–96]. miRNAs affect a variety of biological processes in the body as well as act as oncogenes, tumor-suppressor genes, or regulators of cancer stem cells. Due to their small size, there are established means of miRNA detection methods (traditional and new) in serum, cell lines, and human tissues in esophageal carcinoma [97, 98].

In esophageal adenocarcinomas, expression levels of different sets of miRNAs are altered during the development of adenocarcinoma from Barrett's esophagus. In different studies, miRNAs such as miRNA-192, miRNA-196, and miRNA-21 were frequently upregulated, whereas miRNA-203, miRNA-205, and miR-let-7 were commonly downregulated during the development from Barrett's esophagus to esophageal adenocarcinoma [99]. In addition, changes in the expression of miRNAs are associated with the prediction of metastasis, prognosis, and response to chemoradiation in patients with esophageal adenocarcinoma. Similarly, many miRNAs are involved in the pathogenesis of esophageal squamous cell carcinoma. miRNAs have oncogenic or suppressor roles as well as potential roles as diagnostic and prognostic markers in the cancer. Many more miRNAs have been identified in esophageal squamous cell carcinoma as the carcinoma has a more complex carcinogenesis than esophageal adenocarcinoma [100–102].

Experimental studies to manipulate miRNAs in cancer cell lines may provide new strategies for cancer therapeutics. However, further studies, such as how to deliver miRNAs specifically to cancer tissues, are required in order to be able to apply miRNAs for clinical use.

Cancer Stem Cells

Cancer stem cells (CSCs) are a subgroup of cancer cells with properties resembling the critical properties of embryonic stem cells such as self-renewal and maintenance of stemness [103–106]. Only cancer stem cells have tumor-initiating properties. CSCs are responsible for initiation, progression, metastases, and recurrence in cancer. They play an important role in the resistance of cancer to adjuvant therapies and in cancer recurrence via their activation of different signaling pathways such as Notch, Wnt/β-catenin, TGF-β, hedgehog, PI3K/AKT/mTOR, and JAK/STAT pathways [105, 106]. In addition, epithelial-mesenchymal transition (EMT) may be involved in epithelial cell immortalization and enrichment of stemness. These immortal cells may regain their original properties via mesenchymal-epithelial transition (MET) and maintain epithelial stem cell properties [107].

Identification of cancer stem cells is important in cancer and is challenging. CSCs are most often identified by detecting the expression of their antigens in a group of stem cells [108]. Many surface markers can be used to detect CSCs by directly targeting their specific antigens present in cells. In addition, multiple analytical methods and techniques including functional assays, cell sorting, filtration approaches, and xenotransplantation methods can identify CSCs.

In esophageal squamous cell carcinoma, markers such as CD44, ALDH, Pygo2, MAML1, Twist1, Musashi1, side population (SP), CD271, and CD90 can be used to identify CSCs in individual cancer masses. In addition, stem cell markers like ALDH1, HIWI, OCT3/4, ABCG2, SOX2, SALL4, BMI-1, NANOG, CD133, and podoplanin are associated with patient prognosis, pathological stage, cancer recurrence, and therapy resistance [109]. In esophageal adenocarcinoma, CSCs are responsible for intrinsic and acquired chemotherapy resistance, which is associated with EMT regulation [110]. As in esophageal squamous cell carcinoma, different methods including functional assays, cell sorting using various intracellular & cell surface markers and xenotransplantation techniques can identify and separate out CSCs. None of these methods alone can guarantee complete isolation of the CSC population. Thus, a combination of methods may be used to detect and isolate CSCs.

The development of specific markers and signaling molecules to target esophageal carcinoma CSCs and the validation of these stem cells might provide the basis for a revolutionary treatment approach for the elimination and/or differentiation of CSCs in esophageal cancer. Emerging therapeutic tools based on specific properties and functions of CSCs may improve clinical outcome of esophageal carcinomas. Therefore, innovative insight into the biology of cancer stem cells and therapies targeted to cancer stem cells will help to achieve effective management of esophageal cancers.

Prognostic Information

Predication of Progression

Aneuploidy (detected by FISH/flow cytometry), promoter hypermethylation, and cyclin A protein expression have been shown to correlate with the progression from Barrett's esophagus to esophageal adenocarcinoma [111, 112]. Despite these findings, there is generally a lack of large prospective studies to validate the use of these markers in clinical practice. The most likely candidate for clinical application is p53 protein overexpression as determined by IHC, which correlates with neoplastic progression to esophageal adenocarcinoma. It could be a useful adjunct to determine the grade of dysplasia in Barrett's esophagus. In addition, the results have been validated in some studies and the procedure used is simple.

The expression or identification of cellular and molecular markers can predict the survival of patients with esophageal adenocarcinoma [113, 114]. Some of the more commonly described markers are EGFR1 and 2, transforming growth factor (TGF α and β1), p53, Ki-67, cyclin-dependent kinase inhibitor 1 (p21), B-cell lymphoma 2 (Bcl-2), cyclooxygenase-2 (COX-2), nuclear factor-κB (NF-κB), VEGF, tissue inhibitor of metalloproteinase (TIMP), and microsatellite instability (MSI). At present, there is no routine testing for these markers, as researchers have not validated these markers adequately in prospective studies.

In esophageal squamous cell carcinoma, many molecular and cellular markers are associated with patient prognosis. Expression levels of p21, p53, cyclin D1, Ki-67, and E-cadherin provide some prognostic information [33, 34, 36, 115, 116]. However, this approach is not widely used.

Guidelines for Medical Therapies

Prediction of Response to Medical Therapies

Preoperative chemoradiation is a standard treatment for esophageal cancers. In patients who undergo neoadjuvant chemoradiation therapy, histological regression of the primary cancer, indicated by percentage of residual viable cells, is an important prognostic factor in addition to nodal status and gender [117].

It is thus important to have a means to predict the response to chemoradiation. The grade of esophageal squamous cell carcinoma could potentially predict the response to preoperative chemotherapy [118]. Many molecular makers have been studied [119–122]. p53 protein is expected to be a representative biomarker. The cell cycle markers CDC25B and 14-3-3sigma have potential as response biomarkers independent of the p53 status. The DNA repair markers, p53R2 or ERCC1, VEGF, and hedgehog signaling pathway factor Gli-1 also have potential as predictive biomarkers. However, further studies are required to validate the findings. In esophageal adenocarcinoma, expression of EGFR, VEGF, NF-κB, and cDNA microarray could act as predictive factors for preoperative chemoradiation.

It is important to be aware of the histological changes after preoperative chemoradiation [3]. In the current AJCC (American Joint Committee on Cancer) guidelines for staging of esophageal carcinoma, patients having preoperative chemoradiation have different guidelines for pathological staging than those patients without preoperative therapy [123].

Predictors for Targeted Therapy

Targeted therapy involves targeting a specific gene mutation in the cancer. In clinical settings, oncologists use targeted therapies to treat melanoma, breast cancer, and colorectal cancer with promising results [124–128]. Testing the cancer tissues for molecular markers is useful to predict the response of the patients to these targeted therapies.

Of the potential targets trialed to date in esophageal cancer, EGFR (Her 1 and Her 2) and VEGF surface receptor antagonists have shown the most promising results [129–133]. For instance, overexpression of EGFR-1 is present in 1/3 to 2/3 of esophageal adenocarcinoma and squamous cell carcinoma tissues. Her 2 (also known as c-erbb2, CD340, and Neu) staining has been demonstrated in esophageal squamous cell carcinoma [134].

The most important advance in the molecular biology and oncology of esophageal adenocarcinoma at the gastroesophageal junction is the approval of anti-Her 2 therapy for the treatment of this cancer [135]. On October 20, 2010, the US Food and Drug Administration (FDA) granted approval for the use of trastuzumab (Herceptin), which targets the Her 2 protein. Trastuzumab in combination with other chemotherapy is approved for the treatment of patients with Her 2 overexpressing metastatic esophageal adenocarcinoma at the gastroesophageal junction who have not received prior treatment for metastatic disease. The approval was based on the findings in many clinical trials that trastuzumab-based therapy offered a significant survival advantage for patients with Her 2 overexpressing locally advanced, recurrent, or metastatic gastric and gastroesophageal junctional adenocarcinomas when compared to conventional therapy alone. Approval of the use of trastuzumab by the US FDA was followed by authorities in other countries, e.g., the Therapeutic Goods Administration (TGA) in Australia.

Pathologists are required to determine the Her 2 status in biopsy or resection material from gastroesophageal junction tumors as well as metastatic sites. IHC and in situ hybridization (ISH) testing is used to assess the expression of Her 2. Precise testing of the Her 2 status is important, as Her 2 is the only biomarker established for patients with advanced esophageal adenocarcinoma of the gastroesophageal junction. Pathologists should ensure that biopsies or resection specimens used for testing are properly fixed and pathologically assessed [136]. In many clinical laboratories, the protocol adopted is a combination of testing of Her 2 by IHC and ISH. Her 2 staining is membranous in cancer cells and is scored as "negative, 1+, 2+, and 3+" depending on standard criteria. In many centers, for cases that are negative or "1+" by IHC, the patients are not considered candidates for anti-Her 2 therapy. In cases that are strongly positive (3+, as defined by strong and complete membranous reactivity), patients are candidates for anti-Her 2 therapy. Esophageal adenocarcinomas at the gastroesophageal junction that are equivocal (2+) in staining are typically tested by ISH to reach a decision regarding trastuzumab therapy.

Research Sources for Molecular and Cellular Studies in Esophageal Cancers

Tissue Studies

Human cancer can be studied at the tissue level when tumor tissue is surgically removed from the human body. These cancer tissues are without blood supply and degeneration will quickly occur. Cancer studies on these tissues can be performed in several ways. In clinical settings, cancer tissues are fixed in formalin and embedded in paraffin. Thin sections can be cut from the paraffin-embedded tissues, stained by hematoxylin and eosin, and examined by pathologists under light microscope. These sections are useful for various molecular studies. In fact, many esophageal cancer research findings derived from studies are performed on paraffin-embedded tissues. This approach has the benefit of providing superior morphological features for studying histological features as well as localization of biomarkers at the cellular level when compared with other methods (Fig. 2.2). It is worth noting that histological assessment is important before starting any further molecular research. It is important to confirm the presence of cancer and the proportion of cancer cells on histological examination of the tissue. Proper dissection and histological examination of cancer tissue provides information regarding histological type, grading, and

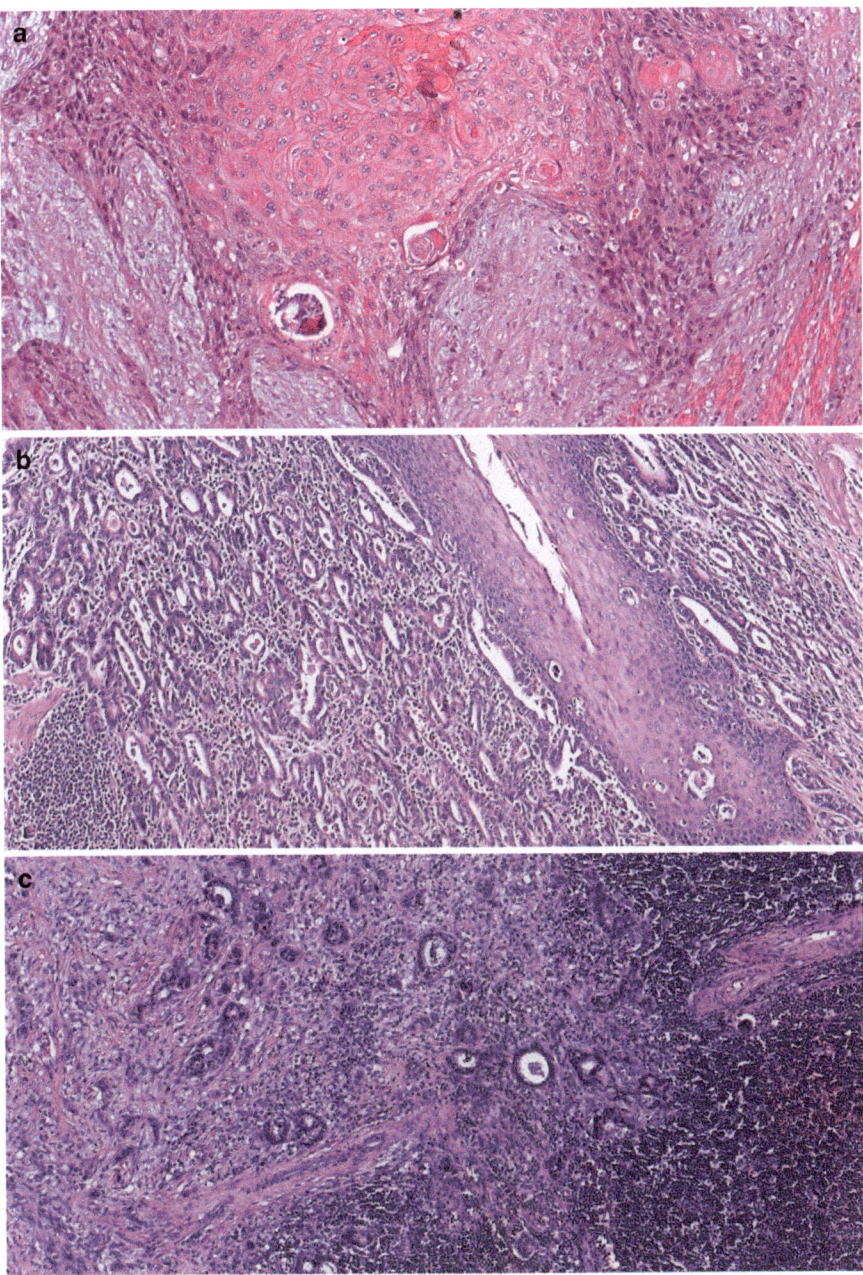

Fig. 2.2 Histological features of carcinomas from formalin-fixed and paraffin-embedded samples. (**a**) Well-differentiated squamous cell carcinoma. (**b**) Well-differentiated adenocarcinoma. (**c**) Lymph node with metastatic esophageal adenocarcinoma

pathological staging which are important parameters to determine the behavior of the cancer as well as the treatment options for esophageal carcinoma [3, 123, 137].

In recent years, the use of tissue microarray (TMA) has increased for testing molecular markers in large numbers of samples by either IHC or ISH (Fig. 2.3). The

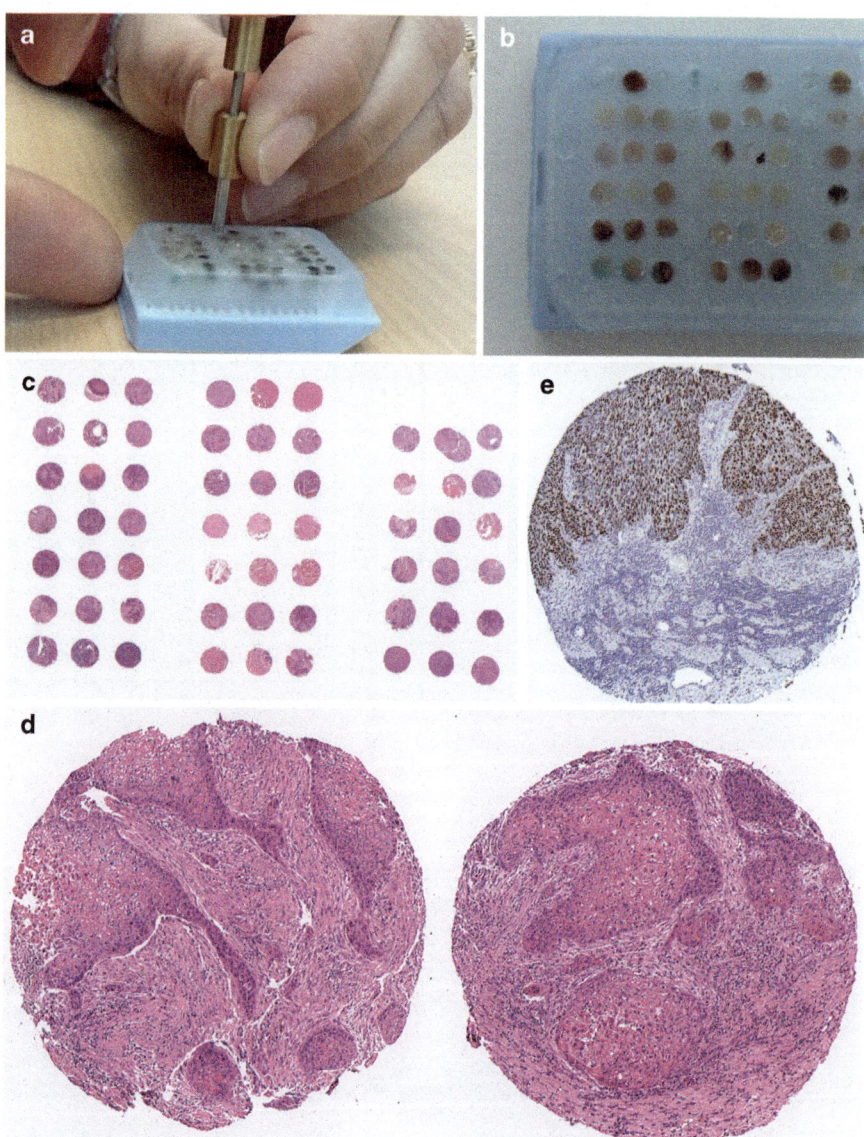

Fig. 2.3 Tissue microarray (TMA) of esophageal carcinoma. (**a**) Making tissue microarray block by manual technique. (**b**) A tissue microarray block with multiple tissue cores in the paraffin. (**c**) Section stained by hematoxylin and eosin taken from the tissue microarray block of esophageal squamous cell carcinoma. (**d**) Higher magnification of two of the cores of 3c. (**e**) The TMA section used to test a biological marker

testing of multiple samples in a block allows rapid screening of large numbers of patient samples and reduces the costs of reagents. The use of tissue in the form of TMA minimizes the amount of invaluable patient tissue used for research tests, making it available for essential clinical use. In the TMA technique, a hollow needle is used to remove tissue cores as small as 0.6 mm in diameter from regions of interest in each paraffin block. These tissue cores are then inserted in a recipient paraffin block in a precisely spaced array pattern [138]. The cores of tissues in the recipient block are from different patients. There are some drawbacks as cancer is heterogeneous, and small samples from a cancer may not represent the information that could be obtained by studying the whole tumor section. In addition, preparation and workup on the TMA blocks require greater technical expertise and time than conventional tissue blocks.

The drawback of working on paraffin-embedded tissues is that formalin irreversibly cross-links proteins via the amino groups, thus preserving the structural integrity of the cells to allow staining with dyes to analyze abnormalities in the tissue that indicate cancer. The effect of these cross-linking fixatives on the nucleic acids and proteins may impair molecular interactions. To overcome this drawback, snap-freezing in liquid nitrogen and storage at -80 °C is used to collect esophageal cancer tissues for use in research. The snap-freezing approach provides tissues that are superior in quality for molecular studies, for instance, whole genome or whole exome studies in esophageal carcinomas; however, the morphological features are inferior to those obtained using paraffin-embedded sections (Fig. 2.4).

The staining of histological sections will fade over time. In addition, storage of large amounts of histological sections is difficult. Whole-slide imaging allows scanning and storage of the histological slides in digital files [139]. This also allows long-term storage of research data as well as computerized analysis of histological parameters (Fig. 2.5). Researchers can share information more easily using digitalized slides.

Blood samples are also important research materials for patients with esophageal carcinomas. Blood can be used to analyze circulating DNA, miRNA, or CTCs in esophageal carcinoma patients [140, 141].

Cancer Cell Lines

It is worth noting that research with removed cancer tissue cannot provide functional dynamic studies of esophageal cancers. For functional studies in esophageal cancer, studies are often performed in cancer cell lines derived from tissues obtained freshly from surgery. Several molecular approaches are used to block the genetic changes in the cancer [142]. For instance, RNA interference (RNAi) is a normal physiological mechanism in which a short effector antisense RNA molecule regulates target gene expression. RNAi can silence a particular gene of interest in a sequence-specific manner and is used to target various molecular pathways in esophageal carcinoma by designing RNAi specific for key pathogenic genes. Several RNAi-based strategies are being explored to develop therapeutics against

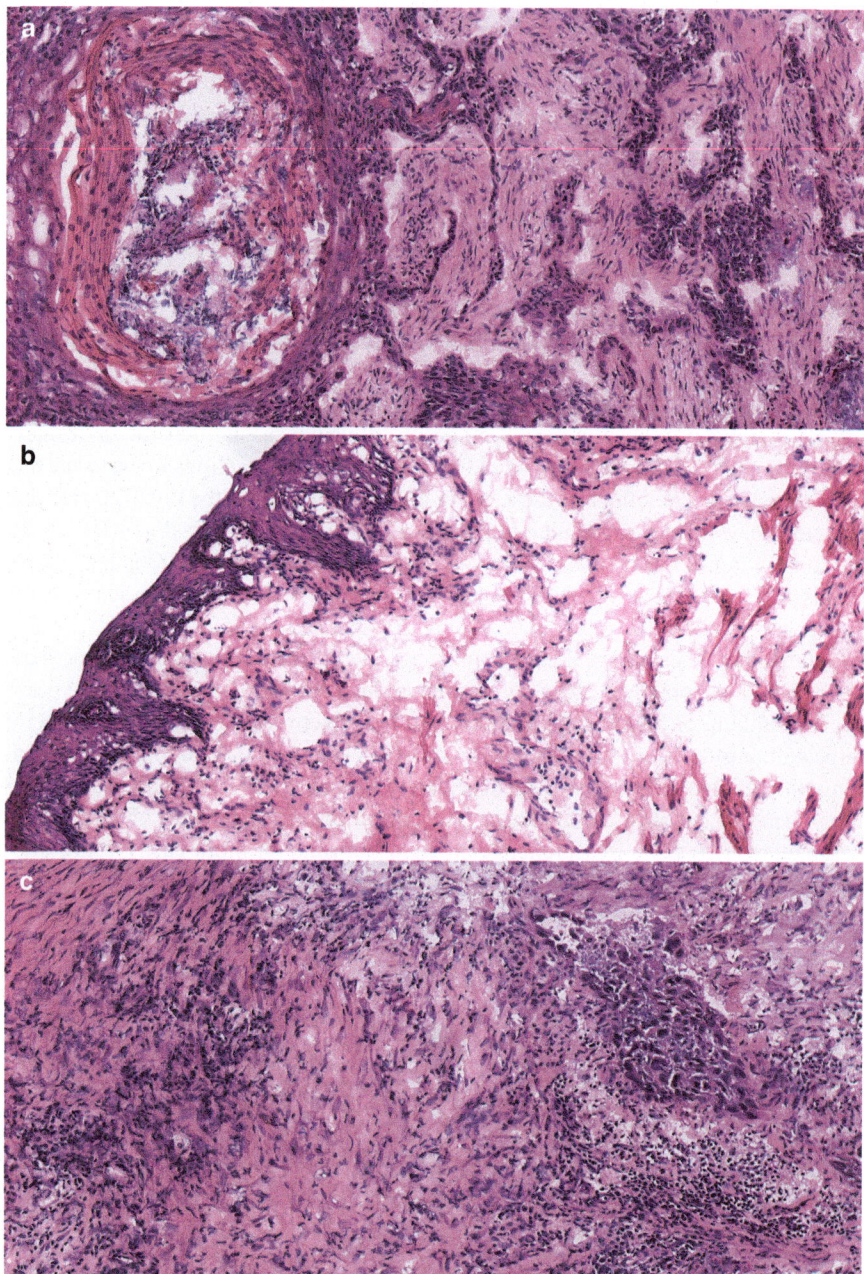

Fig. 2.4 Histological features of esophageal carcinoma prepared by sectioning of frozen tissues. The quality of the morphological features is inferior to those in Fig. 2.2 or 2.3. (**a**) Squamous cell carcinoma of esophagus. (**b**) Non-neoplastic esophageal epithelium (control in research). (**c**) Para-esophageal lymph node infiltrated by squamous cell carcinoma

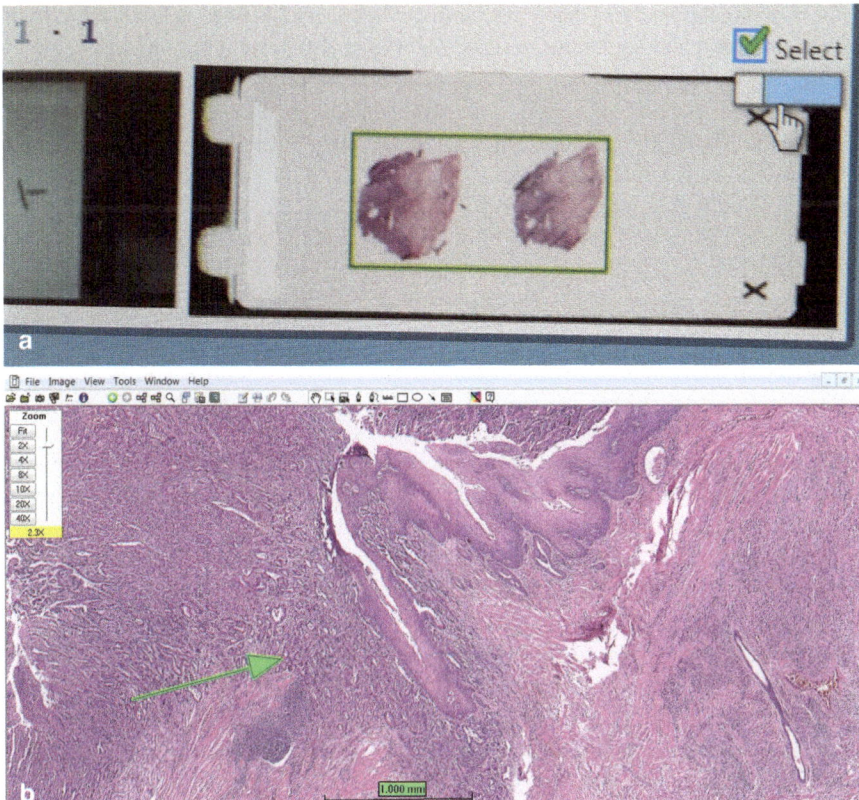

Fig. 2.5 Whole-slide imaging of esophageal carcinoma. (**a**) Capture of the histology of an esoph-ageal squamous cell carcinoma frozen section by scanner. (**b**) Image obtained from scanning of an esophageal adenocarcinoma. Arrow and scale are indicated. Zooming of the image is possible as noted on the right upper corner

esophageal carcinoma, including inhibition of overexpressed oncogenes, blocking cell division by interfering with cyclins and related genes, and enhancing apoptosis by suppressing anti-apoptotic genes.

Cancer cell lines need the appropriate medium to grow. Cancer cell lines often grow without attaching to a surface and they can proliferate to a much higher den-sity in a culture dish. The resulting transformed cancer cell lines, in reciprocal fash-ion, can often cause tumors if injected into a susceptible animal to generate an animal model. Cancer cells can be harvested from the animal and form a more sta-ble cancer cell line. In esophageal cancers, some of the more commonly used cell lines are actually secondary cell lines. Cancer cell lines can allow functional studies to be performed. They can be stored in liquid nitrogen for an indefinite period and retain their viability when thawed.

In esophageal cancers, there are published cancer cell lines available for both adenocarcinoma and squamous carcinoma [143–146]. When compared to esophageal squamous cell carcinoma, esophageal adenocarcinoma is relatively uniform in characteristics as the risk factors and pathogenesis are more established. Model research on esophageal adenocarcinoma relies almost entirely on a relatively small set of established cancer cell lines. The high genomic similarities between the esophageal cell lines and their original cancers provide rationale for their use. Nonetheless, cancer cell lines nearly always differ in important ways from the original cancer from which they were derived.

Animal Models

Animal models are important to study the effects of cancer in vivo and for the production of cancer cell lines. An animal model may be a clinically relevant application for developing therapeutic strategies. Cancer development is a complex process involving the accumulation of genetic alterations and their downstream effects as well as interactions with the microenvironment in different tissues. The cancer microenvironment and its interactions with the cancer are important in determining the growth dynamics of different cancers.

Injection of cancer or cancerous cells in the subcutaneous tissue of the skin of immunodeficient mice is a common practice to produce a cancer model in animals (Fig. 2.6a). In many instances, researchers use a cancer cell line as it is easy to grow. However, to adopt a personalized approach for testing the cancer from a particular group of patients, injection of cancer tissue is required which is labelled as patient-derived xenograft (PDX) model. This approach requires careful planning and highly experience personnel, and there is a high failure rate of growth of the tumor in the animal (when compared to using commercially obtained cancer cell lines).

In esophageal cancers, this approach cannot recapitulate the microenvironment of the esophagus or the response to targeting carcinogens. One approach is to generate an orthotopic (occurring at a normal site) model for esophageal carcinoma [147, 148] (Fig. 2.6b). The orthotopic model provides the optimum environment for cancer growth and drug testing. In the anatomical setting of esophageal cancer, the site is very difficult to approach surgically. Several approaches have been explored, but most of these have some shortcomings. The establishment of these orthotopic models needs to involve radiological guidance (magnetic resonance imaging and fluorescence imaging) so the cancer and the metastases can be visualized in real time [149]. In addition, pathological examination is important to clarify the histological typing, microscopic location, and microenvironment of the cancer in the animal.

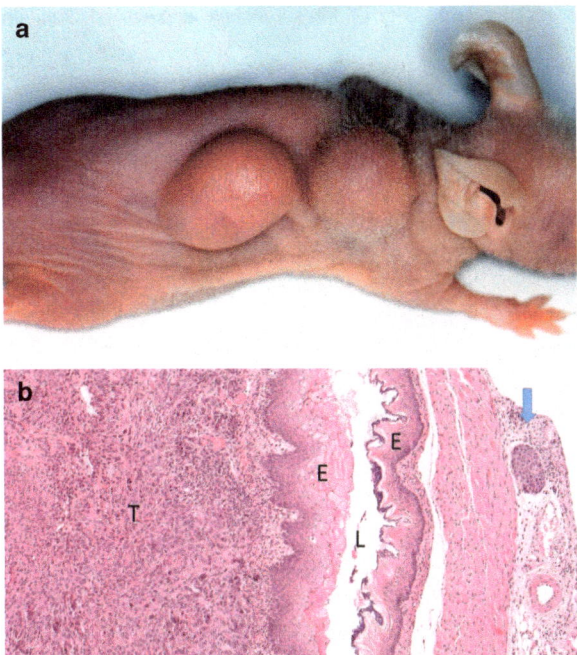

Fig. 2.6 Animal models of esophageal carcinoma. (**a**) Tumor produced in an immunodeficient mouse after subcutaneous injection of primary esophageal squamous cell carcinoma from a patient (courtesy of Dr. Johnny Tang from eHealth Sytle Biotechnology Limited, Hong Kong). (**b**) An orthotopic nude model of esophageal squamous cell carcinoma (courtesy of Professor Maria Lung from the University of Hong Kong, Hong Kong). Histological section of mouse esophagus showing the successful growth of a squamous cell carcinoma (from a cancer cell line surgically implanted in the wall of the esophagus) in the esophagus of the mouse. A carcinoma nodule is present in the lymphatic in the wall of the esophagus (arrow). L: lumen in the esophagus. E: esophageal epithelium. T: carcinoma

References

1. Lam KY, Ma L. Pathology of esophageal cancers: local experience and current insights. Chin Med J. 1997;110:459–64.
2. Lam AKY. Critical review: molecular biology of esophageal squamous cell carcinoma. Crit Rev Oncol Hematol. 2000;33:71–90.
3. Lam AK. Histopathological assessment for esophageal adenocarcinoma. Methods Mol Biol. 2018;1756:67–76.
4. Lam KY, Law S, Tung PH, Wong J. Esophageal basaloid squamous cell carcinoma: an unique clinicopathological entity with telomerase activity as a prognostic indicator. J Pathol. 2001;195:435–42.

5. Lam KY, Law SYK, Loke SL, Fok M, Ma LT. Double sarcomatoid carcinomas of the esophagus. Pathol Res Pract. 1996;192:604–9.
6. Lam KY, Dickens P, Loke SL, Fok M, Ma L, Wong J. Squamous cell carcinoma of the esophagus with mucin-secreting component (mucoepidermoid carcinoma and adenosquamous cell carcinoma): a clinicopathologic study and a review of literature. Eur J Surg Oncol. 1994;20: 25–31.
7. Law SYK, Fok M, Lam KY, Loke SL, Ma LT, Wong J. Small cell carcinoma of the esophagus. Cancer. 1994;73:2894–9.
8. Chow V, Law S, Lam KY, Luk JM, Wong J. Telomerase activity in small cell esophageal carcinoma. Dis Esophagus. 2001;14:139–42.
9. Lam KY, Law S, Tung PH, Wong J. Esophageal small cell carcinoma: clinicopathologic parameters, p53 overexpression, proliferative marker, and their impact on pathogenesis. Arch Pathol Lab Med. 2000;124:228–33.
10. Lam AK. Introduction: esophageal adenocarcinoma: updates of current status. Methods Mol Biol. 1756;2018:1–6.
11. Juckett G, Hartman-Adams H. Human papillomavirus: clinical manifestations and prevention. Am Fam Physician. 2010;82:1209–13.
12. Husain N, Neyaz A. Human papillomavirus associated head and neck squamous cell carcinoma: controversies and new concepts. J Oral Biol Craniofac Res. 2017;7:198–205.
13. Shaikh MH, Khan AI, Sadat A, Chowdhury AH, Jinnah SA, Gopalan V, Lam AK, Clarke DTW, McMillan NAJ, Johnson NW. Prevalence and types of high-risk human papillomaviruses in head and neck cancers from Bangladesh. BMC Cancer. 2017;17:792.
14. He D, Zhang DK, Lam KY, Ma L, Ngan HYS, Liu SS, Tsao SW. Prevalence of HPV infection in esophageal squamous cell carcinoma in Chinese patients and its relationship to the p53 gene mutation. Int J Cancer. 1997;72:959–64.
15. Lam KY, He D, Ma L, Zhang D, Ngan HYS, Wan TSK, Tsao SW. Presence of human papillomavirus in esophageal squamous cell carcinomas of Hong Kong Chinese and its relationship with p53 gene mutation. Hum Pathol. 1997;28:657–63.
16. Li X, Gao C, Yang Y, Zhou F, Li M, Jin Q, Gao L. Systematic review with meta-analysis: the association between human papillomavirus infection and oesophageal cancer. Aliment Pharmacol Ther. 2014;39:270–81.
17. Rajendra S, Yang T, Xuan W, Sharma P, Pavey D, Lee CS, Le S, Collins J, Wang B. Active human papillomavirus involvement in Barrett's dysplasia and oesophageal adenocarcinoma is characterized by wild-type p53 and aberrations of the retinoblastoma protein pathway. Int J Cancer. 2017;141:2037–49.
18. Antonsson A, Knight L, Whiteman DC. Human papillomavirus not detected in esophageal adenocarcinoma tumor specimens. Cancer Epidemiol. 2016;41:96–8.
19. Löfdahl HE, Du J, Näsman A, Andersson E, Rubio CA, Lu Y, Ramqvist T, Dalianis T, Lagergren J, Dahlstrand H. Prevalence of human papillomavirus (HPV) in oesophageal squamous cell carcinoma in relation to anatomical site of the tumour. PLoS One. 2012;7:e46538.
20. Wang WJ, Wu MJ, Ren JL, Xie P, Chang J, Hu GM, Wu HF. p16INK4a is not a reliable screening marker of HPV infection in esophageal squamous cell carcinoma:evidence from a meta-analysis. Int J Biol Markers. 2016;31:e431–9.
21. Bucchi D, Stracci F, Buonora N, Masanotti G. Human papillomavirus and gastrointestinal cancer: a review. World J Gastroenterol. 2016;22:7415–30.
22. Xi R, Pan S, Chen X, Hui B, Zhang L, Fu S, Li X, Zhang X, Gong T, Guo J, Zhang X, Che S. HPV16 E6-E7 induces cancer stem-like cells phenotypes in esophageal squamous cell carcinoma through the activation of PI3K/Akt signaling pathway in vitro and in vivo. Oncotarget. 2016;7:57050–65.
23. Zhang D, Zhang W, Liu W, Mao Y, Fu Z, Liu J, Huang W, Zhang Z, An D, Li B. Human papillomavirus infection increases the chemoradiation response of esophageal squamous cell carcinoma based on P53 mutation. Radiother Oncol. 2017;124:155–60.
24. Wang WL, Wang YC, Lee CT, Chang CY, Lo JL, Kuo YH, Hsu YC, Mo LR. The impact of human papillomavirus infection on the survival and treatment response of patients with esophageal cancers. J Dig Dis. 2015;16:256–63.

25. da Costa AM, Fregnani JHTG, Pastrez PRA, Mariano VS, Silva EM, Neto CS, Guimarães DP, Villa LL, Sichero L, Syrjanen KJ, Longatto-Filho A. HPV infection and p53 and p16 expression in esophageal cancer: are they prognostic factors? Infect Agent Cancer. 2017;12:54.

26. Pouyanfard S, Müller M. Human papillomavirus first and second generation vaccines-current status and future directions. Biol Chem. 2017;398:871–89.

27. Al-Haddad S, El-Zimaity H, Hafezi-Bakhtiari S, Rajendra S, Streutker CJ, Vajpeyi R, Wang B. Infection and esophageal cancer. Ann N Y Acad Sci. 2014;1325:187–96.

28. Lam KY, Srivastava G, Leung ML, Ma L. Absence of Epstein-Barr virus in esophageal squamous cell carcinoma: a study of 74 cases using in-situ hybridization. J Clin Pathol Mol Pathol. 1995;48:M188–90.

29. Xu W, Liu Z, Bao Q, Qian Z. Viruses, other pathogenic microorganisms and esophageal cancer. Gastrointest Tumors. 2015;2:2–13.

30. Wang ZK, Yang YS. Upper gastrointestinal microbiota and digestive diseases. World J Gastroenterol. 2013;19:1541–50.

31. Gibson MK, Dhaliwal AS, Clemons NJ, Phillips WA, Dvorak K, Tong D, Law S, Pirchi ED, Räsänen J, Krasna MJ, Parikh K, Krishnadath KK, Chen Y, Griffiths L, Colleypriest BJ, Farrant JM, Tosh D, Das KM, Bajpai M. Barrett's esophagus: cancer and molecular biology. Ann N Y Acad Sci. 2013;1300:296–314.

32. Li B, Xu WW, Lam AKY, Wang Y, Hu HF, Guan XY, Qin YR, Saremi N, Tsao SW, He QY, Cheung ALM. Significance of PI3K/AKT signaling pathway in metastasis of esophageal squamous cell carcinoma and its potential as a target for anti-metastasis therapy. Oncotarget. 2017;8:38755–66.

33. Yu VZ, Wong VC, Dai W, Ko JM, Lam AK, Chan KW, Samant RS, Lung HL, Shuen WH, Law S, Chan YP, Lee NP, Tong DK, Law TT, Lee VH, Lung ML. Nuclear localization of DNAJB6 is associated with survival of patients with esophageal cancer and reduces AKT signaling and proliferation of cancer cells. Gastroenterology. 2015;149:1825–36.

34. Chung Y, Lam AK, Luk JM, Law S, Chan KW, Lee PY, Wong J. Altered E-cadherin expression and p120 catenin localization in esophageal squamous cell carcinoma. Ann Surg Oncol. 2007;14:3260–7.

35. Xu WW, Li B, Lam AK, Tsao SW, Law SY, Chan KW, Yuan QJ, Cheung AL. Targeting VEGFR1- and VEGFR2-expressing non-tumor cells is essential for esophageal cancer therapy. Oncotarget. 2015;6:1790–805.

36. Chan D, Tsoi MY, Liu CD, Chan SH, Law SY, Chan KW, Chan YP, Gopalan V, Lam AK, Tang JC. Oncogene GAEC1 regulates CAPN10 expression which predicts survival in esophageal squamous cell carcinoma. World J Gastroenterol. 2013;19:2772–80.

37. Chai AW, Cheung AK, Dai W, Ko JM, Ip JC, Chan KW, Kwong DL, Ng WT, Lee AW, Ngan RK, Yau CC, Tung SY, Lee VH, Lam AK, Pillai S, Law S, Lung ML. Metastasis-suppressing NID2, an epigenetically-silenced gene, in the pathogenesis of nasopharyngeal carcinoma and esophageal squamous cell carcinoma. Oncotarget. 2016;7:78859–71.

38. Lam KY, Tsao SW, Zhang D, Law S, He D, Ma L, Wong J. Prevalence and predictive value of p53 mutation in patients with esophageal squamous cell carcinomas: a prospective clinicopathological study and survival analysis of 70 patients. Int J Cancer. 1997;74:212–9.

39. Appelman HD, Matejcic M, Parker MI, Riddell RH, Salemme M, Swanson PE, Villanacci V. Progression of esophageal dysplasia to cancer. Ann N Y Acad Sci. 2014;1325:96–107.

40. Lee KTW, Gopalan V, Lam AK. Somatic DNA copy number alterations detection for oesophageal adenocarcinoma using digital polymerase chain reaction. Methods Mol Biol. 2018;1756:195–212.

41. Islam F, Tang JC, Gopalan V, Lam AK. Epigenetics: DNA methylation analysis in esophageal adenocarcinoma. Methods Mol Biol. 2018;1756:247–56.

42. Haque MH, Islam MN, Islam F, Gopalan V, Nguyen NT, Lam AK, Shiddiky MJ. Electrochemical detection of FAM134B mutations in oesophageal cancer based on DNA-gold affinity interactions. Electroanalysis. 2017;29:1359–67.

43. Haque MH, Gopalan V, Islam MN, Masud MK, Bhattacharjee R, Hossain MSA, Nguyen NT, Lam AK, Shiddiky MJA. Quantification of gene-specific DNA methylation in oesophageal cancer via electrochemistry. Anal Chim Acta. 2017;976:84–93.

44. Pack SD, Karkera JD, Zhuang Z, Pak ED, Balan KV, Hwu P, Park WS, Pham T, Ault DO, Glaser M, Liotta L, Detera-Wadleigh SD, Wadleigh RG. Molecular cytogenetic fingerprinting of esophageal squamous cell carcinoma by comparative genomic hybridization reveals a consistent pattern of chromosomal alterations. Genes Chromosomes Cancer. 1999;25:160–8.

45. Walch AK, Zitzelsberger HF, Bruch J, Keller G, Angermeier D, Aubele MM, Mueller J, Stein H, Braselmann H, Siewert JR, Höfler H, Werner M. Chromosomal imbalances in Barrett's adenocarcinoma and the metaplasia-dysplasia-carcinoma sequence. Am J Pathol. 2000;156:555–66.

46. Kwong D, Lam A, Guan X, Law S, Tai A, Wong J, Sham J. Chromosomal aberrations in esophageal squamous cell carcinoma among Chinese: gain of 12p predicts poor prognosis after surgery. Hum Pathol. 2004;35:309–16.

47. Qin YR, Wang LD, Fan ZM, Kwong D, Guan XY. Comparative genomic hybridization analysis of genetic aberrations associated with development of esophageal squamous cell carcinoma in Henan, China. World J Gastroenterol. 2008;14:1828–35.

48. Tang JCO, Lam KY, Law S, Wong J, Srivastava G. Detection of genetic alterations in esophageal squamous cell carcinomas and adjacent normal epithelia by comparative DNA fingerprinting using inter-simple sequence repeat PCR. Clin Cancer Res. 2001;7:1539–45.

49. Hu YC, Lam KY, Law S, Wong J, Srivastava G. Identification of differentially expressed in esophageal squamous cell carcinoma (ESCC) by cDNA expression array: overexpression of Fra-1, Neogenin, Id-1 and CDC25B genes in ESCC. Clin Cancer Res. 2001;7:2213–21.

50. Fatima S, Chui CH, Tang WK, Hui KS, Au HW, Li WY, Wong MM, Cheung F, Tsao SW, Lam KY, Beh PS, Wong J, Law S, Srivastava G, Ho KP, Chan AS, Tang JC. Transforming capacity of two novel genes JS-1 and JS-2 located in chromosome 5p and their overexpression in human esophageal squamous cell carcinoma. Int J Mol Med. 2006;17:159–70.

51. Tang WK, Chui CH, Fatima S, Kok SH, Pak KC, Ou TM, Hui KS, Wong MM, Wong J, Law S, Tsao SW, Lam KY, Beh PS, Srivastava G, Chan AS, Ho KP, Tang JC. Oncogenic properties of a novel gene JK-1 located in chromosome 5p and its overexpression in human esophageal squamous cell carcinoma. Int J Mol Med. 2007;19:915–23.

52. Goh XY, Rees JR, Paterson AL, Chin SF, Marioni JC, Save V, O'Donovan M, Eijk PP, Alderson D, Ylstra B, Caldas C, Fitzgerald RC. Integrative analysis of array-comparative genomic hybridisation and matched gene expression profiling data reveals novel genes with prognostic significance in oesophageal adenocarcinoma. Gut. 2011;60:1317–26.

53. Law FB, Chen YW, Wong KY, Ying J, Tao Q, Langford C, Lee PY, Law S, Cheung RW, Chui CH, Tsao SW, Lam KY, Wong J, Srivastava G, Tang JC. Identification of a novel tumor transforming gene GAEC1 at 7q22 which encodes a nuclear protein and is frequently amplified and overexpressed in esophageal squamous cell carcinoma. Oncogene. 2007;26:5877–88.

54. Haque MH, Gopalan V, Chan KW, Shiddiky MJ, Smith RA, Lam AK. Identification of novel FAM134B (JK1) mutations in oesophageal squamous cell carcinoma. Sci Rep. 2016;6:29173.

55. Lee KT, Smith RA, Gopalan V, Lam AK. Targeted single gene mutation in oesophageal adenocarcinoma. Methods Mol Biol. 1756;2018:213–29.

56. Pillai S, Gopalan V, Lam AK. DNA genome sequencing in oesophageal adenocarcinoma. Methods Mol Biol. 2018;1756:231–46.

57. Pillai S, Gopalan V, Lam AK. Review of sequencing platforms and their applications in phaeochromocytoma and paragangliomas. Crit Rev Oncol Hematol. 2017;116:58–67.

58. Lin DC, Hao JJ, Nagata Y, Xu L, Shang L, Meng X, Sato Y, Okuno Y, Varela AM, Ding LW, Garg M, Liu LZ, Yang H, Yin D, Shi ZZ, Jiang YY, Gu WY, Gong T, Zhang Y, Xu X, Kalid O, Shacham S, Ogawa S, Wang MR, Koeffler HP. Genomic and molecular characterization of esophageal squamous cell carcinoma. Nat Genet. 2014;46:467–73.

59. Wang Q, Bai J, Abliz A, Liu Y, Gong K, Li J, Shi W, Pan Y, Liu F, Lai S, Yang H, Lu C, Zhang L, Chen W, Xu R, Cai H, Ke Y, Zeng C. An old story retold: loss of G1 control defines a distinct genomic subtype of esophageal squamous cell carcinoma. Genomics Proteomics Bioinformatics. 2015;13:258–70.

60. Stachler MD, Taylor-Weiner A, Peng S, McKenna A, Agoston AT, Odze RD, Davison JM, Nason KS, Loda M, Leshchiner I, Stewart C, Stojanov P, Seepo S, Lawrence MS, Ferrer-Torres

D, Lin J, Chang AC, Gabriel SB, Lander ES, Beer DG, Getz G, Carter SL, Bass AJ. Paired exome analysis of Barrett's esophagus and adenocarcinoma. Nat Genet. 2015;47:1047–55.

61. Rajendra S, Wang B, Merrett N, Sharma P, Humphris J, Lee HC, Wu J. Genomic analysis of HPV-positive versus HPV-negative oesophageal adenocarcinoma identifies a differential mutational landscape. J Med Genet. 2016;53:227–31.

62. Findlay JM, Castro-Giner F, Makino S, Rayner E, Kartsonaki C, Cross W, Kovac M, Ulahannan D, Palles C, Gillies RS, MacGregor TP, Church D, Maynard ND, Buffa F, Cazier JB, Graham TA, Wang LM, Sharma RA, Middleton M, Tomlinson I. Differential clonal evolution in oesophageal cancers in response to neo-adjuvant chemotherapy. Nat Commun. 2016;7:11111.

63. Liu W, Snell JM, Jeck WR, Hoadley KA, Wilkerson MD, Parker JS, Patel N, Mlombe YB, Mulima G, Liomba NG, Wolf LL, Shores CG, Gopal S, Sharpless NE. Subtyping sub-Saharan esophageal squamous cell carcinoma by comprehensive molecular analysis. JCI Insight. 2016;1:e88755.

64. Hao JJ, Lin DC, Dinh HQ, Mayakonda A, Jiang YY, Chang C, Jiang Y, Lu CC, Shi ZZ, Xu X, Zhang Y, Cai Y, Wang JW, Zhan QM, Wei WQ, Berman BP, Wang MR, Koeffler HP. Spatial intratumoral heterogeneity and temporal clonal evolution in esophageal squamous cell carcinoma. Nat Genet. 2016;48:1500–7.

65. Chen XX, Zhong Q, Liu Y, Yan SM, Chen ZH, Jin SZ, Xia TL, Li RY, Zhou AJ, Su Z, Huang YH, Huang QT, Huang LY, Zhang X, Zhao YN, Yun JP, Wu QL, Lin DX, Bai F, Zeng MS. Genomic comparison of esophageal squamous cell carcinoma and its precursor lesions by multi-region whole-exome sequencing. Nat Commun. 2017;8:524.

66. Forouzanfar N, Baranova A, Milanizadeh S, Heravi-Moussavi A, Jebelli A, Abbaszadegan MR. Novel candidate genes may be possible predisposing factors revealed by whole exome sequencing in familial esophageal squamous cell carcinoma. Tumour Biol. 2017;39:1010428317699115.

67. Dai W, Ko JMY, Choi SSA, Yu Z, Ning L, Zheng H, Gopalan V, Chan KT, Lee NP, Chan KW, Law SY, Lam AK, Lung ML. Whole-exome sequencing reveals critical genes underlying metastasis in oesophageal squamous cell carcinoma. J Pathol. 2017;242:500–10.

68. Zhang J, Baran J, Cros A, Guberman JM, Haider S, Hsu J, Liang Y, Rivkin E, Wang J, Whitty B, Wong-Erasmus M, Yao L, Kasprzyk A. International cancer genome consortium data portal—a one-stop shop for cancer genomics data. Database (Oxford). 2011;2011:bar026.

69. Dulak AM, Stojanov P, Peng S, Lawrence MS, Fox C, Stewart C, Bandla S, Imamura Y, Schumacher SE, Shefler E, McKenna A, Carter SL, Cibulskis K, Sivachenko A, Saksena G, Voet D, Ramos AH, Auclair D, Thompson K, Sougnez C, Onofrio RC, Guiducci C, Beroukhim R, Zhou Z, Lin L, Lin J, Reddy R, Chang A, Landrenau R, Pennathur A, Ogino S, Luketich JD, Golub TR, Gabriel SB, Lander ES, Beer DG, Godfrey TE, Getz G, Bass AJ. Exome and whole-genome sequencing of esophageal adenocarcinoma identifies recurrent driver events and mutational complexity. Nat Genet. 2013;45:478–86.

70. Song Y, Li L, Ou Y, Gao Z, Li E, Li X, Zhang W, Wang J, Xu L, Zhou Y, Ma X, Liu L, Zhao Z, Huang X, Fan J, Dong L, Chen G, Ma L, Yang J, Chen L, He M, Li M, Zhuang X, Huang K, Qiu K, Yin G, Guo G, Feng Q, Chen P, Wu Z, Wu J, Ma L, Zhao J, Luo L, Fu M, Xu B, Chen B, Li Y, Tong T, Wang M, Liu Z, Lin D, Zhang X, Yang H, Wang J, Zhan Q. Identification of genomic alterations in oesophageal squamous cell cancer. Nature. 2014;509:91–5.

71. Nones K, Waddell N, Wayte N, Patch AM, Bailey P, Newell F, Holmes O, Fink JL, MCJ Q, Tang YH, Lampe G, Quek K, Loffler KA, Manning S, Idrisoglu S, Miller D, Xu Q, Waddell N, Wilson PJ, TJC B, Christ AN, Harliwong I, Nourse C, Nourbakhsh E, Anderson M, Kazakoff S, Leonard C, Wood S, Simpson PT, Reid LE, Krause L, Hussey DJ, Watson DI, Lord RV, Nancarrow D, Phillips WA, Gotley D, Smithers BM, Whiteman DC, Hayward NK, Campbell PJ, Pearson JV, Grimmond SM, Barbour AP. Genomic catastrophes frequently arise in esophageal adenocarcinoma and drive tumorigenesis. Nat Commun. 2014;5:5224.

72. Weaver JMJ, Ross-Innes CS, Shannon N, Lynch AG, Forshew T, Barbera M, Murtaza M, Ong CJ, Lao-Sirieix P, Dunning MJ, Smith L, Smith ML, Anderson CL, Carvalho B, O'Donovan M, Underwood TJ, May AP, Grehan N, Hardwick R, Davies J, Oloumi A, Aparicio S, Caldas C, Eldridge MD, PAW E, Rosenfeld N, Tavaré S, Fitzgerald RC, OCCAMS consortium.

Ordering of mutations in preinvasive disease stages of esophageal carcinogenesis. Nat Genet. 2014;46:837–43.

73. Paterson AL, Weaver JM, Eldridge MD, Tavaré S, Fitzgerald RC, Edwards PA, OCCAMs Consortium. Mobile element insertions are frequent in oesophageal adenocarcinomas and can mislead paired-end sequencing analysis. BMC Genomics. 2015;16:473.

74. Ross-Innes CS, Becq J, Warren A, Cheetham RK, Northen H, O'Donovan M, Malhotra S, di Pietro M, Ivakhno S, He M, Weaver JMJ, Lynch AG, Kingsbury Z, Ross M, Humphray S, Bentley D, Fitzgerald RC. Whole-genome sequencing provides new insights into the clonal architecture of Barrett's esophagus and esophageal adenocarcinoma. Nat Genet. 2015;47:1038–46.

75. Zhang L, Zhou Y, Cheng C, Cui H, Cheng L, Kong P, Wang J, Li Y, Chen W, Song B, Wang F, Jia Z, Li L, Li Y, Yang B, Liu J, Shi R, Bi Y, Zhang Y, Wang J, Zhao Z, Hu X, Yang J, Li H, Gao Z, Chen G, Huang X, Yang X, Wan S, Chen C, Li B, Tan Y, Chen L, He M, Xie S, Li X, Zhuang X, Wang M, Xia Z, Luo L, Ma J, Dong B, Zhao J, Song Y, Ou Y, Li E, Xu L, Wang J, Xi Y, Li G, Xu E, Liang J, Yang X, Guo J, Chen X, Zhang Y, Li Q, Liu L, Li Y, Zhang X, Yang H, Lin D, Cheng X, Guo Y, Wang J, Zhan Q, Cui Y. Genomic analyses reveal mutational signatures and frequently altered genes in esophageal squamous cell carcinoma. Am J Hum Genet. 2015;96:597–611.

76. Qin HD, Liao XY, Chen YB, Huang SY, Xue WQ, Li FF, Ge XS, Liu DQ, Cai Q, Long J, Li XZ, Hu YZ, Zhang SD, Zhang LJ, Lehrman B, Scott AF, Lin D, Zeng YX, Shugart YY, Jia WH. Genomic characterization of esophageal squamous cell carcinoma reveals critical genes underlying tumorigenesis and poor prognosis. Am J Hum Genet. 2016;98:709–27.

77. Sawada G, Niida A, Uchi R, Hirata H, Shimamura T, Suzuki Y, Shiraishi Y, Chiba K, Imoto S, Takahashi Y, Iwaya T, Sudo T, Hayashi T, Takai H, Kawasaki Y, Matsukawa T, Eguchi H, Sugimachi K, Tanaka F, Suzuki H, Yamamoto K, Ishii H, Shimizu M, Yamazaki H, Yamazaki M, Tachimori Y, Kajiyama Y, Natsugoe S, Fujita H, Mafune K, Tanaka Y, Kelsell DP, Scott CA, Tsuji S, Yachida S, Shibata T, Sugano S, Doki Y, Akiyama T, Aburatani H, Ogawa S, Miyano S, Mori M, Mimori K. Genomic landscape of esophageal squamous cell carcinoma in a Japanese population. Gastroenterology. 2016;150:1171–82.

78. Secrier M, Li X, de Silva N, Eldridge MD, Contino G, Bornschein J, MacRae S, Grehan N, O'Donovan M, Miremadi A, Yang TP, Bower L, Chettouh H, Crawte J, Galeano-Dalmau N, Grabowska A, Saunders J, Underwood T, Waddell N, Barbour AP, Nutzinger B, Achilleos A, Edwards PA, Lynch AG, Tavaré S, Fitzgerald RC, Oesophageal Cancer Clinical and Molecular Stratification (OCCAMS) Consortium. Mutational signatures in esophageal adenocarcinoma define etiologically distinct subgroups with therapeutic relevance. Nat Genet. 2016;48:1131–41.

79. Cheng C, Zhou Y, Li H, Xiong T, Li S, Bi Y, Kong P, Wang F, Cui H, Li Y, Fang X, Yan T, Li Y, Wang J, Yang B, Zhang L, Jia Z, Song B, Hu X, Yang J, Qiu H, Zhang G, Liu J, Xu E, Shi R, Zhang Y, Liu H, He C, Zhao Z, Qian Y, Rong R, Han Z, Zhang Y, Luo W, Wang J, Peng S, Yang X, Li X, Li L, Fang H, Liu X, Ma L, Chen Y, Guo S, Chen X, Xi Y, Li G, Liang J, Yang X, Guo J, Jia J, Li Q, Cheng X, Zhan Q, Cui Y. Whole-genome sequencing reveals diverse models of structural variations in esophageal squamous cell carcinoma. Am J Hum Genet. 2016;98:256–74.

80. Cheng C, Cui H, Zhang L, Jia Z, Song B, Wang F, Li Y, Liu J, Kong P, Shi R, Bi Y, Yang B, Wang J, Zhao Z, Zhang Y, Hu X, Yang J, He C, Zhao Z, Wang J, Xi Y, Xu E, Li G, Guo S, Chen Y, Yang X, Chen X, Liang J, Guo J, Cheng X, Wang C, Zhan Q, Cui Y. Genomic analyses reveal FAM84B and the NOTCH pathway are associated with the progression of esophageal squamous cell carcinoma. Gigascience. 2016;5:1.

81. Fels Elliott DR, Perner J, Li X, Symmons MF, Verstak B, Eldridge M, Bower L, O'Donovan M, Gay NJ, OCCAMS Consortium, Fitzgerald RC. Impact of mutations in toll-like receptor pathway genes on esophageal carcinogenesis. PLoS Genet. 2017;13:e1006808.

82. Noorani A, Bornschein J, Lynch AG, Secrier M, Achilleos A, Eldridge M, Bower L, Weaver JMJ, Crawte J, Ong CA, Shannon N, MacRae S, Grehan N, Nutzinger B, O'Donovan M, Hardwick R, Tavaré S. Fitzgerald RC; oesophageal cancer clinical and molecular stratification (OCCAMS) consortium. A comparative analysis of whole genome sequencing of esophageal adenocarcinoma pre- and post-chemotherapy. Genome Res. 2017;27:902–12.

83. Liu X, Zhang M, Ying S, Zhang C, Lin R, Zheng J, Zhang G, Tian D, Guo Y, Du C, Chen Y, Chen S, Su X, Ji J, Deng W, Li X, Qiu S, Yan R, Xu Z, Wang Y, Guo Y, Cui J, Zhuang S, Yu H, Zheng Q, Marom M, Sheng S, Zhang G, Hu S, Li R, Su M. Genetic alterations in esophageal tissues from squamous dysplasia to carcinoma. Gastroenterology. 2017;153: 166–77.

84. Mamoori A, Wahab R, Islam F, Lee K, Vider J, Lu CT, Gopalan V, Lam AK. Clinical and biological significance of miR-193a-3p targeted KRAS in colorectal cancer pathogenesis. Hum Pathol. 2018;71:145–56.

85. Mamoori A, Gopalan V, Lu CT, Chua TC, Morris DL, Smith RA, Lam AK. Expression pattern of miR-451 and its target MIF (macrophage migration inhibitory factor) in colorectal cancer. J Clin Pathol. 2017;70:308–12.

86. Pillai S, Lo CY, Liew V, Lalloz M, Smith RA, Gopalan V, Lam AK. microRNA 183 family profiles in pheochromocytomas are related to clinical parameters and SDHB expression. Hum Pathol. 2017;64:91–7.

87. Islam F, Gopalan V, Vider J, Wahab R, Ebrahimi F, Lu CT, Kasem K, Lam AKY. MicroRNA-186-5p overexpression modulates colon cancer growth by repressing the expression of the FAM134B tumour inhibitor. Exp Cell Res. 2017;357:260–70.

88. Lee KT, Tan JK, Lam AK, Gan SY. MicroRNAs serving as potential biomarkers and therapeutic targets in nasopharyngeal carcinoma: a critical review. Crit Rev Oncol Hematol. 2016;103:1–9.

89. Gopalan V, Smith RA, Lam AK. Downregulation of microRNA-498 in colorectal cancers and its cellular effects. Exp Cell Res. 2015;330:423–8.

90. Salajegheh A, Vosgha H, Md Rahman A, Amin M, Smith RA, Lam A. Modulatory role of miR-205 in angiogenesis and progression of thyroid cancer. J Mol Endocrinol. 2015;55: 183–96.

91. Ebrahimi F, Gopalan V, Wahab R, Lu CT, Anthony Smith R, Lam AK. Deregulation of miR-126 expression in colorectal cancer pathogenesis and its clinical significance. Exp Cell Res. 2015;339:333–41.

92. Gopalan V, Pillai S, Ebrahimi F, Salajegheh A, Lam TC, Le TK, Langsford N, Ho YH, Smith RA, Lam AK. Regulation of microRNA-1288 in colorectal cancer: altered expression and its clinicopathological significance. Mol Carcinog. 2014;53:E36–44.

93. Ebrahimi F, Gopalan V, Smith RA, Lam AK. miR-126 in human cancers: clinical roles and current perspectives. Exp Mol Pathol. 2014;96:98–107.

94. Maroof H, Salajegheh A, Smith RA, Lam AK. Role of microRNA-34 family in cancer with particular reference to cancer angiogenesis. Exp Mol Pathol. 2014;97:298–304.

95. Vosgha H, Salajegheh A, Smith RA, Lam AK. The important roles of miR-205 in normal physiology, cancers and as a potential therapeutic target. Curr Cancer Drug Targets. 2014;14:621–37.

96. Maroof H, Salajegheh A, Smith RA, Lam AK. MicroRNA-34 family, mechanisms of action in cancer: a review. Curr Cancer Drug Targets. 2014;14:737–51.

97. Amin M, Islam F, Gopalan V, Lam AK. Detection and quantification of microRNAs in in oesophageal adenocarcinoma. Methods Mol Biol. 1756;2018:257–68.

98. Kamal Masud M, Islam MN, Haque MH, Tanaka S, Gopalan V, Alici G, Nguyen NT, Lam AK, Hossain MSA, Yamauchi Y, Shiddiky MJA. Gold-loaded nanoporous superparamagnetic nanocubes for catalytic signal amplification in detecting miRNA. Chem Commun (Camb). 2017;53:8231–4.

99. Amin M, Lam AK. Current perspectives of mi-RNA in oesophageal adenocarcinoma: roles in predicting carcinogenesis, progression and values in clinical management. Exp Mol Pathol. 2015;98:411–8.

100. Mei LL, Qiu YT, Zhang B, Shi ZZ. MicroRNAs in esophageal squamous cell carcinoma: potential biomarkers and therapeutic targets. Cancer Biomark. 2017;19:1–9.

101. Islam F, Gopalan V, Law S, Tang JC, Chan KW, Lam AK∗. MiR-498 in oesophageal squamous cell carcinoma: clinicopathological impacts and functional interactions. Hum Pathol. 2017;62:141–51.

102. Gopalan V, Islam F, Pillai S, Tang JC, Tong DK, Law S, Chan KW, Lam AK. Overexpression of microRNA-1288 in oesophageal squamous cell carcinoma. Exp Cell Res. 2016;348:146–54.
103. Islam F, Qiao B, Smith RA, Gopalan V, Lam AK. Cancer stem cell: fundamental experimental pathological concepts and updates. Exp Mol Pathol. 2015;98:184–91.
104. Wahab SMR, Islam F, Gopalan V, Lam AK. The identifications and clinical implications of cancer stem cells in colorectal cancer. Clin Colorectal Cancer. 2017;16:93–102.
105. Islam F, Gopalan V, Smith RA, Lam AK. Translational potential of cancer stem cells: a review of the detection of cancer stem cells and their roles in cancer recurrence and cancer treatment. Exp Cell Res. 2015;335:135–47.
106. Chruścik A, Gopalan V, Lam AK. The clinical and biological roles of transforming growth factor beta in colon cancer stem cells: a systematic review. Eur J Cell Biol. 2018;97:15–22.
107. Qiao B, Gopalan V, Chen Z, Smith RA, Tao Q, Lam AKY. Epithelial-mesenchymal transition and mesenchymal-epithelial transition are essential for the acquisition of stem cell properties in hTERT-immortalised oral epithelial cells. Bio Cell. 2012;104:476–89.
108. Gopalan V, Islam F, Lam AK. Surface markers for the identification of cancer stem cells. Methods Mol Biol. 1692;2018:17–29.
109. Islam F, Gopalan V, Wahab R, Smith RA, Lam AK. Cancer stem cells in oesophageal squamous cell carcinoma: identification, prognostic and treatment perspectives. Crit Rev Oncol Hematol. 2015;96:9–19.
110. Islam F, Gopalan V, Lam AK. Identification of cancer stem cells in esophageal adenocarcinoma. Methods Mol Biol. 2018;1756:165–76.
111. di Pietro M, Alzoubaidi D, Fitzgerald RC. Barrett's esophagus and cancer risk: how research advances can impact clinical practice. Gut Liver. 2014;8:356–70.
112. Ong CAJ, Lao-Sirieix P, Fitzgerald RC. Biomarkers in Barrett's esophagus and esophageal adenocarcinoma: predictors of progression and prognosis. World J Gastroenterol. 2010;16:5669–81.
113. Chen M, Huang J, Zhu Z, Zhang J, Li K. Systematic review and meta-analysis of tumor biomarkers in predicting prognosis in esophageal cancer. BMC Cancer. 2013;13:539.
114. Shang L, Liu HJ, Hao JJ, Jiang YY, Shi F, Zhang Y, Cai Y, Xu X, Jia XM, Zhan QM, Wang MR. A panel of overexpressed proteins for prognosis in esophageal squamous cell carcinoma. PLoS One. 2014;9:e111045.
115. Lam KY, Law S, Lo T, Tung HM, Wong J. The clinicopathological significance of p21 and p53 expression in esophageal squamous cell carcinoma: an analysis of 153 patients. Am J Gastroenterol. 1999;94:2060–8.
116. Lam KY, Law SYK, So MKP, Fok M, Ma LT, Wong J. Prognostic implication of proliferative markers MIB-1 and PC 10 in esophageal squamous cell carcinoma. Cancer. 1996;77:7–13.
117. Tong DK, Law S, Kwong DL, Chan KW, Lam AK, Wong KH. Histological regression of squamous esophageal carcinoma assessed by percentage of residual viable cells after neoadjuvant chemoradiation is an important prognostic factor. Ann Surg Oncol. 2010;17:2184–92.
118. Lam KY, Law S, Ma LT, Ong SK, Wong J. Pre-operative chemotherapy for squamous cell carcinoma of the esophagus: do histological assessment and p53 overexpression predict chemo-responsiveness? Eur J Cancer. 1997;33:1221–5.
119. Okumura H, Uchikado Y, Setoyama T, Matsumoto M, Owaki T, Ishigami S, Natsugoe S. Biomarkers for predicting the response of esophageal squamous cell carcinoma to neoadjuvant chemoradiation therapy. Surg Today. 2014;44:421–8.
120. Zhang SS, Huang QY, Yang H, Xie X, Luo KJ, Wen J, Cai XL, Yang F, Hu Y, Fu JH. Correlation of p53 status with the response to chemotherapy-based treatment in esophageal cancer: a meta-analysis. Ann Surg Oncol. 2013;20:2419–27.
121. Bain GH, Petty RD. Predicting response to treatment in gastroesophageal junction adenocarcinomas: combining clinical, imaging, and molecular biomarkers. Oncologist. 2010;15:270–84.
122. Imdahl A, Jenkner J, Ihling C, Rückauer K, Farthmann EH. Is MIB-1 proliferation index a predictor for response to neoadjuvant therapy in patients with esophageal cancer? Am J Surg. 2000;179:514–20.

123. Lam AK. Application of pathological staging in esophageal adenocarcinoma. Methods Mol Biol. 2018;1756:93–103.
124. Ung L, Lam AK, Morris DL, Chua TC. Tissue-based biomarkers predicting outcomes in metastatic colorectal cancer: a review. Clin Transl Oncol. 2014;16:425–35.
125. Pakneshan S, Salajegheh A, Smith RA, Lam AK. Clinicopathological relevance of BRAF mutations in human cancer. Pathology. 2013;45:346–56.
126. Rahman MA, Salajegheh A, Smith RA, Lam AK. BRAF inhibitors: from the laboratory to clinical trials. Crit Rev Oncol Hematol. 2014;90:220–32.
127. Rahman MA, Salajegheh A, Smith RA, Lam AK. BRAF inhibitor therapy for melanoma, thyroid and colorectal cancers: development of resistance and future prospects. Curr Cancer Drug Targets. 2014;14:128–43.
128. O'Sullivan CC, Connolly RM. Pertuzumab and its accelerated approval: evolving treatment paradigms and new challenges in the management of HER2-positive breast cancer. Oncology (Williston Park). 2014;28:186–94.
129. Wiedmann MW, Mössner J. New and emerging combination therapies for esophageal cancer. Cancer Manag Res. 2013;5:133–46.
130. Kordes S, Cats A, Meijer SL, van Laarhoven HW. Targeted therapy for advanced esophago-gastric adenocarcinoma. Crit Rev Oncol Hematol. 2014;90:68–76.
131. Orditura M, Galizia G, Fabozzi A, Lieto E, Gambardella V, Morgillo F, Del Genio GM, Fei L, Di Martino N, Renda A, Ciardiello F, De Vita F. Preoperative treatment of locally advanced esophageal carcinoma (review). Int J Oncol. 2013;43:1745–53.
132. Nakajima M, Kato H. Treatment options for esophageal squamous cell carcinoma. Expert Opin Pharmacother. 2013;14:1345–54.
133. Boland PM, Burtness B. Esophageal carcinoma: are modern targeted therapies shaking the rock? Curr Opin Oncol. 2013;25:417–24.
134. Lam KY, Tin L, Ma L. C-erbB-2 protein expression in oesophageal squamous epithelium from oesophageal squamous cell carcinomas, with special reference to histological grade of carcinoma and pre-invasive lesions. Eur J Surg Oncol. 1998;24:431–5.
135. Hicks DG, Whitney-Miller C. HER2 testing in gastric and gastroesophageal junction cancers: a new therapeutic target and diagnostic challenge. Appl Immunohistochem Mol Morphol. 2011;19:506–8.
136. Bartley AN, Washington MK, Colasacco C, Ventura CB, Ismaila N, Benson AB 3rd, Carrato A, Gulley ML, Jain D, Kakar S, Mackay HJ, Streutker C, Tang L, Troxell M, Ajani JA. HER2 testing and clinical decision making in gastroesophageal adenocarcinoma: guideline from the College of American Pathologists, American Society for Clinical Pathology, and the American Society of Clinical Oncology. J Clin Oncol. 2017;35:446–64.
137. Kumarasinghe MP, Brown I, Raftopoulos S, Bourke MJ, Charlton A, de Boer WB, Eckstein R, Epari K, Gill AJ, Lam AK, Price T, Streutker C, Lauwers GY. Standardised reporting protocol for endoscopic resection for Barrett oesophagus associated neoplasia: expert consensus recommendations. Pathology. 2014;46:473–80.
138. Saremi N, Lam AK. Application of tissue microarray in esophageal adenocarcinoma. In: Lam AK, editor. Methods in molecular biology: esophageal adenocarcinoma: Springer; 2018. (in press).
139. Lam AK, Leung M. Whole-slide imaging for esophageal adenocarcinoma. Methods Mol Biol. 2018;1756:135–42.
140. Gopalan V, Lam AK. Circulatory tumor cells in esophageal adenocarcinoma. Methods Mol Biol. 2018;1756:177–86.
141. Smith RA, Lam AK. Liquid biopsy for investigation of cancer DNA in oesophageal adenocarcinoma: cell free plasma DNA and exosome associated DNA. Methods Mol Biol. 2018;1756:187–94.
142. Islam F, Gopalan V. Lam AK. RNA interference mediated genes silencing in oesophageal adenocarcinoma. Methods Mol Biol. 2018;1756:269–79.
143. Tang JCO, Wan TSK, Wong N, Pang E, Lam KY, Law SYK, Chow LMC, Ma ESK, Chan LC, Wong J, Srivastava G. Establishment and characterization of a new xenograft-derived

human esophageal squamous cell line SLMT-1 of Chinese origin. Cancer Genet Cytogenet. 2001;124:36–41.

144. Hu YC, Lam KY, Wan TSK, Fang WG, Ma ESK, Chan LC, Srivastava G. Establishment and characterization of HKESC-1, a new cancer cell line from human esophageal squamous cell carcinoma. Cancer Genet Cytogenet. 2000;118:112–20.

145. Hu YC, Lam KY, Law SYK, Wan TSK, Ma ESK, Kwong YL, Chan LC, Wong J, Srivastava G. Establishment, characterization, karyotyping, and comparative genomic hybridization analysis of HKESC-2 and HKESC-3: two newly established human esophageal squamous cell lines. Cancer Genet Cytogenet. 2002;135:120–7.

146. Boonstra JJ, Tilanus HW, Dinjens WN. Translational research on esophageal adenocarcinoma: from cell line to clinic. Dis Esophagus. 2015;28:90–6.

147. Ip JC, Ko JM, Yu VZ, Chan KW, Lam AK, Law S, Tong DK, Lung ML. A versatile orthotopic nude mouse model for study of esophageal squamous cell carcinoma. Biomed Res Int. 2015;2015:910715.

148. Furihata T, Sakai T, Kawamata H, Omotehara F, Shinagawa Y, Imura J, Ueda Y, Kubota K, Fujimori T. A new in vivo model for studying invasion and metastasis of esophageal squamous cell carcinoma. Int J Oncol. 2001;19:903–7.

149. Hori T, Yamashita Y, Ohira M, Matsumura Y, Muguruma K, Hirakawa K. A novel orthotopic implantation model of human esophageal carcinoma in nude rats: CD44H mediates cancer cell invasion in vitro and in vivo. Int J Cancer. 2001;92:489–96.

Pathology of Premalignant and Malignant Disease of the Esophagus

3

Jessica Tracht, Brian S. Robinson, and Alyssa M. Krasinskas

Introduction

Like most structures of the alimentary canal, the esophagus is a tubular muscular structure that contains a mucosa, submucosa, muscularis propria, and surrounding connective tissue (termed adventitia in the esophagus) (Fig. 3.1). Anatomically, the esophagus extends from the cricopharyngeal muscle, which forms the upper esophageal sphincter, to the lower esophageal junction, where the stomach originates. Histologically, the mucosa consists of a stratified non-keratinizing squamous epithelium, lamina propria and muscularis mucosae. The squamous epithelium sits atop a basement membrane that separates it from the lamina propria. The lamina propria is composed of loose fibroconnective tissue, lymphatic spaces, and capillary vessels. The muscularis mucosa is a thin muscular layer that separates the mucosa from the submucosa. The submucosa is composed of dense irregular fibrovascular connective tissue admixed with scattered mucin-producing glands (esophageal submucosal glands) and ducts, which aid in the passage of food. Deep to the submucosa is the muscularis propria, which is primarily composed of striated muscle in the upper 1/3 of the esophagus, smooth muscle in the lower 1/3 of the esophagus, and a mixture of both in the mid esophagus. Finally, deep to the muscularis propria is the adventitia, a layer of connective tissue and adipose tissue that helps link the esophagus to adjacent structures. The esophagus, unlike most tubular structures of the alimentary canal, lacks a serosa (Fig. 3.1).

Neoplastic transformation can involve any of the cell types found in the esophagus. However, the vast majority of malignant tumors that arise from the esophagus are epithelial in origin. This review will focus on the malignant

J. Tracht · B. S. Robinson · A. M. Krasinskas (✉)
Department of Pathology and Laboratory Medicine, Emory University, Atlanta, GA, USA
e-mail: jtracht@auroradx.com; bsrobin@emory.edu; akrasin@emory.edu

© Springer Nature Switzerland AG 2020
N. F. Saba, B. F. El-Rayes (eds.), *Esophageal Cancer*,
https://doi.org/10.1007/978-3-030-29832-6_3

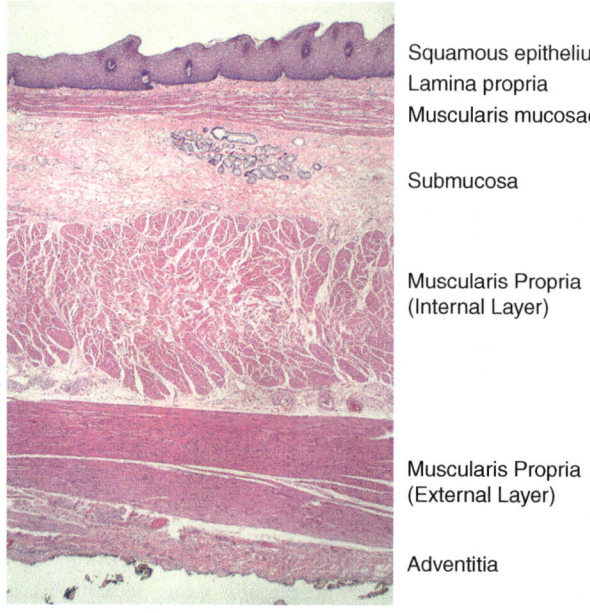

Squamous epithelium
Lamina propria
Muscularis mucosae

Submucosa

Muscularis Propria
(Internal Layer)

Muscularis Propria
(External Layer)

Adventitia

Fig. 3.1 Structural layers of the esophagus (H&E stain). The innermost layer (or tunica) is the mucosa. The mucosa is composed of an epithelial lining (squamous epithelium), the underlying lamina propria (loose connective tissue that supports the epithelium), and the muscularis mucosae (a thin layer of smooth muscle). Deep to the mucosa is the submucosa, which contains more cellular connective tissues, prominent blood vessels (with muscularized arteries), nerve fibers (Meissner plexus), and submucosal mucus (exocrine) glands. A submucosal gland is present in this figure. The thick outer muscular layer is called the muscularis mucosa (or muscularis externa) and in the distal esophagus (as shown in this figure) is composed of an inner circular layer and an outer longitudinal layer of smooth muscle; they layers are separated by the myenteric plexus. Skeletal muscle is admixed with smooth muscle of the muscularis propria in the mid esophagus, and in the proximal esophagus, the outer muscular layers are primarily composed of skeletal muscle. The outermost layer of the esophagus is the adventitia, which is composed of loose connective tissue and helps to anchor the esophagus in place (H&E stain, 20×)

epithelial lesions of the esophagus, namely, adenocarcinoma and squamous cell carcinoma, and their precursor lesions.

Esophageal cancer affects more than 450,000 people worldwide and squamous cell carcinoma is the predominant histologic type [1]. In the United States, Australia, the United Kingdom, and some Western European countries, the incidence of adenocarcinoma is increasing rapidly and now exceeds that of squamous cell carcinoma [1]. The estimated number of new cases of esophageal cancer in the United States in 2019 is 17,650, and the vast majority (13,750) will affect men [2]. Esophageal cancer is estimated to be the seventh leading cause of cancer deaths in men in 2019 in the United States, accounting for 13,020 or 4% of all cancer deaths (following lung, prostate, colorectal, pancreatic, liver cancer and leukemia) [2].

Pathology of Adenocarcinoma and Its Precursor Lesions

Adenocarcinoma typically arises in the distal third of the esophagus and is associated clinically with dysphagia and weight loss. Several risk factors have been described for esophageal adenocarcinoma, including increased age, male gender, white ethnicity, high body mass index, low fruit and vegetable intake, absence of *Helicobacter pylori* infection, the presence of a hiatal hernia, and history of reflux disease [3–10]. Clinical observations and studies in animal models suggest a linear sequence in the development of esophageal adenocarcinoma. Initially, the replacement of the normal squamous epithelium by glandular mucosa (gastric type or intestinal type) occurs secondary to repeated injury from bile and acid reflux. This is followed by dysplastic change within this metaplastic tissue, leading to the development of invasive carcinoma after molecular evolution of the dysplastic epithelium.

Precursor Lesions of Esophageal Adenocarcinoma: Barrett's Esophagus and Barrett's Esophagus-Associated Dysplasia

As recommended by the American College of Gastroenterology in 2016, Barrett's esophagus (BE) "should be diagnosed when there is extension of salmon-colored mucosa into the tubular esophagus extending ≥1 cm proximal to the gastroesophageal junction (GEJ) with biopsy confirmation of intestinal metaplasia (IM)" [11]. Of note, not all professional organizations or countries, including the British Society of Gastroenterology and Japan, require the histologic documentation of intestinal metaplasia [12, 13].

Macroscopically, Barrett's esophagus appears as a well-demarcated area of erythematous or "velvety" mucosa within the squamous-lined tubular esophagus. Histologically, three different types of columnar or glandular metaplasia can be seen on biopsies from patients with "Barrett's" esophagus: (1) gastric cardia-type mucosa (composed of mucin secreting glands); (2) gastric oxyntic (or fundus)-type mucosa composed of parietal cells, chief cells, and mucus secreting cells; and (3) specialized columnar epithelium or intestinal metaplasia containing round, bluish, barrel-shaped cells called goblet cells, often admixed with gastric cardia-type glands (Fig. 3.2). From the pathologist's perspective, the gastric-type mucosa +/− goblet cells seen in the tubular esophagus is indistinguishable from the true gastric mucosa seen in the cardia. Because intestinal metaplasia is commonly seen in the cardia of the stomach in the general population without Barrett's esophagus [14], the American College of Gastroenterology guidelines recommend that biopsies only be taken if there is macroscopic evidence of Barret's esophagus. Biopsies should not be performed in the presence of a normal Z line or a Z line with <1 cm of variability as sampling of gastric cardia with intestinal metaplasia may occur [11]. If the pathologist does not see submucosal glands on a biopsy and does not know what the endoscopist observed at the time of biopsy, a diagnosis of "gastric-type mucosa with intestinal metaplasia" may be rendered instead of a diagnosis of "Barrett's esophagus."

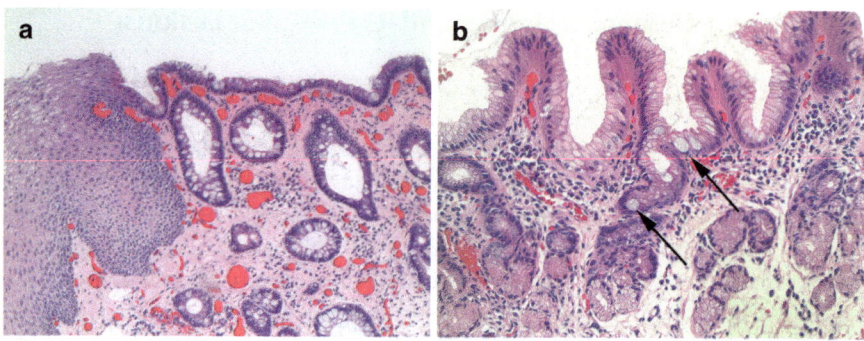

Fig. 3.2 Intestinal metaplasia. (**a**) In this example, the squamous mucosa has been replaced by glandular mucosa of intestinal type. Some intact squamous epithelium is present on the left. All of the glands present on the right contain goblet cells (specialized columnar epithelium or intestinal metaplasia). If this biopsy was obtained ≥1 cm proximal to the GEJ, these findings are consistent with Barrett's esophagus (H&E stain, 100×). (**b**) Gastric-type mucosa with rare goblet cells (focal intestinal metaplasia). Many biopsies from islands of velvety mucosa within the tubular esophagus contain gastric cardiac-type glands. If even one goblet cell is identified, a diagnosis of (focal) intestinal metaplasia can be rendered. As shown in this example, there are about five goblet cells (two are highlighted by arrows) present within gastric-type mucosa. If this biopsy was obtained ≥1 cm proximal to the GEJ, these findings are consistent with Barrett's esophagus (H&E stain, 100×)

It is worth noting that, in addition to designating the presence and/or absence of intestinal metaplasia, pathology reports may detail several other histologic mimics of metaplasia. "Pseudogoblet cells" refer to barrel-shaped gastric foveolar cells that may look like goblet cells on low magnification but have an eosinophilic tinge and do not stain for Alcian blue due to a production of neutral mucins. The term "columnar blues" refers to the identification of mucus cells that contain bluish mucin on the H&E stain and stain positive for Alcian blue but lack goblet cell morphology. The term "multilayered epithelium" may be noted in reports. This finding refers to the identification of an epithelium that contains flattened squamous-appearing cells in the basal layers with an overlying columnar mucus cell layer. Studies have shown that this epithelium can show immunohistochemical features similar to intestinal-type epithelium, indicating that it may represent an early or intermediate phase in the development of intestinal metaplasia and Barrett's esophagus [15]. Finally, pathologists may report the presence of "subsquamous intestinal metaplasia" (also called "buried Barrett's" or "squamous overgrowth"), particularly in endoscopic mucosal resection specimens. Although subsquamous intestinal metaplasia is present in the majority of endoscopic mucosal resection specimens and is no longer felt to be a post-ablative phenomenon, the long-term clinical significance is uncertain and histologic evaluation of squamous-lined mucosa adjacent to areas of BE may be indicated [16, 17].

Once a diagnosis of Barrett's esophagus has been rendered, increased surveillance is indicated at intervals of 3–5 years to monitor for the presence of dysplasia and/or adenocarcinoma. Studies have shown 0.12–0.38% of patients with nondysplastic Barrett's esophagus will develop adenocarcinoma each year [18]; thus

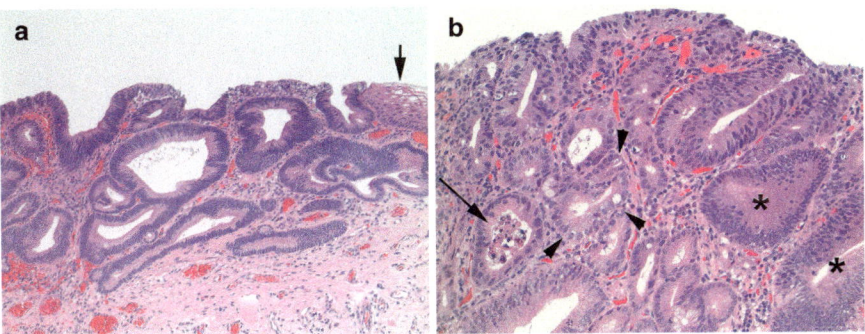

Fig. 3.3 Dysplasia in Barrett's esophagus. (**a**) Low-grade dysplasia. All of the glandular epithelium in this example is involved by low-grade dysplasia; there is a small portion of intact squamous mucosa present (arrow). When dysplasia develops in Barrett's esophagus, the normal goblet cells are often lost because they are replaced by neoplastic epithelial cells that are replicating without normal inhibition and maturation. Characteristic features of low-grade dysplasia include elongation and crowding of the cell nuclei (penicillate nuclei) and increased nuclear-cytoplasmic ratios. These features are typically present from the deep glands all the way to the luminal surface, indicating the lack of maturation. As opposed to high-grade dysplasia, the cell nuclei are still basally oriented (nuclear polarity is maintained), the nuclei are not round, and nucleoli are inconspicuous (H&E stain, 100×). (**b**) High-grade dysplasia. All of the glands in this example show evidence of dysplasia; two glands (∗) show features of low-grade dysplasia, but most of the remaining glands, especially towards the left and towards the luminal surface, show features of high-grade dysplasia. In high-grade dysplasia, there are both cytologic changes and architectural changes. Cytologically, the nuclear-cytoplasmic ratio is increased and the nuclei "round up" often contain prominent nucleoli and lose polarity (several nuclei appear detached from the basal aspect of the cells and are present towards the luminal surface of the glands). Architecturally, the cells proliferate within the lumens of the dysplastic glands, creating cribriform architecture or "gland-within-gland" morphology (arrowheads). Necrotic and apoptotic cells are also often present within glandular lumens (arrow) (H&E stain, 100×)

screening efforts have focused largely on identifying metaplasia in at-risk individuals. Definitive dysplastic change falls into one of two general categories: low-grade or high-grade dysplasia. Features of low-grade dysplasia (Fig. 3.3a) include increased epithelial proliferation characterized by nuclear crowding and minimal distortion of glandular architecture. Mild cytologic atypia and nuclear enlargement, hyperchromasia, stratification, and irregular nuclear contours are also observed. Nuclear-to-cytoplasmic ratios and mitotic counts remain low, basal nuclear polarity is preserved, and in general, the glandular architecture is retained, though there may be increased glandular crowding. Low-grade dysplasia in Barrett's esophagus may resemble the epithelium of a colonic-type adenoma or may be composed of foveolar or gastric-type neoplastic cells. For a diagnosis of low-grade dysplasia, the cytologic atypia should extend to the surface. When surface involvement is not present or cannot be evaluated (for example, due to squamous overgrowth), the term "indefinite for dysplasia" may be used.

In contrast to low-grade dysplasia, high-grade dysplasia (Fig. 3.3b) is characterized by increased cellular atypia and complex architecture. Cells have high

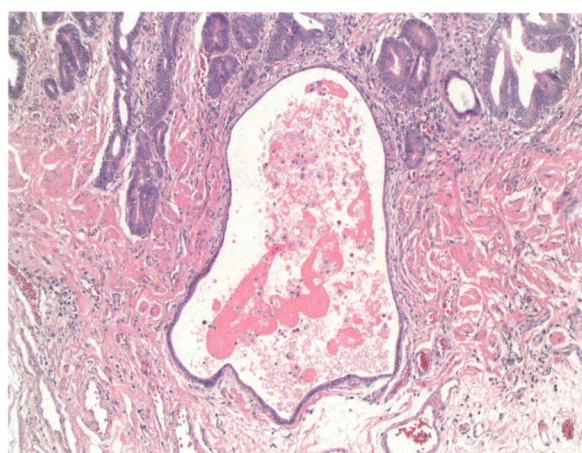

Fig. 3.4 Attenuated gland in the background of high-grade dysplasia. Even though the epithelial lining of the dilated gland is flat and appears bland, the presence of luminal necrotic debris and its presence within muscle bundles make this gland suspicious for attenuated high-grade dysplasia, and it may actually represent early intramucosal adenocarcinoma. If present in the submucosa or within the muscularis propria, attenuated glands with these same histologic features would be diagnostic of invasive adenocarcinoma (H&E stain, 100×)

nuclear-to-cytoplasmic ratios, and there is a loss of basal nuclear polarity with the large often rounded nuclei containing prominent nucleoli. There is also distortion of the normal glandular architecture, often with intraglandular bridging or cribriforming. Cellular or apoptotic debris may be found within glandular lumens. Mitotic activity is evident and often extends beyond the deep proliferative zone and may reach the luminal surface. Deep glands with dilated lumens lined by attenuated epithelium may also indicate the presence of high-grade dysplasia or a lesion of greater clinical significance (Fig. 3.4). In the seventh edition of the AJCC staging manual, the term "Tis" (or "carcinoma in situ") was removed from all epithelial neoplasia of the gastrointestinal tract and was replaced by "high-grade dysplasia" [19]. This distinction is unchanged in the eighth edition of the AJCC staging manual [20]. Since there are some cases of intraepithelial neoplasia that are more atypical than expected for high-grade dysplasia, or cases where definitive invasion cannot be documented, some pathologists may use the term "carcinoma in situ" or "at least high-grade dysplasia." If these terms are noted in the pathology report without an explanatory comment, a discussion with the pathologist may help clarify its meaning in individual cases.

Ancillary studies to aid in the detection of goblet cells and/or dysplasia in Barrett's esophagus are of limited utility at this time. Goblet cells produce acid-rich mucins and thus stain intensely blue with an Alcian blue stain at a pH of 2.5. In addition, the intestinal mucosa stains positive for immunohistochemical stains such as CDX2, villin, and MUC-2 (markers of intestinal differentiation) [21–24]. Although ancillary stains can detect goblet cells and intestinalized epithelium, these stains are not required for a diagnosis of intestinal metaplasia, as the goblet cells can often be readily identified on the routine hematoxylin and eosin (H&E) stain (Fig. 3.2) [25]. Immunohistochemistry to detect aberrant p53 expression in dysplasia and/or as an indicator of malignancy risk may be performed by pathologists; however, its utility in complementing routine histology remains uncertain. Some studies indicate that p53 may be useful in the identification of dysplasia and malignant progression [26, 27]. Immunohistochemistry for p53 is used occasionally by pathologists as an adjunct to diagnosis in select cases. However, based on the review by the Rodger C. Haggitt Gastrointestinal Pathology Society, routine use of ancillary studies is not recommended for the diagnosis of Barrett's esophagus, dysplasia in Barrett's esophagus, or for the final determination of high risk of malignant progression [25]. Further larger prospective studies are needed before p53 or other biomarkers are recommended for this purpose [25].

As recommended by the American College of Gastroenterology, a diagnosis of dysplasia of any grade within Barrett's esophagus should be rendered after review by two separate pathologists, and ideally, this review would include at least one pathologist with expertise in gastrointestinal pathology [11]. This is due to the high interobserver variability seen in the diagnosis of dysplasia in Barrett's epithelium. Such variability is seen most often in the categories of low-grade dysplasia and indeterminate for dysplasia [28]. Variability is also seen between academic and community-centered practices. Recent studies have demonstrated a large percentage of diagnoses of low-grade and indeterminate for dysplasia rendered at community-based practices are downgraded when reviewed by a pathologist with gastrointestinal pathology training [29–31]. However, a pathologist with this specialized gastrointestinal training may not always be available in all settings, and in some settings a second pathologist may not be available for additional review. Therefore, it is important to communicate with the pathologist to determine how to approach these instances in which a new diagnosis of dysplasia in Barrett's esophagus is made.

Esophageal Adenocarcinoma

Once adenocarcinoma develops, it can be managed by different modalities. Small early lesions may be amenable to endoscopic mucosal resection. Surgery +/− neoadjuvant therapy is the treatment of choice for more deeply invasive or more advanced lesions. Grossly, esophageal adenocarcinoma often appears as an infiltrative mass in the distal third of the esophagus, although fungating, polypoid, and flat growths can be seen (Fig. 3.5a). Histologically, adenocarcinoma is characterized by invasion beyond the basement membrane. Invasion beyond the basement membrane into the lamina propria of the esophagus is a significant development, as it allows access to lymphatic channels that are not found in other areas of the alimentary track, such as the colon. Hence, as per the AJCC staging recommendations, early esophageal adenocarcinoma is staged as either T1a (intramucosal invasion) or T1b (submucosal invasion) [20].

In pathology, most early adenocarcinomas are evaluated on either small biopsies or endoscopic mucosal resection (EMR) specimens. Determining the depth of

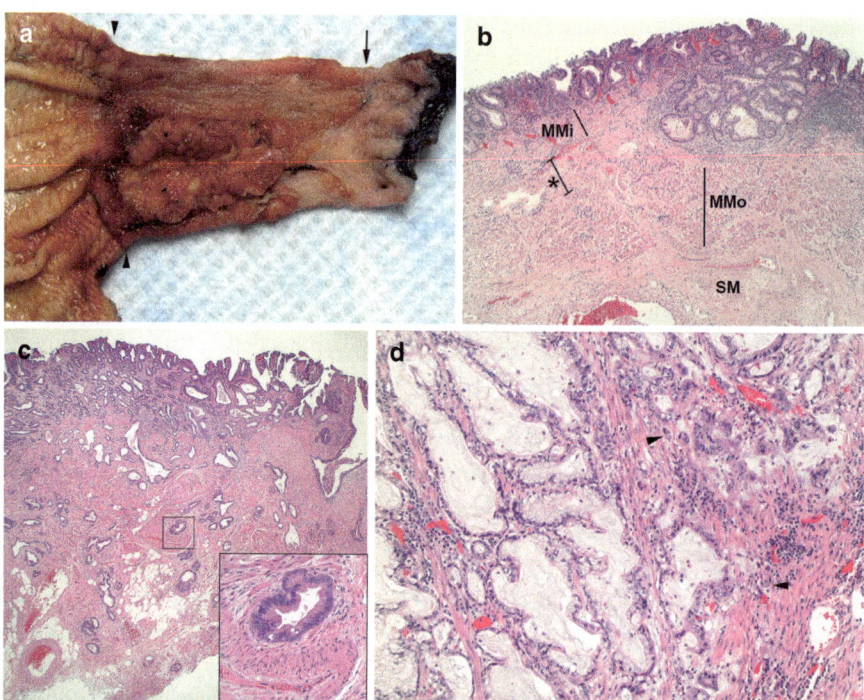

Fig. 3.5 Adenocarcinoma. (**a**) Esophagogastrectomy specimen with adenocarcinoma. The stomach, with normal rugal folds, is towards the left, while the inked squamous-lined esophageal margin is towards the right. The arrowheads highlight the esophagogastric junction. The majority of the esophagus is lined by velvety-appearing mucosa, which represents Barrett's esophagus. The arrow indicates the squamocolumnar junction, which is several centimeters from the esophagogastric junction. Within the distal esophagus and within Barrett's segment, there is an exophytic mass that is an adenocarcinoma. This patient did not receive neoadjuvant therapy prior to the resection. (**b**) Intramucosal adenocarcinoma. A small focus of adenocarcinoma is invading with a pushing border into the space (∗) between the two layers of the duplicated muscularis mucosae, making this a pT1a adenocarcinoma. Even though this tumor has invaded through the internal layer of the muscularis mucosae (MMi), it has not invaded through the outer (duplicated) layer (MMo), so this is not invasive into the submucosa (SM) (H&E stain, 40×). (**c**) Well-differentiated adenocarcinoma. This endoscopic mucosal resection specimen shows dysplasia towards the luminal surface and glandular structures "dripping" through the muscularis mucosae into the submucosa. On low magnification (H&E stain, 20×), there is no obvious desmoplastic response. On high magnification (inset, H&E stain, 200×), if taken out of context, the malignant gland could represent a dysplastic gland, but its presence in the submucosa (as noted by the large muscular artery adjacent to the gland) indicates that this is invasive adenocarcinoma present in the submucosa. (**d**) Invasive adenocarcinoma. This example is primarily well differentiated as most of the malignant cells are forming glands. There is not much desmoplasia in this example, but the malignant glands are present within the muscularis propria and the smooth muscle fibers can be seen in the background stroma. Compared to high-grade dysplasia, there is a bit more cytologic and nuclear atypia in this example of adenocarcinoma, including more nuclear pleomorphism, as well as irregularly shaped glands (upper right corner) and some small nests and single cell infiltration (arrowheads) (H&E stain, 100×)

invasion can be challenging on such specimens because of a phenomenon known as duplication of the muscularis mucosae. For unknown mechanistic reasons, in areas of intestinal metaplasia (Barrett's esophagus), a new internal layer of the muscularis mucosa is created (Fig. 3.5b) [32, 33]. In order to become a T1b lesion, an adenocarcinoma arising in these areas needs to invade through three layers: the "new" superficial muscularis mucosae, the loose connective tissue between the two layers, and then the deep or true muscularis mucosae. Hence, true submucosal invasion is difficult to determine on small biopsies or superficial EMR specimens.

Since EMR specimens are small but contain pertinent information, recommendations for the handling of such specimens have been reported [34]. Ideally, fresh specimens should be pinned to cork or foam prior to formalin fixation. Photographic documentation is recommended. Then the entire specimen should be submitted for histologic evaluation. In addition to reporting the main pathologic findings (dysplasia or intramucosal carcinoma), pathologists must comment on the status of the lateral (mucosal) and deep margins. If an adenocarcinoma is present, the depth of invasion must be assessed. As noted above, the pitfall of overcalling a T1a lesion as a T1b tumor due to a duplicated muscularis mucosae must be avoided. The AJCC further subdivides both intramucosal (m1, m2, and m3) and submucosal (sm1, sm2, sm3) invasion [20]. Although the AJCC does not take into account the different layers of the duplicated MM, other studies have [35]. Hence, pathologists should attempt to describe the specific depth of invasion, for example, "intramucosal adenocarcinoma, invasive into the superficial muscularis mucosal layer." However, only the depth of mucosal invasion may be discernable on biopsies or small EMR specimens. Determining the different levels of submucosal invasion (i.e., sm1, sm2, sm3) is not practical in biopsies or small EMR specimens where the outer limit of the measurement (border of the muscularis propria) is absent. However, given the high risk of nodal involvement with submucosal invasion, the precise depth of invasion on these types of specimens should not alter patient management.

Grading of adenocarcinoma has prognostic significance and falls into one of three categories: well (G1), moderately (G2), or poorly (G3) differentiated; undifferentiated tumors are uncommon, often cannot be subtyped as squamous or glandular, and are considered to be grade 4 (G4) tumors. The importance of accurate tumor grading is critical for clinical management, as AJCC guidelines for clinical staging of adenocarcinoma integrate tumor grade into the algorithm for determining clinical stage (Table 3.1) [20]. For example, a well or moderately differentiated T2 N0 M0 tumor is stage IC, while a poorly differentiated T2 N0 M0 tumor is stage IIA. For adenocarcinoma, grading involves determining the percent of tumor that is composed of glands: well-differentiated tumors contain >95% glands, moderately differentiated tumors contain 50–95% glands, and poorly differentiated tumors display <50% glandular architecture [36]. When tumors contain areas of multiple grades, the highest grade is documented. Histologically, well-differentiated tumors are composed of glands with irregular shapes or profiles (often with focal cribriform formation) lined by cuboidal to columnar cells with mild to moderate atypia. Not all adenocarcinomas illicit a desmoplastic response. In the absence of desmoplasia, a well-differentiated

Table 3.1 Influence of grade on clinical stage for esophageal adenocarcinoma and squamous cell carcinoma

T	Grade	Clinical stage
Adenocarcinoma		
T1	1 or X	IA
T1a	2	IB
T1b	1, 2 or X	IB
T1	3	IC
T2	1 or 2	IC
T2	3 or X	IIA
Squamous cell carcinoma		
T1a	1 or X	IA
	2 or 3	IB
T2	1	IB
	2, 3 or X	IIA
T3	1	IIA
	2, 3 or X	IIB

Note: For all entries above, the N stage is N0 and the M stage is M0. Grade 1 is well differentiated, grade 2 is moderately differentiated, and grade 3 is poorly differentiated

adenocarcinoma could be easily misdiagnosed as dysplasia if assessed out of context. Hence, even the most bland-appearing glands are adenocarcinoma if they are present in the submucosa or muscularis propria (Fig. 3.5c). Esophageal adenocarcinomas are often well-to-moderately differentiated (Fig. 3.5d). As tumors become more poorly differentiated, a more sheetlike appearance is identified. Signet-ring cells, single infiltrating cells, and/or wildly atypical tumor cells may be present. Often, poorly differentiated tumors elicit a strong desmoplastic response from neighboring stromal cells. When dealing with a poorly differentiated adenocarcinoma on biopsy specimens, metastatic disease should be considered and excluded, either clinically or immunohistochemically (for example, immunostains for breast markers could help diagnose metastatic breast carcinoma). Unfortunately, there are no immunomarkers that are diagnostic of esophageal adenocarcinoma, although most tumors express CK7 and may express CDX2 and CK20.

Pathology of Squamous Cell Carcinoma and Its Precursor Lesions

The development of invasive squamous cell carcinoma in the esophagus, like squamous cell carcinoma at other sites, is thought to arise from progression of a dysplastic epithelium [37, 38]. The sequence of events leading to squamous dysplasia and squamous cell carcinoma is ill defined. However, it is clear from association studies that chronic irritation, inflammation, and/or genetic factors are contributory. In the United States, several risk factors for squamous cell carcinoma have been documented including alcohol consumption, smoking, lye exposure, hot beverage consumption, exposure to nitrates/nitrosamines, male gender, increased age (with peak incidence in seventh decade), as well as African-American race [39, 40].

A synergistic relationship between alcohol consumption and smoking is well documented, though the precise molecular basis for this association remains uncertain [41]. Medical conditions that predispose the esophagus to chronic irritation, including achalasia and diverticula, are associated with increased risk [42]. Non-epidermolytic palmoplantar keratoderma, a disease associated with hyperkeratosis as a result of keratin gene mutations, is also associated with increased risk and patients are often counseled about increased screening [43]. Finally, with the rather recent acknowledgment that human papillomavirus (HPV) infection is a risk factor for oropharyngeal squamous cell carcinoma, the association between HPV infection and esophageal squamous cell carcinoma has been studied. However, while HPV has been shown to be causative in some cases of esophageal disease in high prevalence areas, there are cases that do not show any association with HPV infection [44]. Hence the development of esophageal squamous cell carcinoma appears to be multifactorial.

Precursor Lesions of Esophageal Squamous Cell Carcinoma

Squamous dysplasia is uncommonly detected when there is not a concomitant carcinoma. Endoscopically, dysplastic epithelium may appear friable and erythematous. Because squamous dysplasia is difficult to observe grossly, special stains may be used to highlight areas concerning for dysplasia, including toluidine blue (a basic dye which binds to nucleic acids and highlights areas with increased nuclear content common in dysplasia) and Lugol's iodine stain (which highlights areas with decreased glycogen content seen in dysplasia). Cytologically, dysplastic cells are indistinguishable from those observed in invasive disease, but they are confined to the epithelium by an intact basement membrane. Histologic features of squamous dysplasia include increased nuclear-to-cytoplasmic ratios, nuclear hyperchromasia, and pleomorphism. Premature keratinization (e.g., dyskeratosis) may be observed in the cytoplasm and an increased mitotic activity is typically present. Cells lose their polarity and may display increased crowding. Squamous dysplasia is separated into two categories: low-grade intraepithelial neoplasia (LG-IEN), which includes mild and moderate dysplasia, and high-grade intraepithelial neoplasia (HG-IEN), which includes severe dysplasia and squamous cell carcinoma in situ (WHO 5th ed.) [45]. With LG-IEN, the above neoplastic changes are generally confined to the lower third of the epithelium, whereas with HG-IEN, these features extend to the surface. As with adenocarcinoma, high-grade lesions portend a higher risk towards developing invasive disease.

Esophageal Squamous Cell Carcinoma

Squamous cell carcinoma typically arises as a mass in the middle third of the esophagus, although an estimated 30% of cases can arise in the distal third of the esophagus [46]. Typically, squamous cell carcinoma appears as a firm, white flat mucosal

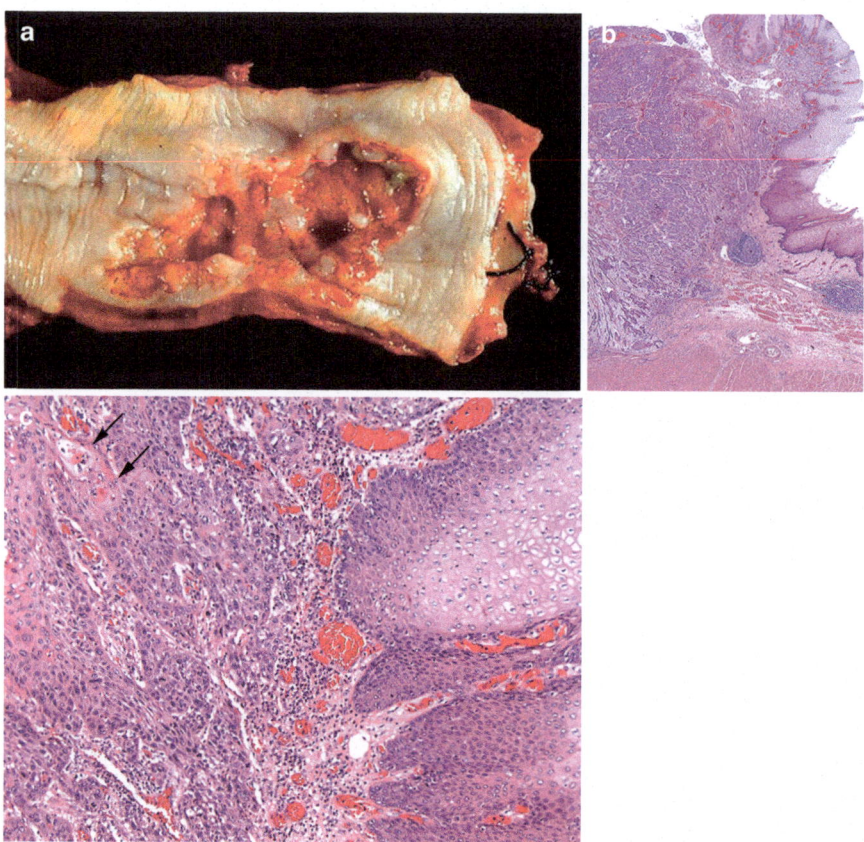

Fig. 3.6 Squamous cell carcinoma. (**a**) Esophagogastrectomy specimen (only the esophagus is shown with the esophageal margin towards the right). A large ulcerating tumor with heaped-up edges is present within the squamous-lined esophagus. (**b**) Histologically, this low-magnification image shows the invasive squamous cell carcinoma (towards the left) undermining the squamous mucosa (to the right) and invading down into the muscularis propria (H&E stain, 20×). (**c**) Histologically, at higher magnification, the invasive squamous cell carcinoma on the left is attempting to recapitulate normal squamous epithelium (present on the right). Although there is a suggestion of keratin formation within the tumor (arrows), overall this tumor is moderately differentiated (H&E stain, 100×)

lesion, as an exophytic ulcerated mass or as polypoid projections, that latter presentation being associated with a spindled morphology (Fig. 3.6a). Surface ulceration is often present.

Squamous cell carcinomas are graded as either well (G1), moderate (G2), or poorly (G3) differentiated based on their ability to recapitulate squamous epithelial cells (Fig. 3.6b,c); undifferentiated tumors are uncommon, often cannot be subtyped as squamous or glandular, and are considered to be grade 4 (G4) tumors. As with adenocarcinoma, accurate grading of specimens is critical as AJCC guidelines for clinical staging likewise integrate tumor grade into the algorithm for tumor staging

(Table 3.1); of note, the change in clinical stage occurs between well and moderately differentiated, which is different than for adenocarcinomas, where the cutoff is between moderately and poorly differentiated [20, 36]. Well-differentiated lesions will display the nuclear features of dysplastic change and maintain an increased nuclear-to-cytoplasmic ratio, but will have intracellular bridges and/or bright eosinophilic swirls of keratin (e.g., keratin pearls). Often, an intense desmoplastic reaction is observed in the surrounding stroma. As lesions become less differentiated, more varied histologic features will be observed, often with sheets or nests of basophilic cells. Frequently, single cell invasion can be identified. Rare intercellular bridge and keratin pearl formation may be identified, but are not abundant. In poorly differentiated tumors, immunohistochemical stains for CK5/6, p63, and p40 may prove useful. In the case of undifferentiated squamous cell carcinoma, they prove diagnostic.

Assessment of Specimens

Beyond indicating histologic subtype and tumor grade, special care must be taken to detail additional factors that will impact patient prognosis. These include margin status; tumor size and location; depth of invasion (e.g., pathologic T stage); presence of lymphatic, vascular, or perineural invasion; and lymph node status (if lymph nodes are present in the specimen). Additionally, if neoadjuvant therapy is administered, assessment of therapy effect is warranted.

Tumors that are not amenable to endoluminal therapy will likely require partial or complete esophagectomy, which should include a portion of the proximal stomach and the adjacent soft tissue and/or lymph nodes. When received in the pathology laboratory, the entire radial/adventitial margin is inked allowing for assessment of margin status. The serosal surface of the stomach should also be inked (typically, with distinct colors) to allow for orientation and to assess for serosal involvement. Once inked, the specimen is opened longitudinally. Appropriate sections should include the esophageal and gastric margins, full thickness sections of the lesion at the point of greatest depth of invasion (with inked adventitial margin), and representative sections of tumor in relation to the proximal (esophageal) and distal (e.g., gastric) mucosa. For cases with preoperative chemotherapy and/or radiation therapy, the lesion typically appears as an excavated scar and should be entirely submitted to allow for assessment of treatment effect. All lymph nodes identified by either palpation of direct visualization should be submitted and evaluated for metastatic disease. The National Comprehensive Cancer Network currently specifies that at least 15 lymph nodes should be examined after esophagectomy [47]. Regional lymph nodes extend from periesophageal cervical nodes for the cervical esophagus to celiac lymph nodes for the distal esophagus. Anatomic dissection should include upper mediastinal and perigastric lymph nodes if possible (in addition to periesophageal lymph nodes) as recent anatomic and clinical studies suggest that submucosal lymphatic vessels connect longitudinally to the superior mediastinal and the paracardial lymphatics, while lymphatic routes to periesophageal nodes originate from the muscle layer [47].

Current staging guidelines for esophageal carcinoma follow the TNM staging system detailed in the eighth edition of AJCC guidelines published in 2017 [20]. This system applies to those lesions which arise primarily in the esophagus, including those involving the esophagogastric junction with or without proximal stomach involvement. As mentioned before, unlike most clinical staging systems, the clinical staging of esophageal carcinomas integrates tumor grade for both squamous and adenocarcinoma (Table 3.1). Adenosquamous carcinomas (e.g., those lesions with both glandular and squamous differentiation) are staged according to squamous protocols. Primary pathologic tumor staging (e.g., pT staging) involves assessing the depth of invasion and is the same for both squamous and adenocarcinoma. High-grade lesions confined to the epithelial basement membrane are classified as pTis (this includes high-grade dysplasia in Barrett's esophagus and HG-IEN squamous dysplasia). pT1 lesions include those lesions in which lamina propria, muscularis mucosae, or submucosal invasion can be demonstrated, with invasion into the lamina propria or muscularis mucosae being classified as pT1a and invasion into the submucosa classified as pT1b. Adventitial involvement is classified as pT3 lesions, while involvement of adjacent structures (e.g., aorta, pleura, pericardium, diaphragm) is classified as pT4. The eighth edition of the AJCC guidelines split pT4 lesions into two stages: those that are resectable (pT4a) and those that are deemed unresectable (pT4b). Finally, lymph node involvement is divided into 5 categories: pNX, pN0, pN1, pN2, or pN3. pNX is used for specimens in which lymph nodes cannot be assessed or were not removed (e.g., EMR specimens, by default, will not have lymph nodes). pN1 designates involvement in 1–2 lymph nodes, while pN2 represents involvement in 3–6 lymph nodes. Involvement of 7 or more lymph nodes is classified as pN3. Extranodal extension, in which metastatic deposits erode the lymph node capsule and extend into the perinodal space, is associated with poor prognosis and may be indicated in reports when present.

Finally, since esophageal cancer has a poor 5-year survival rate of only 17% for all stages [48], some patients are offered neoadjuvant chemotherapy and/or radiation therapy prior to surgery. Similar to other tumor sites, such as rectum and pancreas, this approach has several theoretical benefits. Neoadjuvant therapy may (1) improve symptoms, such as dysphagia, (2) downstage the tumor with the hope of increasing resection rates, (3) treat micrometastatic disease that is not detected on imaging studies, and (4) indicate the biologic behavior of the tumor by its response to treatment that may help guide further therapy [49].

In the TNM classification, specimens that have received neoadjuvant chemotherapy and/or radiation therapy should be designated with a "y" prefix (e.g., ypT3, ypN2). Studies have shown that the pathologic responses in the tumor to primary therapy are important predictors of local recurrence and long-term survival [50–52]. The College of American Pathologists' Protocol for the Examination of Specimens from Patients with Carcinoma of the Esophagus recommends the reporting of response to prior chemotherapy or radiation therapy (www.CAP.org). Although other grading systems exist [50, 52, 53], the CAP assigns response to one of four tumor regression grades. According to this system, those specimens in which no viable cancer cells can be found and are suggestive of complete response are classified as grade 0. When single cells or small groups of cancer cells are identified, response is deemed "moderate" and is given a tumor regression grade of 1. Minimal response (e.g., grade 2 response) represents those specimens in which residual cancer shows extensive fibrosis, while grade 3 lesions (e.g., poor response) represent those lesions in which minimal tumor lysis is observed and extensive residual cancer remains. Sometimes sizable pools of acellular mucin are observed after treatment; importantly, these acellular pools of mucin should not be interpreted as residual disease.

HER2-Neu Testing

In October 2010, the FDA granted approval for trastuzumab for the first-line treatment of HER2+ metastatic esophagogastric adenocarcinoma in combination with cisplatin and capecitabine or 5-fluorouracil. This approval followed the publication of the results of the ToGA trial that showed a 2.7-month prolongation of medial overall survival in patients with advanced gastric, esophageal, or esophagogastric adenocarcinomas that overexpressed HER2 [54]. In 2016, the College of American Pathologists, the American Society for Clinical Pathology, and the American Society of Clinical Oncology issued guidelines for HER2 testing and clinical decision making for patients with esophageal or gastroesophageal junction adenocarcinoma [55]. These guidelines recommend assessment of HER2 overexpression in patients with locally advanced, recurrent, or metastatic adenocarcinoma of the esophagus/gastroesophageal junction. Per these recommendations, assessment of HER2 overexpression can be performed on biopsy or resection specimens prior to initiation of treatment with trastuzumab. The use of cell blocks prepared from cytologic preparations to assess for HER2 overexpression is also deemed acceptable, though not ideal. HER2 assessment can also be performed in metastatic lesions if needed. It is suggested that the tissue block containing the lowest grade of tumor should be used for HER2 assessment. The recommendations further state that appropriately validated HER2 immunohistochemistry (IHC) be performed initially. Of note, the scoring system for HER2 positivity in gastric or gastroesophageal junction cancer is different from the scoring used in breast cancer [54, 55]. Cases showing 3+ IHC expression are interpreted as positive, 2+ expression as equivocal, and both 1+ and 0 expression as negative. According to the 2016 recommendations and NCCN guidelines, samples with equivocal (2+) IHC expression must then be examined by HER2 in situ hybridization [55, 56]. Cases with 3+ overexpression by IHC (Fig. 3.7a) or cases showing ISH positivity (a HER2:CEP17 ratio of ≥2) are considered positive. These patients are then eligible for combination chemotherapy and trastuzumab. It is important to realize, though, that only a relatively small number of esophageal adenocarcinomas overexpress the HER2 protein on the surface of their cells; the positivity rate ranges from 17% to 22% [57].

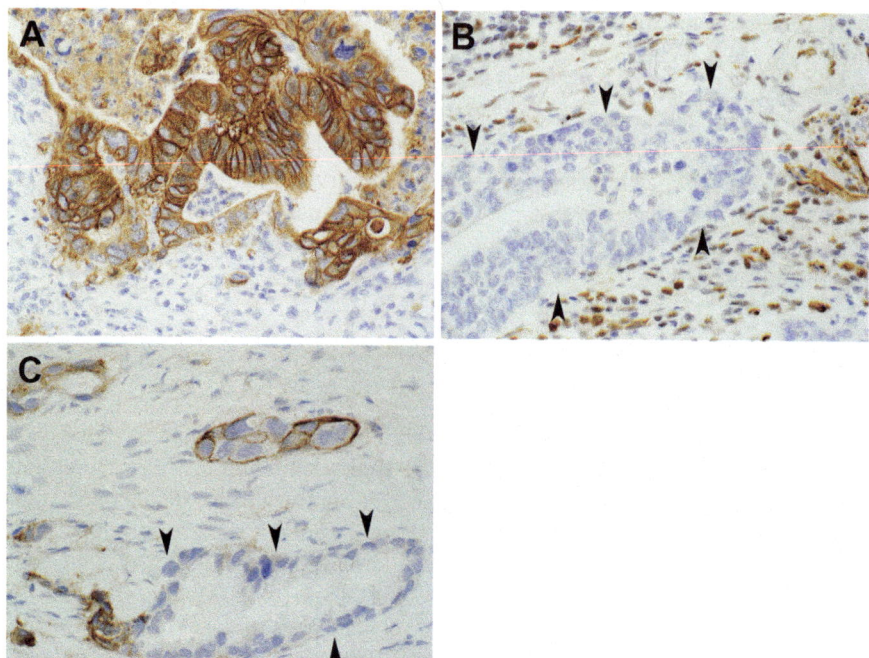

Fig. 3.7 Her2, MLH1 and PD-L1 testing by immunohistochemistry. (**a**) This is an example of Her2 overexpression in esophageal adenocarcinoma. There is strong, complete basolateral membranous (brown) staining in ≥10% of the tumor cells (HER2 immunohistochemical stain, 400×). (**b**) This is an example of loss of MLH-1 in adenocarcinoma. The background inflammatory and stromal cells show scattered nuclear staining. However, the cells within the malignant gland (arrowhead) show complete loss of nuclear staining for the mismatch repair protein. PMS2 would also be lost in this case (MLH-1 immunohistochemical stain, 400×). (**c**) This is an example of PD-L1 expression in adenocarcinoma of the gastroesophageal junction. There is strong membranous (dark brown) staining of some tumor cells, as well as negative staining in tumor cells (arrowheads), with a resultant combined positive score (CPS) of ≥1 (PD-L1 immunohistochemical stain, 400×)

Microsatellite Instability Testing

In May 2017, the FDA granted accelerated approval for pembrolizumab, a PD-1 inhibitor, for the treatment of unresectable or metastatic solid tumors that are microsatellite instability-high (MSI-H) or mismatch repair deficient (dMMR). This includes solid tumors that have progressed despite previous chemotherapeutic treatment and for which there is determined to be no other adequate therapeutic treatment option. Microsatellite instability and/or mismatch repair deficiency can occur at relatively high frequencies in colorectal, gastric, esophageal, and pancreatic adenocarcinomas and at lower frequencies in endometrial, bladder, ovarian, and other carcinomas [58, 59]. This approval by the FDA is unprecedented and unique because treatment parameters are not defined as site or tumor specific, but are rather based on the presence of a molecular abnormality in potentially any tumor type in any location. Based on the results of five single-arm multicohort multicenter trials (KEYNOTE-016, KEYNOTE-164, KEYNOTE-012, KEYNOTE-028, and KEYNOTE-158), the NCCN guidelines recommend pembrolizumab for second-line or subsequent therapy for MSI-H or dMMR for esophageal and esophagogastric junction adenocarcinomas [56, 58, 60].

Microsatellite instability testing can be performed either molecularly, to detect patterns of microsatellites in key genes, or immunohistochemically, to detect loss of protein expression as a surrogate marker of an abnormally functioning gene. Microsatellites are simple (1 or more base pair) units that may be repeated up to 100 times and are scattered throughout the genome. Due to their redundancy, errors, such as DNA slippage, can occur during DNA replication. Mismatch repair genes play a critical role in the identification and correction of these errors. Failure of the mismatch repair apparatus leads to persistence of errors and an alteration in the length of a microsatellite sequence. Persistence of such errors leads to frameshift mutations with loss of the normal function of the involved genes, which can lead to tumorigenesis. MSI is defined as a change of any length due to either insertion or deletion of repeating units in a microsatellite within a tumor when compared to normal tissue. MSI can be detect by PCR using a validated panel of microsatellites or as part of a validated next-generation sequencing panel.

Currently, many pathology laboratories routinely use immunohistochemistry as the test of choice to determine the microsatellite status of a tumor. The DNA mismatch repair system requires the cooperation of many genes, including *MLH1*, *PMS2*, *MSH2*, and *MSH6*. Biochemically, the MSH2 protein recognizes and binds directly to the mismatched DNA sequence and then forms a heterodimer with MSH6. Binding of a second heterodimer, MLH1 and PMS2, is needed for proper function of the MMR complex to adequately excise and repair the mismatched nucleotides. Intact staining of all four proteins indicates that the tumor is mismatch repair protein proficient and therefore microsatellite stable. Loss of staining for one or two paired proteins indicates that the tumor is dMMR and therefore MSI (Fig. 3.7b).

PD-L1 Testing

In September of 2017, the FDA granted accelerated approval of pembrolizumab for the treatment of recurrent locally advanced or metastatic, gastric, or gastroesophageal junction adenocarcinoma that expresses PD-L1. Patients are eligible for treatment as a third-line or subsequent therapy if disease progression occurs after two attempts with fluoropyrimidine- and platinum-containing chemotherapy and/or HER2/neu-targeted therapy [56, 61]. The FDA-approved immunohistochemical stain for the determination of PD-L1 status is the 22C3 pharmDx antibody kit by Dako. Expression of PD-L1 within adenocarcinoma is determined by calculation of a combined positive score (CPS), which is assessed by positive membranous staining of PD-L1 within tumor cells and tumoral or peri-tumoral lymphocytes and macrophages; a total number of 100 tumor cells must be present. This total is divided by the total number of cells examined, then divided by 100. A CPS of ≥ 1 is considered positive (Fig. 3.7c) and the tumor eligible for third-line treatment with pembrolizumab [56]. Initial diagnostic tissue prior to the initial attempts of treatment can be used to evaluate for PD-L1 expression. However, additional tissue can be obtained if indicated.

References

1. Pennathur A, Gibson MK, Jobe BA, Luketich JD. Oesophageal carcinoma. Lancet. 2013;381(9864):400–12. https://doi.org/10.1016/S0140-6736(12)60643-6.
2. American Cancer Society. Cancer Facts & Figures 2019. Atlanta: American Cancer Society; 2019.
3. Avidan B, Sonnenberg A, Schnell TG, Chejfec G, Metz A, Sontag SJ. Hiatal hernia size, Barrett's length, and severity of acid reflux are all risk factors for esophageal adenocarcinoma. Am J Gastroenterol. 2002;97(8):1930–6. https://doi.org/10.1111/j.1572-0241.2002.05902.x.
4. Cheng KK, Sharp L, McKinney PA, Logan RF, Chilvers CE, Cook-Mozaffari P, Ahmed A, et al. A case-control study of oesophageal adenocarcinoma in women: a preventable disease. Br J Cancer. 2000;83(1):127–32. https://doi.org/10.1054/bjoc.2000.1121.
5. Cook MB, Kamangar F, Whiteman DC, Freedman ND, Gammon MD, Bernstein L, Brown LM, et al. Cigarette smoking and adenocarcinomas of the esophagus and esophagogastric junction: a pooled analysis from the international BEACON consortium. J Natl Cancer Inst. 2010;102(17):1344–53. https://doi.org/10.1093/jnci/djq289.
6. de Jonge PJ, van Blankenstein M, Looman CW, Casparie MK, Meijer GA, Kuipers EJ. Risk of malignant progression in patients with Barrett's oesophagus: a Dutch nationwide cohort study. Gut. 2010;59(8):1030–6. https://doi.org/10.1136/gut.2009.176701.
7. el-Serag HB. The epidemic of esophageal adenocarcinoma. Gastroenterol Clin N Am. 2002;31(2):421–40. viii.
8. Hampel H, Abraham NS, El-Serag HB. Meta-analysis: obesity and the risk for gastroesophageal reflux disease and its complications. Ann Intern Med. 2005;143(3):199–211.
9. Islami F, Kamangar F. Helicobacter pylori and esophageal cancer risk: a meta-analysis. Cancer Prev Res (Phila). 2008;1(5):329–38. https://doi.org/10.1158/1940-6207.CAPR-08-0109.
10. Pohl H, Wrobel K, Bojarski C, Voderholzer W, Sonnenberg A, Rosch T, Baumgart DC. Risk factors in the development of esophageal adenocarcinoma. Am J Gastroenterol. 2013;108(2):200–7. https://doi.org/10.1038/ajg.2012.387.
11. Shaheen NJ, Falk GW, Iyer PG, Gerson LB. ACG clinical guideline: diagnosis and Management of Barrett's Esophagus. Am J Gastroenterol. 2016;111(1):30–50.; quiz 1. https://doi.org/10.1038/ajg.2015.322.
12. Fitzgerald RC, di Pietro M, Ragunath K, Ang Y, Kang JY, Watson P, Trudgill N, et al. British Society of Gastroenterology guidelines on the diagnosis and management of Barrett's oesophagus. Gut. 2014;63(1):7–42. https://doi.org/10.1136/gutjnl-2013-305372.
13. Takubo K, Vieth M, Aida J, Sawabe M, Kumagai Y, Hoshihara Y, Arai T. Differences in the definitions used for esophageal and gastric diseases in different countries: endoscopic definition of the esophagogastric junction, the precursor of Barrett's adenocarcinoma, the definition of Barrett's esophagus, and histologic criteria for mucosal adenocarcinoma or high-grade dysplasia. Digestion. 2009;80(4):248–57. https://doi.org/10.1159/000235923.
14. Byrne JP, Bhatnagar S, Hamid B, Armstrong GR, Attwood SE. Comparative study of intestinal metaplasia and mucin staining at the cardia and esophagogastric junction in 225 symptomatic patients presenting for diagnostic open-access gastroscopy. Am J Gastroenterol. 1999;94(1):98–103. https://doi.org/10.1111/j.1572-0241.1999.00778.x.

15. Glickman JN, Spechler SJ, Souza RF, Lunsford T, Lee E, Odze RD. Multilayered epithelium in mucosal biopsy specimens from the gastroesophageal junction region is a histologic marker of gastroesophageal reflux disease. Am J Surg Pathol. 2009;33(6):818–25. https://doi.org/10.1097/PAS.0b013e3181984697.

16. Anders M, Lucks Y, El-Masry MA, Quaas A, Rosch T, Schachschal G, Bahr C, et al. Subsquamous extension of intestinal metaplasia is detected in 98% of cases of neoplastic Barrett's esophagus. Clinical Gastroenterol Hepatol. 2014;12(3):405–10. https://doi.org/10.1016/j.cgh.2013.07.013.

17. Yachimski P, Shi C, Slaughter JC, Washington MK. Endoscopic mucosal resection of Barrett's esophagus detects high prevalence of subsquamous intestinal metaplasia. World J Gastrointest Endosc. 2013;5(12):590–4. https://doi.org/10.4253/wjge.v5.i12.590.

18. Dunbar KB, Spechler SJ. Controversies in Barrett esophagus. Mayo Clin Proc. 2014;89(7):973–84. https://doi.org/10.1016/j.mayocp.2014.01.022.

19. Edge SB, Byrd DR, Carducci MA, Compton CC, Fritz AG, Greene FL, Trotti A, editors. AJCC cancer staging manual. 7th ed. New York, NY: Springer; 2009.

20. Amin MB, Edge SB, Greene F, Byrd DR, Brookland RK, Washington MK, Gershenwald JE, et al., editors. AJCC cancer staging manual. 8th ed. New York, NY: Springer; 2017.

21. Chinyama CN, Marshall RE, Owen WJ, Mason RC, Kothari D, Wilkinson ML, Sanderson JD. Expression of MUC1 and MUC2 mucin gene products in Barrett's metaplasia, dysplasia and adenocarcinoma: an immunopathological study with clinical correlation. Histopathology. 1999;35(6):517–24.

22. Groisman GM, Amar M, Meir A. Expression of the intestinal marker Cdx2 in the columnar-lined esophagus with and without intestinal (Barrett's) metaplasia. Mod Pathol. 2004;17(10):1282–8. https://doi.org/10.1038/modpathol.3800182.

23. Guillem P, Billeret V, Buisine MP, Flejou JF, Lecomte-Houcke M, Degand P, Aubert JP, et al. Mucin gene expression and cell differentiation in human normal, premalignant and malignant esophagus. Int J Cancer. 2000;88(6):856–61.

24. Phillips RW, Frierson HF Jr, Moskaluk CA. Cdx2 as a marker of epithelial intestinal differentiation in the esophagus. Am J Surg Pathol. 2003;27(11):1442–7.

25. Srivastava A, Appelman H, Goldsmith JD, Davison JM, Hart J, Krasinskas AM. The use of ancillary stains in the diagnosis of Barrett esophagus and Barrett Esophagus-associated dysplasia: recommendations from the Rodger C. Haggitt gastrointestinal pathology society. Am J Surg Pathol. 2017;41(5):e8–e21. https://doi.org/10.1097/pas.0000000000000819.

26. Murray L, Sedo A, Scott M, McManus D, Sloan JM, Hardie LJ, Forman D, et al. TP53 and progression from Barrett's metaplasia to oesophageal adenocarcinoma in a UK population cohort. Gut. 2006;55(10):1390–7. https://doi.org/10.1136/gut.2005.083295.

27. Kaye PV, Haider SA, James PD, Soomro I, Catton J, Parsons SL, Ragunath K, et al. Novel staining pattern of p53 in Barrett's dysplasia – the absent pattern. Histopathology. 2010;57(6):933–5. https://doi.org/10.1111/j.1365-2559.2010.03715.x.

28. Kerkhof M, van Dekken H, Steyerberg EW, Meijer GA, Mulder AH, de Bruine A, Driessen A, et al. Grading of dysplasia in Barrett's oesophagus: substantial interobserver variation between general and gastrointestinal pathologists. Histopathology. 2007;50(7):920–7. https://doi.org/10.1111/j.1365-2559.2007.02706.x.

29. Curvers WL, ten Kate FJ, Krishnadath KK, Visser M, Elzer B, Baak LC, Bohmer C, et al. Low-grade dysplasia in Barrett's esophagus: overdiagnosed and underestimated. Am J Gastroenterol. 2010;105(7):1523–30. https://doi.org/10.1038/ajg.2010.171.

30. Duits LC, Phoa KN, Curvers WL, Ten Kate FJ, Meijer GA, Seldenrijk CA, Offerhaus GJ, et al. Barrett's oesophagus patients with low-grade dysplasia can be accurately risk-stratified after histological review by an expert pathology panel. Gut. 2015;64(5):700–6. https://doi.org/10.1136/gutjnl-2014-307278.

31. Alikhan M, Rex D, Khan A, Rahmani E, Cummings O, Ulbright TM. Variable pathologic interpretation of columnar lined esophagus by general pathologists in community practice. Gastrointest Endosc. 1999;50(1):23–6.

32. Abraham SC, Krasinskas AM, Correa AM, Hofstetter WL, Ajani JA, Swisher SG, Wu TT. Duplication of the muscularis mucosae in Barrett esophagus: an underrecognized feature and its implication for staging of adenocarcinoma. Am J Surg Pathol. 2007;31(11):1719–25. https://doi.org/10.1097/PAS.0b013e318093e3bf.

33. Mandal RV, Forcione DG, Brugge WR, Nishioka NS, Mino-Kenudson M, Lauwers GY. Effect of tumor characteristics and duplication of the muscularis mucosae on the endoscopic staging of superficial Barrett esophagus-related neoplasia. Am J Surg Pathol. 2009;33(4):620–5. https://doi.org/10.1097/PAS.0b013e31818d632f.

34. Kumarasinghe MP, Brown I, Raftopoulos S, Bourke MJ, Charlton A, de Boer WB, Eckstein R, et al. Standardised reporting protocol for endoscopic resection for Barrett oesophagus associated neoplasia: expert consensus recommendations. Pathology. 2014;46(6):473–80. https://doi.org/10.1097/PAT.0000000000000160.

35. Vieth M, Stolte M. Pathology of early upper GI cancers. Best Pract Res Clin Gastroenterol. 2005;19(6):857–69. https://doi.org/10.1016/j.bpg.2005.02.008.

36. Edge SB, Compton CC, et al., editors. AJCC cancer staging manual. New York: Springer-Verlag; 2009.

37. Dry SM, Lewin KJ. Esophageal squamous dysplasia. Semin Diagn Pathol. 2002;19(1):2–11.

38. Shimizu M, Ban S, Odze RD. Squamous dysplasia and other precursor lesions related to esophageal squamous cell carcinoma. Gastroenterol Clin N Am. 2007;36(4):797–811., v-vi. https://doi.org/10.1016/j.gtc.2007.08.005.

39. Daly JM, Fry WA, Little AG, Winchester DP, McKee RF, Stewart AK, Fremgen AM. Esophageal cancer: results of an American College of Surgeons patient care evaluation study. J Am Coll Surg. 2000;190(5):562–72; discussion 72-3

40. Dawsey SM, Fagundes RB, Jacobson BC, Kresty LA, Mallery SR, Paski S, van den Brandt PA. Diet and esophageal disease. Ann N Y Acad Sci. 2014;1325(1):127–37. https://doi.org/10.1111/nyas.12528.

41. Prabhu A, Obi KO, Rubenstein JH. The synergistic effects of alcohol and tobacco consumption on the risk of esophageal squamous cell carcinoma: a meta-analysis. Am J Gastroenterol. 2014;109(6):822–7. https://doi.org/10.1038/ajg.2014.71.

42. O'Neill OM, Johnston BT, Coleman HG. Achalasia: a review of clinical diagnosis, epidemiology, treatment and outcomes. World J Gastroenterol: WJG. 2013;19(35):5806–12. https://doi.org/10.3748/wjg.v19.i35.5806.

43. Iwaya T, Maesawa C, Ogasawara S, Tamura G. Tylosis esophageal cancer locus on chromosome 17q25.1 is commonly deleted in sporadic human esophageal cancer. Gastroenterology. 1998;114(6):1206–10.

44. Al-Haddad S, El-Zimaity H, Hafezi-Bakhtiari S, Rajendra S, Streutker CJ, Vajpeyi R, Wang B. Infection and esophageal cancer. Ann N Y Acad Sci. 2014;1325(1):187–96. https://doi.org/10.1111/nyas.12530.

45. Takubo K, Fujii S. Squamous cell carcinoma of the oesophagus. In: WHO Classification of Tumours Editorial Board, editor. WHO classification of tumors: digestive system. 5th ed. Lyon: WHO Press; 2019. p. 36–7.

46. Ando N, Ozawa S, Kitagawa Y, Shinozawa Y, Kitajima M. Improvement in the results of surgical treatment of advanced squamous esophageal carcinoma during 15 consecutive years. Ann Surg. 2000;232(2):225–32.

47. Tachimori Y, Nagai Y, Kanamori N, Hokamura N, Igaki H. Pattern of lymph node metastases of esophageal squamous cell carcinoma based on the anatomical lymphatic drainage system. Dis Esophagus. 2011;24(1):33–8. https://doi.org/10.1111/j.1442-2050.2010.01086.x.

48. Howlader N, Noone AM, Krapcho M, Garshell J, Neyman N, Altekruse SF, Kosary CL, et al. SEER cancer statistics review 1975–2010. Bethesda, MD: National Cancer Institute. (http://seer.cancer.gov/csr/1975_2010/, based on November 2012 SEER data submission, posted to the SEER Web site, April 2013)

49. Shah RD, Cassano AD, Neifeld JP. Neoadjuvant therapy for esophageal cancer. World J Gastrointest Oncol. 2014;6(10):403–6. https://doi.org/10.4251/wjgo.v6.i10.403.

50. Brucher BL, Becker K, Lordick F, Fink U, Sarbia M, Stein H, Busch R, et al. The clinical impact of histopathologic response assessment by residual tumor cell quantification in esophageal squamous cell carcinomas. Cancer. 2006;106(10):2119–27. https://doi.org/10.1002/cncr.21850.
51. Chang F, Deere H, Mahadeva U, George S. Histopathologic examination and reporting of esophageal carcinomas following preoperative neoadjuvant therapy: practical guidelines and current issues. Am J Clin Pathol. 2008;129(2):252–62. https://doi.org/10.1309/CCR3QN4874YJDJJ7.
52. Wu TT, Chirieac LR, Abraham SC, Krasinskas AM, Wang H, Rashid A, Correa AM, et al. Excellent interobserver agreement on grading the extent of residual carcinoma after preoperative chemoradiation in esophageal and esophagogastric junction carcinoma: a reliable predictor for patient outcome. Am J Surg Pathol. 2007;31(1):58–64. https://doi.org/10.1097/01.pas.0000213312.36306.cc.
53. Hermann RM, Horstmann O, Haller F, Perske C, Christiansen H, Hille A, Schmidberger H, et al. Histomorphological tumor regression grading of esophageal carcinoma after neoadjuvant radiochemotherapy: which score to use? Dis Esophagus. 2006;19(5):329–34. https://doi.org/10.1111/j.1442-2050.2006.00589.x.
54. Bang YJ, Van Cutsem E, Feyereislova A, Chung HC, Shen L, Sawaki A, Lordick F, et al. Trastuzumab in combination with chemotherapy versus chemotherapy alone for treatment of HER2-positive advanced gastric or gastro-oesophageal junction cancer (ToGA): a phase 3, open-label, randomised controlled trial. Lancet. 2010;376(9742):687–97. https://doi.org/10.1016/S0140-6736(10)61121-X.
55. Bartley AN, Washington MK, Colasacco C, Ventura CB, Ismaila N, Benson AB 3rd, Carrato A, et al. HER2 testing and clinical decision making in gastroesophageal adenocarcinoma: guideline from the College of American Pathologists, American Society for Clinical Pathology, and the American Society of Clinical Oncology. J Clin Oncol. 2017;35(4):446–64. https://doi.org/10.1200/JCO.2016.69.4836.
56. National Comprehensive Cancer Network. Clinical Practice Guidelines in Oncology: Esophageal and Esophagogastric Junction Cancers. , V.4.2017. http://www.nccn.org. Accessed 10 Feb 2018.
57. Yoon HH, Shi Q, Sukov WR, Wiktor AE, Khan M, Sattler CA, Grothey A, et al. Association of HER2/ErbB2 expression and gene amplification with pathologic features and prognosis in esophageal adenocarcinomas. Clin Cancer Res. 2012;18(2):546–54. https://doi.org/10.1158/1078-0432.CCR-11-2272.
58. Le DT, Uram JN, Wang H, Bartlett BR, Kemberling H, Eyring AD, Skora AD, et al. PD-1 blockade in Tumors with mismatch-repair deficiency. N Engl J Med. 2015;372(26):2509–20. https://doi.org/10.1056/NEJMoa1500596.
59. Meltzer SJ, Yin J, Manin B, Rhyu MG, Cottrell J, Hudson E, Redd JL, et al. Microsatellite instability occurs frequently and in both diploid and aneuploid cell populations of Barrett's-associated esophageal adenocarcinomas. Cancer Res. 1994;54(13):3379–82.
60. Le DT, Durham JN, Smith KN, Wang H, Bartlett BR, Aulakh LK, Lu S, et al. Mismatch repair deficiency predicts response of solid tumors to PD-1 blockade. Science. 2017;357(6349):409–13. https://doi.org/10.1126/science.aan6733.
61. Curea FG, Hebbar M, Ilie SM, Bacinschi XE, Trifanescu OG, Botnariuc I, Anghel RM. Current targeted therapies in HER2-positive gastric adenocarcinoma. Cancer Biother Radiopharm. 2017;32(10):351–63. https://doi.org/10.1089/cbr.2017.2249.

Barrett's Esophagus: Diagnosis and Management

4

Adam Templeton, Andrew Kaz, Erik Snider, and William M. Grady

Introduction

Esophageal adenocarcinoma (EAC) is one of the most rapidly increasing cancers in developed countries. EAC is thought to arise from a specialized intestinal metaplasia in the esophagus, called Barrett's esophagus (BE), which forms in the lower esophagus in response to chronic acid reflux injury [1]. Barrett's esophagus occurs in 1–6.4% of the US population and is the strongest risk factor for EAC [2]. As such, people with BE are placed in surveillance programs with the intent to decrease EAC-associated mortality. Unfortunately, despite years of study of BE and EAC, it is still controversial whether current BE surveillance programs effectively decrease mortality from EAC. The controversy likely stems from low-sensitivity methods for identifying people with BE, the modest accuracy of current surveillance methods to identify people with BE at increased risk of EAC, and the morbidity of historical

A. Templeton · E. Snider
Department of Medicine, Division of Gastroenterology, University of Washington School of Medicine, Seattle, WA, USA

A. Kaz
Department of Medicine, Division of Gastroenterology, University of Washington School of Medicine, Seattle, WA, USA

Clinical Research Division, Fred Hutchinson Cancer Research Center, Seattle, WA, USA

Gastroenterology Section, VA Puget Sound Healthcare System, Seattle, WA, USA

W. M. Grady (✉)
Department of Medicine, Division of Gastroenterology, University of Washington School of Medicine, Seattle, WA, USA

Clinical Research Division, Fred Hutchinson Cancer Research Center, Seattle, WA, USA
e-mail: wgrady@fredhutch.org

© Springer Nature Switzerland AG 2020
N. F. Saba, B. F. El-Rayes (eds.), *Esophageal Cancer*,
https://doi.org/10.1007/978-3-030-29832-6_4

83

treatments for high-grade dysplasia and EAC. Recent advances have been made or are being made that address all these issues; thus, BE continues to be a promising target for screening and surveillance [3, 4].

The asymptomatic nature of BE and the current requirement for endoscopic biopsies and histologic assessment of the biopsies to diagnose BE pose several challenges to the use of BE for early cancer detection and treatment. These challenges include: (1) What is the optimal way to identify patients with BE and appropriately risk-stratify identified BE patients for surveillance? (2) What is the optimal surveillance program for a particular patient with BE, including issues related to surveillance intervals and methods used for surveillance? (3) What are the indications for endoscopic or surgical treatment? In this chapter we will review Barrett's esophagus with a special focus on the diagnosis and management of this condition.

Natural History and Risk Factors

Natural History

Norman Barrett was the first to describe the clinical finding of a columnar-lined epithelium that extended proximal to the gastroesophageal (GE) junction. The condition that bears his name is now recognized as the replacement of the normal esophageal squamous mucosa with a columnar-lined metaplastic epithelium [5]. Metaplasia is thought to arise as a response to esophageal reflux of hydrochloric acid and bile acids that damage the esophageal mucosa [6]. The subsequent progression of BE to dysplasia and eventually EAC is felt to involve the accumulation of a series of genetic and epigenetic alterations that are also likely driven in part by genotoxic damage secondary to reflux of gastric fluids [7]. As with other premalignant conditions such as colonic adenomas, Barrett's esophagus is asymptomatic, and clinically important only because of its malignant potential. As an identifiable precursor to cancer, BE is a logical target for screening and surveillance programs aiming to decrease EAC-associated morbidity and mortality through the prevention of EAC or the detection and treatment of early-stage EAC. Unfortunately, the utility of these programs is suboptimal because of our incomplete understanding of the epidemiology, biology, and natural history of BE and EAC. Although it presumably requires many years for BE to transform into EAC, it is unclear how long BE to EAC progression takes and how variable the progression sequence is between different patients. Nonetheless, data from patients in surveillance programs suggest that when high-grade dysplasia arises, there is often concurrent EAC or a high risk of progression to EAC during the next 6 months to 2 years [8–11]. It also appears unlikely that BE can spontaneously regress once it has formed.

Risk Factors for BE and EAC

Risk Factors for BE and Strategies to Identify a Screening Population

The true prevalence of BE is unclear; however, estimates range from 1% to 18%. The marked variability in prevalence estimates is presumably secondary to the variability of the underlying populations studied. In studies of patients referred for endoscopic evaluation of reflux symptoms or dyspepsia, BE can be found in between 6–18% of patients, with higher percentages reflective of more stringent criteria for symptomatic reflux disease [12–14]. In studies in the United States of patients referred for screening colonoscopy that additionally underwent upper endoscopy, BE was found in 6–8% of patients [15, 16]. In the two largest population-based studies from Sweden and Italy, the incidence appears to be closer to 1–2% [17, 18].

Because gastroesophageal reflux disease (GERD) is thought to be the major mechanism driving the formation of BE, the presence of chronic symptomatic GERD has become a central clinical indication for BE screening. Yet reflux symptoms have poor sensitivity and specificity for identifying patients with BE. In some of the larger population studies noted above, less than 50% of those with BE reported reflux symptoms prior to their diagnosis [17, 18]. In other studies, those with symptomatic reflux disease and erosive changes on endoscopy were found to have a five-fold increased risk of developing BE in the following 5 years when compared to patients with nonerosive reflux disease [19]. In addition, symptomatic GERD may best predict those with long-segment BE as opposed to those with short-segment BE [20]. Notably, the longer reflux symptoms have been present, the greater the relative risk of BE [12]. However, the low prevalence of BE even in the setting of chronic GERD does not support the use of chronic reflux symptoms alone as an indication for BE screening, which has led to the use of a combination of demographic risk factors (e.g., older age, Caucasian race, obesity) in addition to chronic GERD to identify candidates for BE screening exams [19, 21–23].

Aside from chronic gastroesophageal reflux, several demographic features are associated with an increased risk for intestinal metaplasia and dysplasia of the esophagus. BE has a higher incidence in Caucasians, males, and those with central adiposity. The incidence of BE also increases with age [24, 25]. With few exceptions, BE is uncommon in the young (in men below age 20, in women below age 40), African Americans, Asians, or women [24]. Other associated clinical risk factors include the presence of a hiatal hernia [12], obstructive sleep apnea [26], possibly diets low in fruit, and cigarette smoking [27]. The contribution of *H. pylori* remains unclear; however, there is some evidence that gastric infection with *H. pylori* may decrease the risk of developing BE [28], possibly through gastric mucosal atrophy and decreased parietal cell hydrochloric acid production.

Risk Factors for the Progression of BE to EAC

Once it develops, the time course for progression of BE to EAC is variable. Currently, the most accepted clinical risk factor for progression to adenocarcinoma is the degree of dysplasia present in BE. In the absence of dysplasia, large population studies suggest that the annual risk of progression to EAC is low, approximately 0.12–0.40% [8, 29, 30]. Those with low-grade dysplasia (LGD) have an annual risk of progression from 0.6% to 13.4% [8–10, 31–33]. Studies are markedly divergent in the estimate of the annual risk of high-grade dysplasia progression, with the lowest estimates being 2% per year and the highest reported risk at 59% per year [34–38].

Among those diagnosed with BE, several risk factors are clearly associated with an increased risk for progression to EAC. In the largest reported population study, de Jonge assessed 42,207 Dutch patients with BE. EAC was found to be most closely associated with age >75 (hazard ratio (HR) 12), male sex (HR 2.01), and presence of LGD at the time of the baseline exam (HR 1.91) [30]. Additionally, a longer duration of heartburn symptoms and increased frequency of reflux symptoms were associated with a five-fold increased risk for the development of EAC [39].

Histological stability of BE over time also associates with a decreased risk of progression of BE to EAC. In a multicenter cohort of patients with BE, those who had persistent nondysplastic BE were least likely to develop EAC or progress to HGD at a median of 5 years of follow-up [40]. Prevalent cases are more likely to progress than incident cases. In a study of a series of patients with BE from Cleveland ($N = 299$), patients with BE and LGD or indefinite for dysplasia (IND) had an annual incidence rate of HGD or EAC of 2.4% and 0.6%, respectively. Within this group, the greatest risk for progression to HGD or EAC was for male patients, those patients with longer length of BE, and those patients with multifocal dysplasia and nodules seen on endoscopy. The median time after diagnosis of BE to diagnosis of HGD was 63.1 months and for EAC was 53 months. In this group, 58.5% regressed to nondysplastic BE (NDBE). Notably, prevalent cases of BE (those within 1 year from their BE diagnosis) had an increased risk of progression to EAC compared to incident cases [33]. These findings suggest that those at highest risk for dysplastic progression devolve to cancer quickly, and those with stable dysplastic changes over a course of years are less likely to progress. This may also explain why in a trial of radiofrequency ablation for dysplasia in BE, 19% of patients with high-grade dysplasia developed cancer at 1 year [41]. As with regression, this may partially represent under-sampling or intra-observer pathologic disagreement; however, it may also indicate that a more dynamic phenotype exists that progresses quickly to cancer in patients with more histologically advanced BE.

Just as there is variability in the likelihood of progression of BE, spontaneous regression of BE to squamous epithelium may occur but appears to do so variably and very infrequently. Some of the studies mentioned above suggest that as many as half of patients diagnosed with LGD may regress to nondysplastic BE [33, 42]. However, due to the known limitations of endoscopic surveillance (e.g., variability in the areas of BE biopsied from endoscopic exam to exam, small proportion of BE sampled) and modest consistency of the pathologic assessment of dysplasia (see further discussion below), it should be noted that some of the reported cases of regression may in fact be due to intra-observer pathologic disagreement or sampling error (i.e., areas of dysplasia not biopsied on follow-up exams). Features associated with regression are short segment of BE [33] and acid suppression with proton-pump inhibitor (PPI) medications [43–45].

Diagnosing Barrett's Esophagus (BE): Current Criteria and Areas of Controversy

Currently, in the United States, the diagnosis of BE requires both endoscopic visualization of columnar mucosa extending above the gastroesophageal junction and biopsies of this region confirming the presence of intestinal metaplasia [21, 22, 46]. Endoscopically, columnar mucosa has a stereotypic appearance of "salmon" or "reddish" appearing tongues or patches, which is distinct from the normal pale-whitish appearance of squamous mucosa (Fig. 4.1). Accurate determination of the location of the GE junction, the diaphragmatic hiatus, and the squamo-columnar junction where the esophageal squamous epithelium meets the gastric mucosa (also known as the Z-line) is critical for determining the length of BE and identifying the presence of a concurrent hiatal hernia. In the United States, the GE junction is classically defined by the top of the gastric folds [21]; however in Japan, endoscopists have used the bottom edge of the palisading esophageal vessels to define the GE junction [47, 48]. It remains to be determined which method is more accurate [21, 48].

Several types of columnar epithelium can be found in the biopsy samples of suspected BE, including gastric-fundic type, cardiac type, and intestinal type [49]. Gastric-fundic type is typically considered as part of a hiatal hernia and not thought to be associated with an increased risk of malignancy. There is controversy regarding whether a pathologic diagnosis of BE requires the presence of goblet cells within the BE segment (i.e., specialized intestinal metaplasia). In the United States,

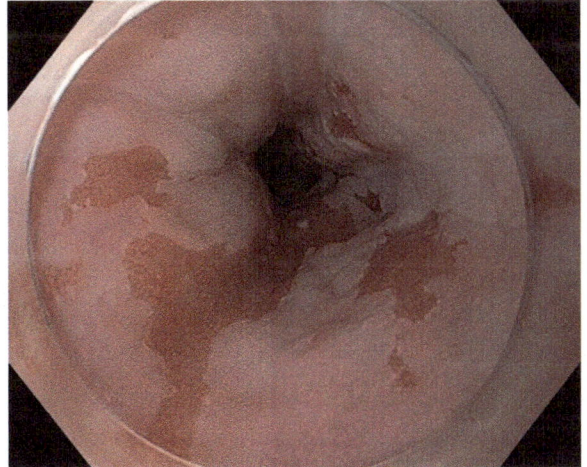

Fig. 4.1 Endoscopic image demonstrating short segment of Barrett's esophagus without nodularity. Prague C1M2

specialized intestinal metaplasia is considered the hallmark of BE as this is clearly associated with increased risk of malignancy [21, 46]. It is less clear whether there is a risk of malignancy associated with cardiac tissue that extends above the level of the GE junction. The most recent British guidelines propose cardiac-type epithelium be designated BE. These guidelines state that the reason for designating cardiac-type epithelium is the concern that a lack of goblet cells may be a consequence of sampling error and that non-goblet cell specialized intestinal metaplastic (SIM) epithelium may contain molecular features typically observed in goblet-cell epithelium [22]. US societies currently disagree with this designation because of the lack of definitive data supporting the concept that non-goblet cell SIM epithelium carries an increased risk of progressing to EAC, and because of both the financial cost and the negative emotional impact of placing patients with non-goblet cell BE under surveillance for a condition of unclear significance [8, 21, 50, 51].

BE has historically been divided into long-segment BE (>3 cm) and short segment BE (<3 cm), which has been used to stratify BE patients into high-risk (long-segment BE) and low-risk (short segment BE) (Fig. 4.2a–d). While increasing length of BE is clearly associated with increased risk for malignant progression, there is a lack of consensus regarding what differentiates a short segment of Barrett's

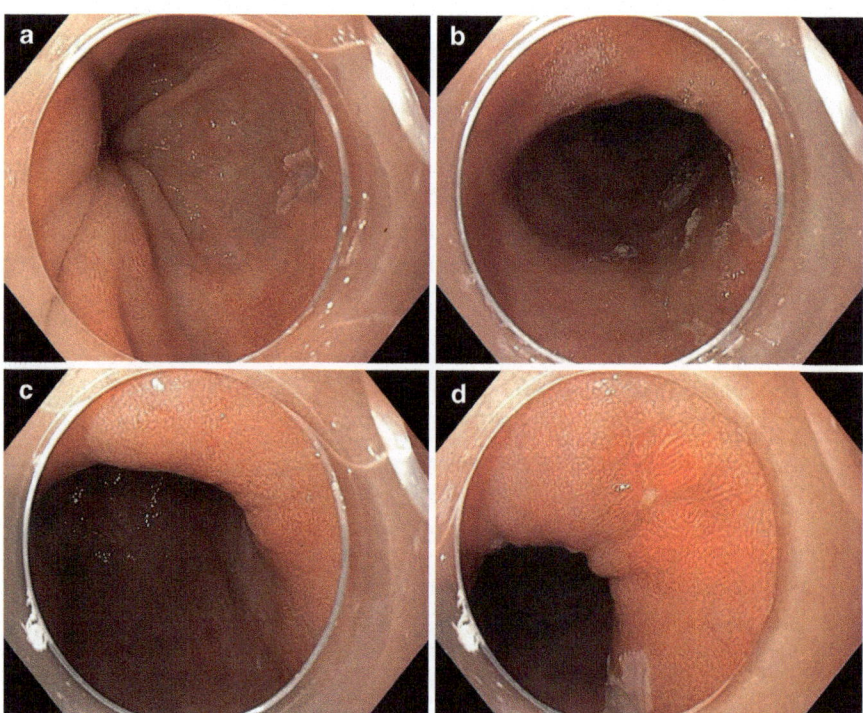

Fig. 4.2 (**a–d**) Endoscopic images demonstrating long segment Barrett's esophagus with low-grade dysplasia. Low-grade dysplasia does not have endoscopic features that can reliably distinguish it from nondysplastic Barrett's esophagus

esophagus (SSBE) from an irregular squamo-columnar junction. The identification of SSBE is clinically important because of the small increased risk of EAC even in people with SSBE [52]. In addition, there are no current guidelines regarding the number of biopsies required to establish an initial diagnosis of BE. Due to the very low risk of malignancy associated with SSBE and ongoing debate regarding the value of current BE surveillance strategies, it is controversial whether an irregular z-line should be biopsied with the intent of making a diagnosis of BE [22].

Tissue-Based Diagnostic and Risk Markers

Broadly speaking, a biomarker is a detectable indicator for the presence or future risk of disease. In the case of Barrett's esophagus, this term encompasses demographic measurements, such as BMI or smoking status; histologic findings such as low-grade dysplasia (LGD) or inflammation; and molecular markers such as aneuploidy or tetraploidy or aberrant DNA methylation [53]. Symptoms of long-standing GERD have historically been the main clinical features used to identify people at risk of having BE, who are then advised to undergo endoscopic assessment. It is clear that many people with BE have no history of GERD, which is one of the reasons behind the lack of clear success of current BE surveillance programs for preventing EAC [7]. With regard to strategies to identify BE at high risk of progressing to EAC, the presence or absence of BE with or without dysplasia on histologic review is currently the only biomarker used clinically for risk stratification and directing treatment [21, 22, 46]. This dearth of well-studied biomarkers and the reliance on reflux symptoms and endoscopic findings of dysplasia had led to what Reid has called the "paradox" of BE management. In this paradox, Reid notes several frustrating epidemiologic facts: (1) a large number of individuals with BE are asymptomatic, (2) nearly 50% develop EAC without associated GERD symptoms, (3) 95% of EACs arise without a prior diagnosis of BE, and (4) nearly 80% of EAC arise without a prior diagnosis of GERD [7]. Furthermore, the vast number of people with BE detected by endoscopy will not progress to EAC and instead will die of unrelated causes, which is a consequence of the late age of occurrence of most EACs. In fact, the majority of people with BE are more likely to die from complications of cardiac disease than from EAC [54]. With these insights, several areas of active research in molecular biology are underway to resolve the "paradox" of BE and may lead to a more effective approach to identifying and managing those patients with BE. A number of promising markers have been identified, however, currently there are only a limited number of biomarkers available to precisely identify patients with BE and BE patients at high risk of progression to EAC.

With recent advances in genomics (i.e., next-generation sequencing), epigenomics, proteomics, and microarray technology, many potential diagnostic and prognostic molecular biomarkers have been identified at the level of DNA, RNA, and individual proteins. Examples of types of prospectively tested molecular biomarkers include chromosomal alterations such as abnormal DNA ploidy and alterations in DNA copy number (based on fluorescence in situ hybridization (FISH)) [55–57], gene mutations, aberrantly methylated genes, loss of heterozygosity of specific DNA loci [42], and measurements of clonal diversity in the BE tissue [58]. These molecular alterations may serve as adjunctive markers to delineate the degree of dysplasia (e.g., use of FISH probes for *C-MYC* to confirm HGD or carcinoma [57]) or to further risk stratify patients at greatest risk for progression to EAC (e.g., loss of ploidy associates with a 38.7% increased relative risk of developing EAC [55]). Other nonprospectively evaluated but promising markers include epigenetic alterations in the form of aberrantly methylated gene panels [59], and alterations in gene mRNA and microRNA expression [60]. Several groups have also explored the use of protein markers to augment endoscopic visualization and diagnosis of BE with dysplasia [56]. At this time, these studies are limited by a lack of suitably large prospective clinical validation trials because of the lack of sufficiently large esophageal tissue repositories from appropriate patient populations [59].

BE Surveillance: Current Clinical Strategies and Features That Affect the Implementation of the Surveillance Program

Once the diagnosis of BE is established, an appropriate assessment should be performed to stratify the patient into a low- or high-risk group for the development of esophageal cancer. Optimal risk stratification dictates specific aspects of the recommended BE surveillance program. Thus, the index endoscopy description should include information on the length of the esophagus involved, the presence or absence of nodularity or other lesions, and whether esophagitis or atypical appearing glands were present [21, 22].

Because the length of BE directly correlates with increasing risk of malignancy, it is recommended that the endoscopist clearly document the length of the visualized BE segment as well as the circumferential extent [21, 22, 46]. In order to improve the consistency of the description of these endoscopic features, there is multi-society support for the use of the "Prague classification" to describe BE. This system mandates that the endoscopist report the length of circumferential involvement and the maximal length of BE measured from the GE junction (e.g., 4 cm of circumferential involvement with a tongue extending an additional 2 cm would be reported as C4M6). Standardization of the description of BE using the Prague classification promises to both facilitate communication between providers and to assist the endoscopist in determining response to therapy. There is reasonable agreement between operators using this classification tool [61, 62].

Another critical feature that governs specific aspects of a BE surveillance program is the presence of dysplasia. It is important to recognize that the presence of esophagitis, either visualized on endoscopy or by histology, impairs the ability of the pathologist to diagnose dysplasia, and may result in a pathologic description of "indefinite for dysplasia (IND)" [22]. In this instance, the patient is advised to comply with aggressive anti-GERD therapy (i.e., twice daily proton pump inhibitor (PPI) therapy) for at least 3 months and then have follow-up endoscopic biopsies performed. It is also important to recognize that esophageal ulceration may represent invasive EAC when high-grade dysplasia (HGD) is present [63].

The presence of mucosal abnormalities such as nodularity, glandular irregularity, or ulceration is concerning for dysplasia, particularly in the absence of esophagitis [64–66]. If these changes are visualized on endoscopy, standard practice is for endoscopic resection (ER) of the affected segment [21, 22] (the techniques of endoscopic mucosal resection (EMR) and endoscopic submucosal dissection (ESD) are discussed below). For staging, these resective techniques provide more tissue than can be obtained with standard endoscopic biopsies. Consequently, ER has proved more useful than adjunctive staging techniques such as CT or endoscopic ultrasound for distinguishing HGD from EAC. The use of ER improves the certainty of pathologic diagnosis and staging of superficial EAC lesions, in part by increased intra-observer agreement and better diagnostic reproducibility when compared to standard biopsy specimens [67–71].

The use of high-definition white light endoscopy (HD-WLE) theoretically improves the endoscopist's ability to identify BE and to identify abnormal and potentially dysplastic glands within the segment of BE, though studies demonstrating the superiority of HD-WLE over conventional "low-resolution" endoscopy are lacking. At the present time, HD-WLE remains the standard of care for the endoscopic management of BE. Adjunctive technologies such as narrow band imaging (NBI), confocal microscopy, chromoendoscopy, volumetric laser-enhanced imaging, and optical coherence technology are still being assessed with regard to their role in the management of BE, as discussed below [21, 22].

The Role of Dysplasia in Risk Stratification in Guiding BE Surveillance and Treatment

Dysplasia is the central factor used currently for determining the risk for EAC and for guiding BE surveillance exam intervals and for selecting patients for EMR/ESD. The Vienna classification system divides BE into five categories: no dysplasia, indefinite for dysplasia, low-grade dysplasia, high-grade dysplasia, and invasive neoplasia [72]. Despite discrete categories, the transformation of BE from LGD to HGD and then to intramucosal carcinoma (IMC) occurs along a spectrum. As such, it is important to note two points: (1) the artificial separation between LGD, HGD, and IMC results in difficulties with intra-observer variability and (2) a single biopsy specimen only samples a small fraction of the larger field of BE and may miss adjacent dysplasia. Because much of the BE management algorithm rests on differentiating subtypes of dysplasia, societal guidelines recommend two expert pathologists review biopsies reported as dysplastic or intramucosal carcinoma to provide confidence in the diagnosis [21, 22, 46]. A challenge in diagnosing BE is the high level of intra- and inter-observer variability for pathologic differentiation of dysplasia. This lack of agreement holds true even between expert gastrointestinal pathologists [10, 72–74] and is thought in part due to the relatively arbitrary nature of the discrete categories placed on the continuum of dysplastic BE. While there is relative consensus for nondysplastic BE and for IMC, separating LGD and HGD remains challenging [75]. Despite this limitation, the degree of dysplasia remains the only clearly identified biomarker which has received support across clinical societies for directing specific treatment regimens [21, 22, 46].

Molecular markers to reliably determine the risk of EAC have recently been validated for clinical use and may help improve our current model of risk stratification. There is now sufficient validation data for p53 immunohistochemistry to support its consideration for clinical use in assessing the significance of LGD and resolving the inter-observer variability seen with histology alone. Nuclear expression of p53 is a surrogate for *TP53* mutations that stabilize the p53 protein, and complete loss of p53 can also indicate a *TP53* mutation that leads to failed translation of the protein. However, this assay is not 100% sensitive for all inactivating genetic alterations[76]. Studies of nuclear p53 expression by IHC conducted in large observational cohorts of patients with BE have shown that this assay can improve inter-observer variability in diagnosing dysplasia and can predict progression risk with an OR of 3–8 [56, 77–83]. However, concerns about the reproducibility of this assay remain, as the reported p53 positivity rate in BE dysplasia ranges from 50% to 89%[79, 80]. This appears to be because p53 immunostaining protocols are not standardized, nor is the interpretation of the results, leading to inter-observer variability and suboptimal reproducibility for a clinical assay. Some authorities in this field have proposed that the addition of p53 immunostaining to the histopathological assessment may improve the diagnostic reproducibility of a diagnosis of dysplasia in BE and should be considered as an adjunct to routine clinical diagnosis. This has led the British Society of Gastroenterology to propose its use in this setting (Grade C recommendation in the most recent BSG Guidelines) [22].

The variability in the reported risk of progression based on dysplasia is relatively striking. It is clear that those with confirmed nondysplastic BE have a relatively low risk of adenocarcinoma; however the reported range of risk of progression to EAC for dysplastic BE between studies is large [6]. One of the explanations given for this variability is the reliance on forceps biopsies to sample the BE field. Within a column or tongue of Barrett's there may be several areas of dysplastic foci, and these areas can be easily missed using standard biopsy forceps. The commonly accepted "Seattle Protocol" relies upon four-quadrant biopsies every 2 cm in nondysplastic BE, or every 1 cm in dysplastic BE. However, even when this aggressive tissue sampling protocol is performed appropriately, small foci of dysplasia may be missed [8].

Novel Screening and Surveillance Methods

As previously discussed, current BE screening and surveillance methods suffer from a number of issues related to cost, procedural risk, and suboptimal detection rates. Therefore, new technologies that can enhance the detection of BE or early EAC, or avoid the cost and risk associated with frequent endoscopy, are an area of considerable research activity. This section will summarize endoscopic and nonendoscopic methods under active investigation. Although several techniques are quite promising, with few exceptions these have not yet been recommended for routine use according to society guidelines [21, 22, 84].

Advances in endoscopic technology, including novel microscopic or imaging modalities, have been developed to supplement or supplant traditional HD-WLE and the Seattle biopsy protocol for the detection of Barrett's metaplasia or dysplasia. These techniques can be divided broadly into wide-field and cross-sectional modalities [85]. Wide-field methods, similar to traditional endoscopy, are employed to survey large mucosal surfaces, while cross-sectional imaging typically only assesses smaller areas but can assess depth of mucosal penetration. The primary wide-field methods currently in use include chromoendoscopy, narrow-band imaging and autofluorescence imaging, while cross-sectional techniques include optical coherence tomography, volumetric laser endomicroscopy, and confocal laser endomicroscopy.

Chromoendoscopy involves the use of topically applied dyes, most commonly methylene blue or acetic acid, to enhance the visible contrast between metaplastic or dysplastic tissue and normal squamous tissue. Advantages of chromoendoscopy include its relatively low cost and lack of need for specialized equipment. Meta-analysis of acetic acid chromoendoscopy for the detection of HGD or EAC demonstrated a sensitivity and specificity of 0.92 and 0.96, respectively. However, the detection of Barrett's metaplasia, while highly sensitive (0.96) was nonspecific (0.69) [86].

Narrow-band imaging (NBI), also known as electronic chromoendoscopy, relies on filtering the visible light spectrum to enhance endoscopic contrast. Optical peaks matching the absorption spectrum of hemoglobin are enhanced, allowing improved visualization of hypervascular tissues, such as BE or areas of dysplasia. Randomized controlled trial data and meta-analyses have demonstrated that NBI may increase the yield of the diagnosis of dysplasia while requiring fewer biopsies [87, 88]. A conditional recommendation for the adjuvant use of this technique was included in the most recent version of the American College of Gastroenterology (ACG) guidelines for the diagnosis and management of BE [84].

Autofluorescence imaging (AFI) uses excitation of endogenous fluorophores to differentiate between metaplastic and dysplastic tissue. Dysplastic or neoplastic tissue excites at difference wavelengths than squamous or metaplastic tissue, allowing the visual differentiation of high-grade dysplasia or EAC. Studies have demonstrated this technology has an increased sensitivity for the detection of HGD or EAC compared to WLE alone, although AFI has not been demonstrated to improve the detection of dysplasia when compared to the Seattle protocol [89, 90].

The combination of the above modalities (WLE, NBI and AFI) has been termed "endoscopic trimodal imaging (ETMI)." This technology, while possibly useful for the detection of dysplasia in a small subset of high-risk patients, has not been demonstrated to increase the diagnostic yield of dysplasia during routine surveillance [91, 92].

Molecular imaging, a process where neoplasia- or dysplasia-specific fluorescent-tagged markers are applied topically to the esophageal mucosa, is still in the initial stages of development. A variety of cell surface moieties, including lectins, peptides, antibodies, and enzymes are under investigation as potential targets, and several have shown promise in ex vivo and pilot studies [93–96].

Optical coherence tomography (OCT) employs differential laser backscattering to provide real-time, cross-sectional, subsurface imaging, similar to ultrasound but with dramatically increased resolution (~10 μM) and lower depth of penetration (1–3 mm) [97]. Second-generation OCT, known as volumetric laser endoscopy (VLE) or optical frequency domain imaging (OFDI), can be used to rapidly acquire 360° cross-sectional imaging of up to 6 cm of esophageal length [98]. Retrospective

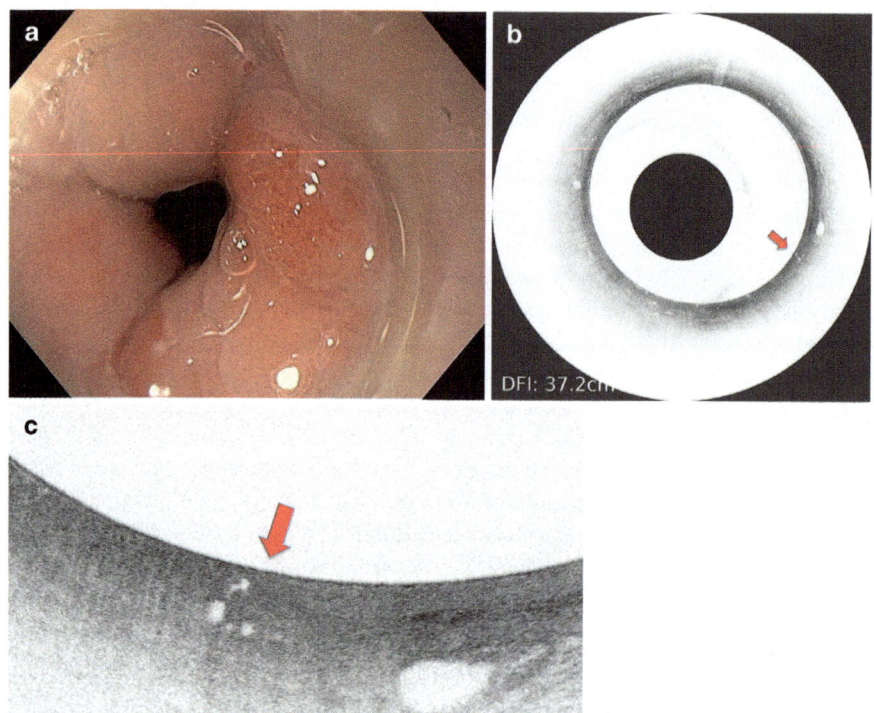

Fig. 4.3 (**a–c**) Endoscopic image demonstrating an irregular GEJ junction. OCT imaging showing atypical glands later demonstrated on EMR to represent high-grade dysplasia

data and ex vivo trials suggest that VLE has an increased rate of dysplasia and neoplasia detection compared to the Seattle protocol in BE surveillance [99, 100] (Fig. 4.3). VLE may also be employed for procedural planning or staging of previously detected BE or EAC, although its clinical role has yet to be firmly established.

Confocal laser endomicroscopy (CLE) provides high-magnification, histology-like images that can be collected during endoscopy. CLE with targeted biopsy had a sensitivity of 89% and specificity of 83% for the detection of neoplasia in meta-analysis, although these values varied significantly between studies, presumably related to technique, operator experience and the type of CLE system used (probe or endoscope based) [101].

In addition to novel esophageal imaging techniques, non-oral approaches to endoscopy are also under investigation. Ultrathin transnasal endoscopy is an alternative screening method that has some advantages over traditional oral endoscopy. The transnasal approach bypasses the root of the tongue and thus avoids the discomfort and gagging associated with oral endoscopy. Transnasal endoscopy can be undertaken in an office setting without sedation, and therefore can be performed by physician extenders [102]. Transnasal endoscopy has a similar sensitivity and specificity to standard endoscopy for the detection of BE, although suffers from reduced optical quality and reduced yield of intestinal metaplasia on biopsy [103]. Although it has not gained widespread acceptance at this point, it has been recommended by the ACG as an acceptable alternative to traditional endoscopy for BE screening [84].

Nonendoscopic methods for BE screening have the advantages of being less invasive and less costly than endoscopic options. One method currently being evaluated is based on retrievable esophageal cytology collection devices, such as the "Cytosponge" or "Esophacap," which are swallowed capsules that degrade in the stomach to release a sponge tethered to a string. As the sponge is pulled back through the esophagus and out of the mouth, it captures esophageal cells which can later be analyzed for particular molecular changes associated with BE and/or dysplasia [2]. The use of the Cytosponge combined with the tissue biomarker trefoil factor 3 (TFF3) had a reasonable sensitivity (87%) and specificity (92%) for detection of BE segments greater than 3 cm in length in a large cross-sectional trial. The device was well tolerated by patients with only minimal anxiety or discomfort reported [104]. Another study determined the Cytosponge was cost-effective, with the potential to reduce mortality from EAC as compared to a no-screening strategy [105]. Additional accurate biomarkers are being sought with this and similar swallowable devices, which may enhance BE detection as well as risk-stratification of known BE [106–108]. For example, the use of a panel of two methylated DNA biomarkers on samples collected by a swallowable balloon device achieved a sensitivity of 90.3% and specificity of 91.7% for the detection of BE in an early clinical trial [108].

Blood, stool, or saliva biomarkers would theoretically provide an ideal screening or surveillance method given their ease and safety of collection. A number of such markers, including circulating microRNAs, metabolite panels, and peptides have been identified in small, retrospective, in vitro, and nonhuman trials, although to date none have been evaluated in prospective clinical trials [109–112].

Treatment of Barrett's Esophagus

The treatment of BE is primarily focused on the prevention of BE progressing to EAC. Until recently, this meant that the focus of BE treatment was on managing risk factors for progression, such as controlling acid reflux, and on endoscopic surveillance to detect HGD or carcinoma, at which point patients were referred for surgical resection of the esophagus. Despite improvements in minimally invasive surgical techniques, the morbidity and mortality of esophagectomy remains high (2–5%) even at expert centers [113]. This high mortality prompted the development of endoscopic treatments for BE. These modalities include ablative techniques such as radiofrequency ablation (RFA), cryotherapy, photodynamic therapy (PDT), and argon plasma coagulation (APC), and resective therapies such as EMR and ESD. While surgical management remains the standard of care for patients with esophageal cancer that has progressed beyond the level of IMC, endoscopic treatments are the new standard of care for patients with dysplastic BE [21, 22, 46, 84].

Nonendoscopic Management of BE

Lifestyle Modifications

The only currently recommended nonendoscopic management strategy for BE is the avoidance of risk factors known to be associated with the risk of progression to EAC. Based on the risk factors described above, it is intuitive, albeit poorly studied, that avoiding smoking, decreasing central adiposity, and consuming a diet high in fruits and vegetables should be recommended to all patients with a diagnosis of BE. Less intuitive is the recommendation that patients with BE have an assessment of their cardiovascular function and/or cardiovascular disease risk factors. In a population-based study from the UK, individuals diagnosed with BE had an increased risk of death from esophageal cancer; however, the largest single cause of death was ischemic heart disease. BE patients had a fourfold increased risk of dying from ischemic heart disease versus esophageal cancer [54]. This raises the interesting question of whether patients diagnosed with BE would be better served by first optimizing their cardiovascular health before embarking on extensive screening and surveillance programs for their BE.

Chemoprevention

There is no proven agent that is effective for primary or secondary chemoprophylaxis for BE. Even though there is considerable data in preclinical models that reflux of acid/bile is a central mechanism for BE formation and progression, there remains no evidence that patients with asymptomatic reflux have a mortality benefit from the use of PPIs or histamine 2 receptor inhibitors [21, 22]. Nonetheless, the use of PPI medications irrespective of symptomatic reflux has been recommended by some authorities [114], although most society position statements do not promote PPI use in the absence of symptomatic reflux. There is relatively strong support for the use of PPIs in BE patients with symptomatic GERD or those patients undergoing endoscopic eradication therapy (EET) [21, 22].

To add to the controversy, there are a number of well-done but conflicting studies regarding the role of acid suppression in BE therapy. A longitudinal study from the Netherlands demonstrated a 75% reduction in the risk of dysplastic progression in patients compliant with PPI therapy [115]. Another large population-based study demonstrated no benefit for PPI therapy in patients with Barrett's and possibly increased risk of advanced disease [116].For patients with symptomatic reflux, there is clearly a role for diet and lifestyle modification and antacid therapy for symptom control. Also, for patients who are undergoing endoscopic therapy of BE, medication nonadherence may contribute to incomplete eradication of BE [117, 118]. A biological explanation for incomplete acid reflux suppression leading to incomplete BE eradication may be in part secondary to the poor barrier function of the neo-squamous epithelium [119]. Data from case-control studies have suggested that the use of nonsteroidal anti-inflammatory medications (NSAIDs) may prevent Barrett's and EAC [120, 121]; however, in aggregate, the studies performed to date have found little to no benefit for the use of NSAIDs for chemoprophylaxis in all patients [122, 123]. Instead, it is typically recommended that individuals with BE undergo evaluation for cardiovascular risk factors, and initiate aspirin therapy based on cardiovascular risk status, under the assumption that they may also benefit from a possible reduction in EAC risk as well.

Surgical Management

Given the putative benefit of acid control in preventing the progression of BE to EAC, fundoplication was previously advocated for individuals with BE to decrease refluxate exposure and thus decrease the risk of BE progression. However, no study to date has shown a clear benefit for fundoplication in decreasing the progression of BE [124, 125]. There may be a role for the use of fundoplication in patients undergoing endoscopic eradication who are unable to achieve eradication in the setting of hiatal hernia or persistent reflux [118].

Endoscopic Management

The success of endoscopic therapy is generally determined by: (1) the removal of dysplastic or nondysplastic BE epithelia (eradication), and (2) the promotion of neo-squamous growth following therapy (remission). To obtain both complete eradication and durable remission, endoscopists generally use a combination of endoscopic resection (EMR or ESD) and ablative therapies (Figs. 4.3 and 4.5). As noted above, EMR provides improved staging capabilities. Appropriate staging is a critical aspect of ER because unlike esophagectomy, endoscopic therapy is limited to mucosal lesions and cannot address locally advanced neoplasms with submucosal involvement or regional lymph node metastasis. If appropriately staged, the risk of lymph node involvement for HGD or IMC is less than 2%. However, lymph node involvement increases to 20% with submucosal invasion [126]. Thus, determination of submucosal involvement plays an important role in determining whether treatment will be primarily endoscopic or surgical.

There are two currently practiced techniques of endoscopic mucosal resection: the cap and snare technique and the band-assisted ligation technique. In the cap and snare technique, a submucosal injection is first performed and then, using a snare fit to the edge of an endoscopic cap, the targeted area of BE is suctioned into the cap. Next, the snare is closed around the suctioned mucosa and cautery is used to resect the targeted mucosa. In the band-assisted technique, a band ligator is attached to the end of the endoscope, and in a similar fashion to endoscopic variceal band ligation, the mucosa is suctioned into the cap, a band is deployed around the suctioned mucosa, and then a snare is used to resect the banded mucosa with cautery (Fig. 4.5).

Endoscopic submucosal dissection for Barrett's remains less common, though has been increasingly described for nodular Barrett's. ESD is an advanced endoscopic technique that permits en bloc resection of mucosal and submucosal lesions. This technique has the benefit of improved histopathologic evaluation with the potential for decreased local recurrence rates due to en bloc curative resection. Widespread uptake of this practice has been limited by a steep learning curve and increased risks of perforation, stricture and bleeding. However, a recent meta-analysis of the limited literature (501 patients, 524 lesions) demonstrated low risk of stricture (11.6%), perforation, or bleeding (1.5% and 1.7%) [127].

The use of resective techniques in combination with effective medical management of reflux can result in durable eradication of BE; however, the use of EMR as monotherapy for BE, particularly when applied circumferentially, has a prohibitively high risk (30–40%) of esophageal stricture without demonstrating any improvement in eradication rates [128–130]. For this reason, in the United States, EMR is generally performed for the staging of nodular BE and, once the nodular area is removed, it is subsequently followed by radio frequency ablation (RFA).RFA is applied under endoscopic visualization using either circumferential balloon catheters or RFA application devices attached to the tip of the endoscope (Fig. 4.4). After initial treatment, patients return for repeat endoscopy every 2–3 months for "touch-up" ablation treatments of persistent BE, as indicated by the appearance of the post-RFA BE (Figs. 4.4 and 4.5). The procedure is widely considered safe and

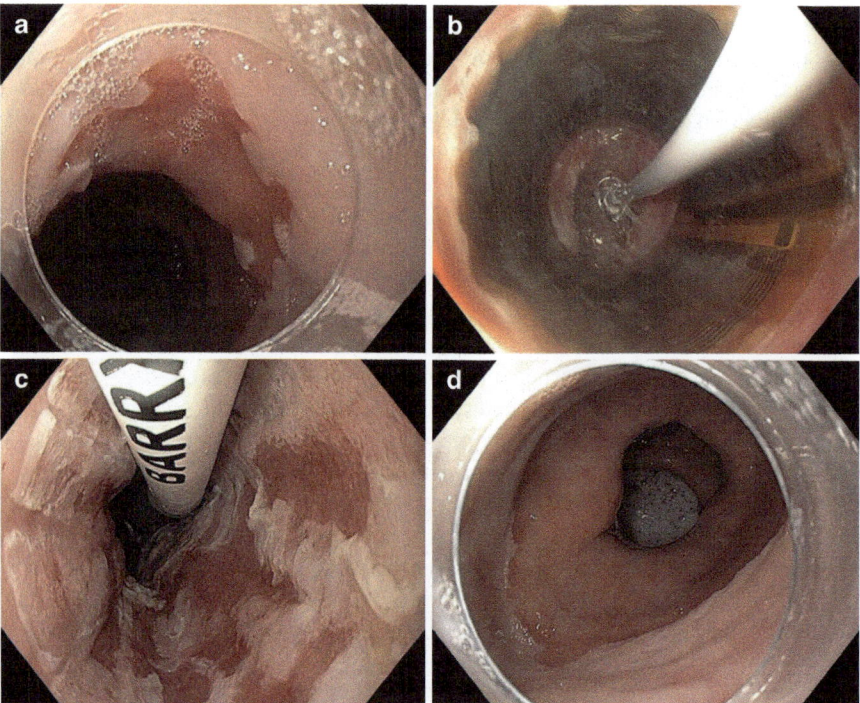

Fig. 4.4 (**a**–**d**) Endoscopic images demonstrating (**a**) short-segment Barrett's esophagus, (**b**) circumferential radio-frequency ablation (RFA) balloon catheter inflated, (**c**) post-RFA treatment appearance of Barrett's esophagus, (**d**) 3-month follow-up of Barrett's esophagus demonstrating ablation of Barrett's esophagus

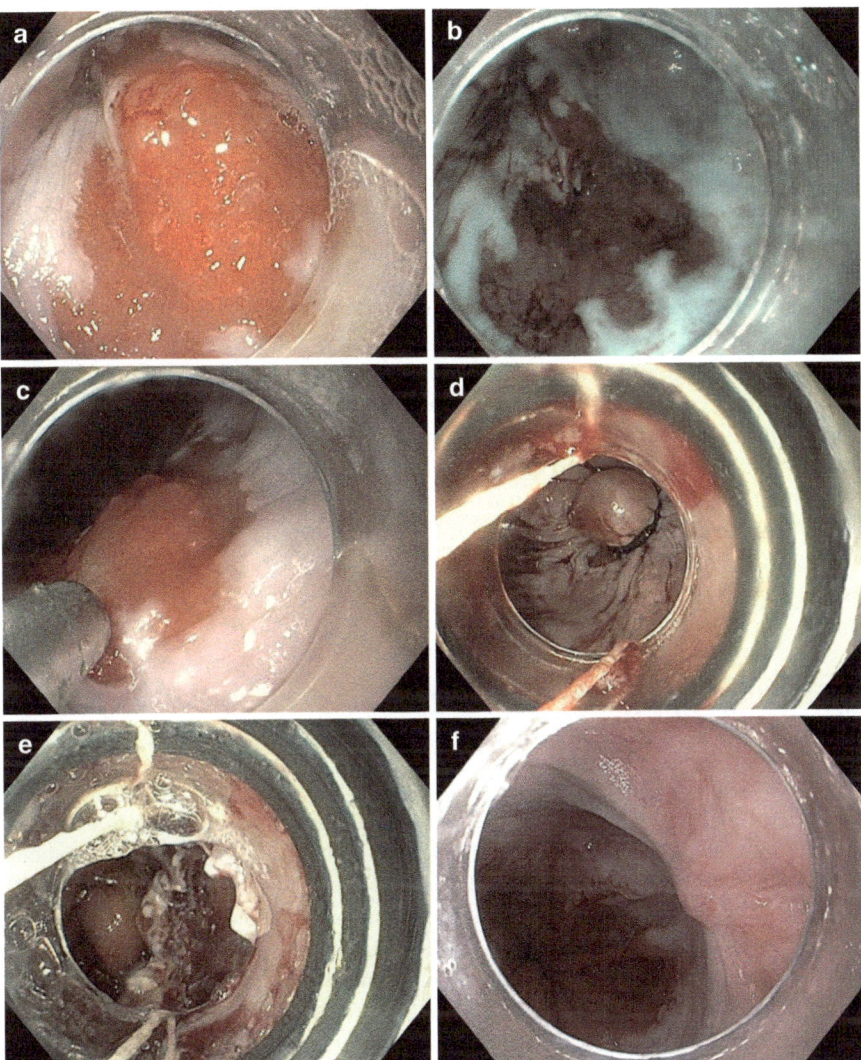

Fig. 4.5 (**a–f**) Endoscopic images demonstrating (**a**) Barrett's with nodule (pathology of nodule: high-grade dysplasia), (**b**) narrow-band imaging (NBI) of nodular lesion, (**c**) submucosal injection of nodule with saline (saline lift) prior to endomucosal resection (EMR), (**d**) EMR using Duette banding kit, (**e**) EMR site after snare removal, (**f**) 3-month follow-up of site with scar and no endoscopically evident Barrett's esophagus

the post-therapy quality of life is substantially better than that after esophageal resection. The major adverse events are stricture formation (4–10%), bleeding (<1%), and perforation (<1/1000) [130, 131]. Randomized controlled studies have shown that use of RFA can result in durable eradication of BE with a relatively infrequent adverse event rate [132, 133]. A large systematic review and meta-analysis of 18 studies involving 3802 patients treated with RFA demonstrated complete eradication of dysplasia in 91% of patients and complete eradication of intestinal metaplasia (IM) in 78% of patients. Notably, progression to cancer only occurred in 0.2% of patients during treatment and 0.7% of patients after complete eradication [131].

Given that the rates of complete eradication of dysplasia and metaplasia remain less than 100%, along with the complication of stricture formation (5% of patients treated with RFA alone, 10–13% in patients treated with RFA and resection), cryotherapy is being explored as an alternative ablative treatment [130, 134]. Unlike RFA, cryoablation is a noncontact method of directing a spray of liquid nitrogen on the Barrett's mucosa. This causes rapid freezing and thawing and resultant cell membrane disruption, apoptosis, thrombosis, and necrosis of the superficial layers of the esophagus, potentially decreasing injury to deeper structures and thus, decreasing stricture formation [135]. Data is limited; however, recently published long-term retrospective data of 40 patients with HGD and IMC demonstrated complete eradication of 98% of HGD, 90% of dysplasia and 60% of IM [136]. This study demonstrates feasibility of cryotherapy, though more work is required to determine if cryotherapy could be used to complement RFA or would replace it.

Determining Candidacy for Endoscopic Management of BE: Issues Surrounding the Use of Ablation Therapy for Low-Risk BE

The success of endoscopic therapy in achieving durable eradication for HGD has resulted in multi-society consensus suggesting the use of endoscopic treatment as first line for patients with HGD [21, 22, 46]. The larger question is whether patients with a lower risk of malignant progression, including those with nondysplastic BE or LGD, should be offered EET followed by surveillance. More recently the ACG recommended that patients with LGD confirmed by two pathologists should undergo EET. This is largely based on the 2014 surveillance versus radiofrequency ablation (SURF) multicenter study[137]. In this study, 136 patients with a confirmed diagnosis of BE with LGD were enrolled and randomized to ablation or surveillance. Notably, the risk of progression to HGD or adenocarcinoma was reduced to 1.5% for ablation versus 26.5% for control (95% CI, 14.1–35.9%; $P < 0.001$). In a recent follow-up report of these patients, Duits et al. found that the number of pathologists confirming LGD as well as patients who had persistence of LGD over time increased the risk for development of HGD or EAC [138].

The issue of treating low-risk BE endoscopically is less a matter of safety than one of cost and necessity. Treating BE with HGD endoscopically is generally considered cost-effective and there are estimates using the most recently revised rates of progression to cancer that suggest that RFA is cost effective for patients with LGD [139, 140]. However, EMR and RFA for nondysplastic BE is generally considered to have an inappropriately high risk:benefit ratio and to be prohibitively expensive from a population-level perspective[139, 141].

Surveillance After Treatment

The main goal of therapy is complete eradication or remission of intestinal metaplasia (CEIM or CRIM), though many argue that a lesser goal, complete eradication of intestinal dysplasia (CEID), or cancer is a reasonable endpoint. CEIM is defined as endoscopic and histologic remission of intestinal metaplasia on follow-up endoscopy.

Multiple studies have shown that despite initial endoscopic and histologic eradication, 12–32% of patients will have recurrence of dysplasia and 0.7–1.4% will experience recurrence of EAC [130, 131, 133]. The greatest probability of recurrence is at 1 year, although those who did not initially recur have a lower but still possible chance of recurrence [133]. Patients with a longer initial segment of Barrett's and more advanced pathology appear to be at greater risk for recurrence [142].

Currently, the ACG is the only professional society to provide practice guidelines for post-EET surveillance. These guidelines recommend a stratified approach, suggesting individuals with baseline HGD undergo endoscopy every 3 months for the first year following CEIM, and those with baseline LGD (or those with HGD in their second year of surveillance) undergo endoscopy every 6 months. For those who have not progressed, annual surveillance is then recommended [84].

Current Controversies Surrounding BE Surveillance and Treatment

Recognition of Barrett's as a marker for EAC led to the early acceptance of endoscopic screening and surveillance. These programs are endoscopically intensive. Individuals with BE are currently advised to undergo endoscopy every 1–5 years depending on the presence and degree of dysplasia. Two studies highlight the controversy regarding screening and surveillance programs. In a study comparing patients with adenocarcinoma from 1995 to 2009 to a matched control population of patients with BE, the authors found that endoscopic surveillance provided no mortality benefit [143]. This study included patients prior to the widespread use of HD-WLE and the use of less morbid endoscopically based treatment, yet the lack of any benefit from screening is concerning. Some of the lack of surveillance benefit may in part be explained by the known poor adherence to the recommended biopsy protocol by community endoscopists [144]. Of interest, this study demonstrated that early cancers were found in the surveyed population, but that there was no mortality benefit in this group. However, a more recent study evaluated all patients diagnosed with EAC between 1999 and 2009 within the Netherlands Cancer Registry for prior surveillance. In this group of 9780 EAC patients, mortality was significantly lower (adjusted HR 0.79; 95% confidence interval (0.64–0.92) when compared to patients with a prior BE diagnosis who did not participate in surveillance [3]. This study highlights the importance of performing surveillance appropriately, but also demonstrated that 90% of all patients with EAC in this group did not have a diagnosis of BE preceding their diagnosis of EAC.

If endoscopic surveillance of BE is challenging to perform in clinical practice and outcomes from clinical trials of ablation demonstrate durable response, it is reasonable to ask whether all BE should be ablated. Again, the clinical issues surrounding ablating all Barrett's include (1) the low absolute risk of BE progressing to EAC; (2) the suboptimal performance of current risk markers; (3) the risks of complications from EMR and RFA; and (4) problems predicting who will achieve a durable response to ablation and who can be successfully discharged from ongoing surveillance. As such, the treatment recommendations for nondysplastic BE remain vague. In very-low-risk cohorts (e.g., short segment of Barrett's, female, slender, and non-Caucasian), there is likely no benefit to treatment or surveillance; however, individuals with multiple risk factors for BE progression might benefit from treatment and ongoing surveillance.

Conclusions

The ultimate goal of the management of BE is to prevent EAC. Recent studies suggest that population-based screening tests utilizing a variety of biomarkers or demographic characteristics that identify those people at risk for BE and that accurately risk stratify could be implemented in the near future. Ideally, these individuals could then undergo simple, noninvasive, or minimally invasive screening tests to confirm the presence of BE. Depending on the risk profile of the individual, appropriate treatment or surveillance could then be performed and tailored to the individual's progression risk. As our prognostic and therapeutic tools continue to improve, it is widely anticipated that the benefits of screening and surveillance in large, multicenter controlled trials of BE will be shown. Since many of the risk factors for the development of BE and EAC are expected to remain static or increase in the coming years, unless we refine our screening and surveillance programs beyond the reliance on a single biomarker (dysplasia), we cannot hope to reduce the upward trend in the incidence of esophageal cancer and EAC-related deaths.

References

1. Paulson TG, Reid BJ. Focus on Barrett's esophagus and esophageal adenocarcinoma. Cancer Cell. 2004;6(1):11–6. https://doi.org/10.1016/j.ccr.2004.06.021.
2. Kadri S, Lao-Sirieix P, Fitzgerald RC. Developing a nonendoscopic screening test for Barrett's esophagus. Biomark Med. 2011;5(3):397–404. https://doi.org/10.2217/bmm.11.40.
3. Verbeek RE, Leenders M, Ten Kate FJ, van Hillegersberg R, Vleggaar FP, van Baal JW, van Oijen MG, Siersema PD. Surveillance of Barrett's esophagus and mortality from esophageal adenocarcinoma: a population-based cohort study. Am J Gastroenterol. 2014;109(8):1215–22. https://doi.org/10.1038/ajg.2014.156.
4. Thrift AP, Whiteman DC. The incidence of esophageal adenocarcinoma continues to rise: analysis of period and birth cohort effects on recent trends. Ann Oncol. 2012;23(12):3155–62. https://doi.org/10.1093/annonc/mds181.
5. Barrett NR. Chronic peptic ulcer of the oesophagus and 'oesophagitis'. Br J Surg. 1950;38(150):175–82.
6. Spechler SJ. Barrett esophagus and risk of esophageal cancer: a clinical review. JAMA. 2013;310(6):627–36. https://doi.org/10.1001/jama.2013.226450.

7. Reid BJ, Li X, Galipeau PC, Vaughan TL. Barrett's oesophagus and oesophageal adenocarcinoma: time for a new synthesis. Nat Rev Cancer. 2010;10(2):87–101. https://doi.org/10.1038/nrc2773.

8. Bhat S, Coleman HG, Yousef F, Johnston BT, McManus DT, Gavin AT, Murray LJ. Risk of malignant progression in Barrett's esophagus patients: results from a large population-based study. J Natl Cancer Inst. 2011;103(13):1049–57. https://doi.org/10.1093/jnci/djr203.

9. Dulai GS, Shekelle PG, Jensen DM, Spiegel BM, Chen J, Oh D, Kahn KL. Dysplasia and risk of further neoplastic progression in a regional veterans administration Barrett's cohort. Am J Gastroenterol. 2005;100(4):775–83.

10. Sharma P, Falk GW, Weston AP, Reker D, Johnston M, Sampliner RE. Dysplasia and cancer in a large multicenter cohort of patients with Barrett's esophagus. ClinGastroenterolHepatol. 2006;4(5):566–72.

11. Bhat SK, McManus DT, Coleman HG, Johnston BT, Cardwell CR, McMenamin U, Bannon F, Hicks B, Kennedy G, Gavin AT, Murray LJ. Oesophageal adenocarcinoma and prior diagnosis of Barrett's oesophagus: a population-based study. Gut 2015;64:20–25. https://doi.org/10.1136/gutjnl-2013-305506.

12. Balasubramanian G, Singh M, Gupta N, Gaddam S, Giacchino M, Wani SB, Moloney B, Higbee AD, Rastogi A, Bansal A, Sharma P. Prevalence and predictors of columnar lined esophagus in gastroesophageal reflux disease (GERD) patients undergoing upper endoscopy. Am J Gastroenterol. 2012;107(11):1655–61. https://doi.org/10.1038/ajg.2012.299.

13. Spechler SJ, Zeroogian JM, Antonioli DA, Wang HH, Goyal RK. Prevalence of metaplasia at the gastro-oesophageal junction. Lancet. 1994;344(8936):1533–6.

14. Connor MJ, Weston AP, Mayo MS, Sharma P. The prevalence of Barrett's esophagus and erosive esophagitis in patients undergoing upper endoscopy for dyspepsia in a VA population. Dig Dis Sci. 2004;49(6):920–4.

15. Rex DK, Cummings OW, Shaw M, Cumings MD, Wong RK, Vasudeva RS, Dunne D, Rahmani EY, Helper DJ. Screening for Barrett's esophagus in colonoscopy patients with and without heartburn. Gastroenterology. 2003;125(6):1670–7.

16. Rubenstein JH, Morgenstern H, Appelman H, Scheiman J, Schoenfeld P, McMahon LF Jr, Metko V, Near E, Kellenberg J, Kalish T, Inadomi JM. Prediction of Barrett's esophagus among men. Am J Gastroenterol. 2013;108(3):353–62. https://doi.org/10.1038/ajg.2012.446.

17. Ronkainen J, Aro P, Storskrubb T, Johansson SE, Lind T, Bolling-Sternevald E, Vieth M, Stolte M, Talley NJ, Agreus L. Prevalence of Barrett's esophagus in the general population: an endoscopic study. Gastroenterology. 2005;129(6):1825–31. https://doi.org/10.1053/j.gastro.2005.08.053.

18. Zagari RM, Fuccio L, Wallander MA, Johansson S, Fiocca R, Casanova S, Farahmand BY, Winchester CC, Roda E, Bazzoli F. Gastro-oesophageal reflux symptoms, oesophagitis and Barrett's oesophagus in the general population: the Loiano-Monghidoro study. Gut. 2008;57(10):1354–9. https://doi.org/10.1136/gut.2007.145177.

19. Ronkainen J, Talley NJ, Storskrubb T, Johansson SE, Lind T, Vieth M, Agreus L, Aro P. Erosive esophagitis is a risk factor for Barrett's esophagus: a community-based endoscopic follow-up study. Am J Gastroenterol. 2011;106(11):1946–52. https://doi.org/10.1038/ajg.2011.326.

20. Taylor JB, Rubenstein JH. Meta-analyses of the effect of symptoms of gastroesophageal reflux on the risk of Barrett's esophagus. Am J Gastroenterol. 2010;105(8):1729., 1730–1727; quiz 1738. https://doi.org/10.1038/ajg.2010.194.

21. American Gastroenterological A, Spechler SJ, Sharma P, Souza RF, Inadomi JM, Shaheen NJ. American Gastroenterological Association medical position statement on the management of Barrett's esophagus. Gastroenterology. 2011;140(3):1084–91. https://doi.org/10.1053/j.gastro.2011.01.030.

22. Fitzgerald RC, di Pietro M, Ragunath K, Ang Y, Kang JY, Watson P, Trudgill N, Patel P, Kaye PV, Sanders S, O'Donovan M, Bird-Lieberman E, Bhandari P, Jankowski JA, Attwood S, Parsons SL, Loft D, Lagergren J, Moayyedi P, Lyratzopoulos G, de Caestecker J, British

Society of G. British Society of Gastroenterology guidelines on the diagnosis and management of Barrett's oesophagus. Gut. 2014;63(1):7–42. https://doi.org/10.1136/gutjnl-2013-305372.

23. Spechler SJ, Souza RF. Barrett's Esophagus. N Engl J Med. 2014;371(9):836–45. https://doi.org/10.1056/NEJMra1314704.

24. de Jonge PJ, van Blankenstein M, Grady WM, Kuipers EJ. Barrett's oesophagus: epidemiology, cancer risk and implications for management. Gut. 2014;63(1):191–202. https://doi.org/10.1136/gutjnl-2013-305490.

25. Rubenstein JH. Risk factors for Barrett's esophagus. Curr Opin Gastroenterol. 2014;30(4):408–14. https://doi.org/10.1097/MOG.0000000000000084.

26. Leggett CL, Gorospe EC, Calvin AD, Harmsen WS, Zinsmeister AR, Caples S, Somers VK, Dunagan K, Lutzke L, Wang KK, Iyer PG. Obstructive sleep apnea is a risk factor for Barrett's esophagus. ClinGastroenterolHepatol. 2014;12(4):583–588.e581. https://doi.org/10.1016/j.cgh.2013.08.043.

27. Anderson LA, Watson RG, Murphy SJ, Johnston BT, Comber H, Mc Guigan J, Reynolds JV, Murray LJ. Risk factors for Barrett's oesophagus and oesophageal adenocarcinoma: results from the FINBAR study. World J Gastroenterol: WJG. 2007;13(10):1585–94.

28. Corley DA, Kubo A, Levin TR, Block G, Habel L, Zhao W, Leighton P, Rumore G, Quesenberry C, Buffler P, Parsonnet J. Helicobacter pylori infection and the risk of Barrett's oesophagus: a community-based study. Gut. 2008;57(6):727–33. doi:gut.2007.132068 [pii]

29. Hvid-Jensen F, Pedersen L, Drewes AM, Sorensen HT, Funch-Jensen P. Incidence of adenocarcinoma among patients with Barrett's esophagus. N Engl J Med. 2011;365(15):1375–83. https://doi.org/10.1056/NEJMoa1103042.

30. de Jonge PJ, van Blankenstein M, Looman CW, Casparie MK, Meijer GA, Kuipers EJ. Risk of malignant progression in patients with Barrett's oesophagus: a Dutch nationwide cohort study. Gut. 2010;59(8):1030–6. https://doi.org/10.1136/gut.2009.176701.

31. Curvers WL, ten Kate FJ, Krishnadath KK, Visser M, Elzer B, Baak LC, Bohmer C, Mallant-Hent RC, van Oijen A, Naber AH, Scholten P, Busch OR, Blaauwgeers HG, Meijer GA, Bergman JJ. Low-grade dysplasia in Barrett's esophagus: overdiagnosed and underestimated. Am J Gastroenterol. 2010;105(7):1523–30. https://doi.org/10.1038/ajg.2010.171.

32. Wani S, Falk GW, Post J, Yerian L, Hall M, Wang A, Gupta N, Gaddam S, Singh M, Singh V, Chuang KY, Boolchand V, Gavini H, Kuczynski J, Sud P, Bansal A, Rastogi A, Mathur SC, Young P, Cash B, Goldblum J, Lieberman DA, Sampliner RE, Sharma P. Risk factors for progression of low-grade dysplasia in patients with Barrett's esophagus. Gastroenterology. 2011;141(4):1179–86,. 1186.e1171. https://doi.org/10.1053/j.gastro.2011.06.055.

33. Thota PN, Lee HJ, Goldblum JR, Liu X, Sanaka MR, Gohel T, Kanadiya M, Lopez R. Risk stratification of patients with Barrett's esophagus and low-grade dysplasia or indefinite for dysplasia. ClinGastroenterolHepatol. 2015;13(3):459–65.e1. https://doi.org/10.1016/j.cgh.2014.07.049.

34. Rastogi A, Puli S, El-Serag HB, Bansal A, Wani S, Sharma P. Incidence of esophageal adenocarcinoma in patients with Barrett's esophagus and high-grade dysplasia: a meta-analysis. Gastrointest Endosc. 2008;67(3):394–8.

35. Schnell TG, Sontag SJ, Chejfec G, Aranha G, Metz A, O'Connell S, Seidel UJ, Sonnenberg A. Long-term nonsurgical management of Barrett's esophagus with high-grade dysplasia. Gastroenterology. 2001;120(7):1607–19.

36. Buttar NS, Wang KK, Sebo TJ, Riehle DM, Krishnadath KK, Lutzke LS, Anderson MA, Petterson TM, Burgart LJ. Extent of high-grade dysplasia in Barrett's esophagus correlates with risk of adenocarcinoma. Gastroenterology. 2001;120(7):1630–9.

37. Weston AP, Sharma P, Topalovski M, Richards R, Cherian R, Dixon A. Long-term follow-up of Barrett's high-grade dysplasia. Am J Gastroenterol. 2000;95(8):1888–93.

38. Rabinovitch PS, Longton G, Blount PL, Levine DS, Reid BJ. Predictors of progression in Barrett's esophagus III: baseline flow cytometric variables. Am J Gastroenterol. 2001;96(11):3071–83.

39. Cook MB, Corley DA, Murray LJ, Liao LM, Kamangar F, Ye W, Gammon MD, Risch HA, Casson AG, Freedman ND, Chow WH, Wu AH, Bernstein L, Nyren O, Pandeya N, Whiteman DC, Vaughan TL. Gastroesophageal reflux in relation to adenocarcinomas of the esophagus: a

pooled analysis from the Barrett's and Esophageal adenocarcinoma consortium (BEACON). PLoS One. 2014;9(7):e103508. https://doi.org/10.1371/journal.pone.0103508.

40. Gaddam S, Singh M, Balasubramanian G, Thota P, Gupta N, Wani S, Higbee AD, Mathur SC, Horwhat JD, Rastogi A, Young PE, Cash BD, Bansal A, Vargo JJ, Falk GW, Lieberman DA, Sampliner RE, Sharma P. Persistence of nondysplastic Barrett's esophagus identifies patients at lower risk for esophageal adenocarcinoma: results from a large multicenter cohort. Gastroenterology. 2013;145(3):548–553.e541. https://doi.org/10.1053/j.gastro.2013.05.040.

41. Shaheen NJ, Sharma P, Overholt BF, Wolfsen HC, Sampliner RE, Wang KK, Galanko JA, Bronner MP, Goldblum JR, Bennett AE, Jobe BA, Eisen GM, Fennerty MB, Hunter JG, Fleischer DE, Sharma VK, Hawes RH, Hoffman BJ, Rothstein RI, Gordon SR, Mashimo H, Chang KJ, Muthusamy VR, Edmundowicz SA, Spechler SJ, Siddiqui AA, Souza RF, Infantolino A, Falk GW, Kimmey MB, Madanick RD, Chak A, Lightdale CJ. Radiofrequency ablation in Barrett's esophagus with dysplasia. N Engl J Med. 2009;360(22):2277–88. https://doi.org/10.1056/NEJMoa0808145.

42. Reid BJ, Blount PL, Rubin CE, Levine DS, Haggitt RC, Rabinovitch PS. Flow-cytometric and histological progression to malignancy in Barrett's esophagus: prospective endoscopic surveillance of a cohort. Gastroenterology. 1992;102(4 Pt 1):1212–9.

43. Weston AP, Krmpotich PT, Cherian R, Dixon A, Topalosvki M. Prospective long-term endoscopic and histological follow-up of short segment Barrett's esophagus: comparison with traditional long segment Barrett's esophagus. Am J Gastroenterol. 1997;92(3):407–13.

44. Horwhat JD, Baroni D, Maydonovitch C, Osgard E, Ormseth E, Rueda-Pedraza E, Lee HJ, Hirota WK, Wong RK. Normalization of intestinal metaplasia in the esophagus and esophagogastric junction: incidence and clinical data. Am J Gastroenterol. 2007;102(3):497–506.

45. Oelschlager BK, Barreca M, Chang L, Oleynikov D, Pellegrini CA. Clinical and pathologic response of Barrett's esophagus to laparoscopic antireflux surgery. Ann Surg. 2003;238(4):458–64;. discussion 464-456. https://doi.org/10.1097/01.sla.0000090443.97693.c3.

46. Committee ASoP, Evans JA, Early DS, Fukami N, Ben-Menachem T, Chandrasekhara V, Chathadi KV, Decker GA, Fanelli RD, Fisher DA, Foley KQ, Hwang JH, Jain R, Jue TL, Khan KM, Lightdale J, Malpas PM, Maple JT, Pasha SF, Saltzman JR, Sharaf RN, Shergill A, Dominitz JA, Cash BD. The role of endoscopy in Barrett's esophagus and other premalignant conditions of the esophagus. Gastrointest Endosc. 2012;76(6):1087–94. https://doi.org/10.1016/j.gie.2012.08.004.

47. Takubo K, Vieth M, Aida J, Sawabe M, Kumagai Y, Hoshihara Y, Arai T. Differences in the definitions used for esophageal and gastric diseases in different countries: endoscopic definition of the esophagogastric junction, the precursor of Barrett's adenocarcinoma, the definition of Barrett's esophagus, and histologic criteria for mucosal adenocarcinoma or high-grade dysplasia. Digestion. 2009;80(4):248–57. https://doi.org/10.1159/000235923.

48. Kusano C, Kaltenbach T, Shimazu T, Soetikno R, Gotoda T. Can Western endoscopists identify the end of the lower esophageal palisade vessels as a landmark of esophagogastric junction? J Gastroenterol. 2009;44(8):842–6. https://doi.org/10.1007/s00535-009-0083-1.

49. Paull A, Trier JS, Dalton MD, Camp RC, Loeb P, Goyal RK. The histologic spectrum of Barrett's esophagus. N Engl J Med. 1976;295(9):476–80. https://doi.org/10.1056/NEJM197608262950904.

50. Westerhoff M, Hovan L, Lee C, Hart J. Effects of dropping the requirement for goblet cells from the diagnosis of Barrett's esophagus. ClinGastroenterolHepatol. 2012;10(11):1232–6. https://doi.org/10.1016/j.cgh.2012.05.013.

51. Chandrasoma P, Wickramasinghe K, Ma Y, DeMeester T. Is intestinal metaplasia a necessary precursor lesion for adenocarcinomas of the distal esophagus, gastroesophageal junction and gastric cardia? DisEsophagus. 2007;20(1):36–41.

52. Gilbert EW, Luna RA, Harrison VL, Hunter JG. Barrett's esophagus: a review of the literature. J Gastrointest Surg. 2011;15(5):708–18. https://doi.org/10.1007/s11605-011-1485-y.

53. Varghese S, Lao-Sirieix P, Fitzgerald RC. Identification and clinical implementation of biomarkers for Barrett's esophagus. Gastroenterology. 2012;142(3):435–441.e432. https://doi.org/10.1053/j.gastro.2012.01.013.

54. Solaymani-Dodaran M, Card TR, West J. Cause-specific mortality of people with Barrett's esophagus compared with the general population: a population-based cohort study. Gastroenterology. 2013;144(7):1375–83,. 1383.e1371. https://doi.org/10.1053/j.gastro.2013.02.050.

55. Galipeau PC, Li X, Blount PL, Maley CC, Sanchez CA, Odze RD, Ayub K, Rabinovitch PS, Vaughan TL, Reid BJ. NSAIDs modulate CDKN2A, TP53, and DNA content risk for progression to esophageal adenocarcinoma. PLoS Med. 2007;4(2):e67. doi:06-PLME-RA-0387R2 [pii]

56. Bird-Lieberman EL, Dunn JM, Coleman HG, Lao-Sirieix P, Oukrif D, Moore CE, Varghese S, Johnston BT, Arthur K, McManus DT, Novelli MR, O'Donovan M, Cardwell CR, Lovat LB, Murray LJ, Fitzgerald RC. Population-based study reveals new risk-stratification biomarker panel for Barrett's esophagus. Gastroenterology. 2012;143(4):927–35e923. https://doi.org/10.1053/j.gastro.2012.06.041.

57. Rygiel AM, Milano F, Ten Kate FJ, Schaap A, Wang KK, Peppelenbosch MP, Bergman JJ, Krishnadath KK. Gains and amplifications of c-myc, EGFR, and 20.q13 loci in the no dysplasia-dysplasia-adenocarcinoma sequence of Barrett's esophagus. Cancer Epidemiol Biomark Prev. 2008;17(6):1380–5. https://doi.org/10.1158/1055-9965.EPI-07-2734.

58. Maley CC, Galipeau PC, Finley JC, Wongsurawat VJ, Li X, Sanchez CA, Paulson TG, Blount PL, Risques RA, Rabinovitch PS, Reid BJ. Genetic clonal diversity predicts progression to esophageal adenocarcinoma. Nat Genet. 2006;38(4):468–73.

59. Kaz AM, Grady WM. Epigenetic biomarkers in esophageal cancer. Cancer Lett. 2014;342(2):193–9. https://doi.org/10.1016/j.canlet.2012.02.036.

60. Revilla-Nuin B, Parrilla P, Lozano JJ, de Haro LF, Ortiz A, Martinez C, Munitiz V, de Angulo DR, Bermejo J, Molina J, Cayuela ML, Yelamos J. Predictive value of MicroRNAs in the progression of Barrett esophagus to adenocarcinoma in a long-term follow-up study. Ann Surg. 2013;257(5):886–93. https://doi.org/10.1097/SLA.0b013e31826ddba6.

61. Alvarez Herrero L, Curvers WL, van Vilsteren FG, Wolfsen H, Ragunath K, Wong Kee Song LM, Mallant-Hent RC, van Oijen A, Scholten P, Schoon EJ, Schenk EB, Weusten BL, Bergman JG. Validation of the Prague C&M classification of Barrett's esophagus in clinical practice. Endoscopy. 2013;45(11):876–82. https://doi.org/10.1055/s-0033-1344952.

62. Vahabzadeh B, Seetharam AB, Cook MB, Wani S, Rastogi A, Bansal A, Early DS, Sharma P. Validation of the Prague C & M criteria for the endoscopic grading of Barrett's esophagus by gastroenterology trainees: a multicenter study. Gastrointest Endosc. 2012;75(2):236–41. https://doi.org/10.1016/j.gie.2011.09.017.

63. Montgomery E, Bronner MP, Greenson JK, Haber MM, Hart J, Lamps LW, Lauwers GY, Lazenby AJ, Lewin DN, Robert ME, Washington K, Goldblum JR. Are ulcers a marker for invasive carcinoma in Barrett's esophagus? Data from a diagnostic variability study with clinical follow-up. Am J Gastroenterol. 2002;97(1):27–31. https://doi.org/10.1111/j.1572-0241.2002.05420.x.

64. Kara MA, Peters FP, Rosmolen WD, Krishnadath KK, ten Kate FJ, Fockens P, Bergman JJ. High-resolution endoscopy plus chromoendoscopy or narrow-band imaging in Barrett's esophagus: a prospective randomized crossover study. Endoscopy. 2005;37(10):929–36. https://doi.org/10.1055/s-2005-870433.

65. Thomas T, Gilbert D, Kaye PV, Penman I, Aithal GP, Ragunath K. High-resolution endoscopy and endoscopic ultrasound for evaluation of early neoplasia in Barrett's esophagus. Surg Endosc. 2010;24(5):1110–6. https://doi.org/10.1007/s00464-009-0737-3.

66. Pech O, Gossner L, Manner H, May A, Rabenstein T, Behrens A, Berres M, Huijsmans J, Vieth M, Stolte M, Ell C. Prospective evaluation of the macroscopic types and location of early Barrett's neoplasia in 380 lesions. Endoscopy. 2007;39(7):588–93. https://doi.org/10.1055/s-2007-966363.

67. Moss A, Bourke MJ, Hourigan LF, Gupta S, Williams SJ, Tran K, Swan MP, Hopper AD, Kwan V, Bailey AA. Endoscopic resection for Barrett's high-grade dysplasia and early esophageal adenocarcinoma: an essential staging procedure with long-term therapeutic benefit. Am J Gastroenterol. 2010;105(6):1276–83. https://doi.org/10.1038/ajg.2010.1.

68. Mino-Kenudson M, Hull MJ, Brown I, Muzikansky A, Srivastava A, Glickman J, Park DY, Zuckerberg L, Misdraji J, Odze RD, Lauwers GY. EMR for Barrett's esophagus-related superficial neoplasms offers better diagnostic reproducibility than mucosal biopsy. Gastrointest Endosc. 2007;66(4):660–6. quiz 767, 769doi:S0016-5107(07)00405-1[pii]

69. Mino-Kenudson M, Brugge WR, Puricelli WP, Nakatsuka LN, Nishioka NS, Zukerberg LR, Misdraji J, Lauwers GY. Management of superficial Barrett's epithelium-related neoplasms by endoscopic mucosal resection: clinicopathologic analysis of 27 cases. Am J Surg Pathol. 2005;29(5):680–6. doi:00000478-200505000-00016[pii]

70. Mandal RV, Forcione DG, Brugge WR, Nishioka NS, Mino-Kenudson M, Lauwers GY. Effect of tumor characteristics and duplication of the muscularis mucosae on the endoscopic staging of superficial Barrett esophagus-related neoplasia. Am J Surg Pathol. 2009;33(4):620–5. https://doi.org/10.1097/PAS.0b013e31818d632f.

71. Wani S, Abrams J, Edmundowicz SA, Gaddam S, Hovis CE, Green D, Gupta N, Higbee A, Bansal A, Rastogi A, Early D, Lightdale CJ, Sharma P. Endoscopic mucosal resection results in change of histologic diagnosis in Barrett's esophagus patients with visible and flat neoplasia: a multicenter cohort study. Dig Dis Sci. 2013;58(6):1703–9. https://doi.org/10.1007/s10620-013-2689-7.

72. Schlemper RJ, Riddell RH, Kato Y, Borchard F, Cooper HS, Dawsey SM, Dixon MF, Fenoglio-Preiser CM, Flejou JF, Geboes K, Hattori T, Hirota T, Itabashi M, Iwafuchi M, Iwashita A, Kim YI, Kirchner T, Klimpfinger M, Koike M, Lauwers GY, Lewin KJ, Oberhuber G, Offner F, Price AB, Rubio CA, Shimizu M, Shimoda T, Sipponen P, Solcia E, Stolte M, Watanabe H, Yamabe H. The Vienna classification of gastrointestinal epithelial neoplasia. Gut. 2000;47(2):251–5. https://doi.org/10.1136/gut.47.2.251.

73. Skacel M, Petras RE, Gramlich TL, Sigel JE, Richter JE, Goldblum JR. The diagnosis of low-grade dysplasia in Barrett's esophagus and its implications for disease progression. Am J Gastroenterol. 2000;95(12):3383–7.

74. Lim CH, Treanor D, Dixon MF, Axon AT. Low-grade dysplasia in Barrett's esophagus has a high risk of progression. Endoscopy. 2007;39(7):581–7. https://doi.org/10.1055/s-2007-966592.

75. Montgomery E, Bronner MP, Goldblum JR, Greenson JK, Haber MM, Hart J, Lamps LW, Lauwers GY, Lazenby AJ, Lewin DN, Robert ME, Toledano AY, Shyr Y, Washington K. Reproducibility of the diagnosis of dysplasia in Barrett esophagus: a reaffirmation. Hum Pathol. 2001;32(4):368–78.

76. Greenblatt MS, Bennett WP, Hollstein M, Harris CC. Mutations in the p53 tumor suppressor gene: clues to cancer etiology and molecular pathogenesis. Cancer Res. 1994;54(18):4855–78.

77. Kaye PV, Haider SA, Ilyas M, James PD, Soomro I, Faisal W, Catton J, Parsons SL, Ragunath K. Barrett's dysplasia and the Vienna classification: reproducibility, prediction of progression and impact of consensus reporting and p53 immunohistochemistry. Histopathology. 2009;54(6):699–712. https://doi.org/10.1111/j.1365-2559.2009.03288.x.

78. Skacel M, Petras RE, Rybicki LA, Gramlich TL, Richter JE, Falk GW, Goldblum JR. p53 expression in low grade dysplasia in Barrett's esophagus: correlation with interobserver agreement and disease progression. Am J Gastroenterol. 2002;97(10):2508–13. https://doi.org/10.1111/j.1572-0241.2002.06032.x.

79. Kaye PV, Haider SA, James PD, Soomro I, Catton J, Parsons SL, Ragunath K, Ilyas M. Novel staining pattern of p53 in Barrett's dysplasia – the absent pattern. Histopathology. 2010;57(6):933–5. https://doi.org/10.1111/j.1365-2559.2010.03715.x.

80. Khan S, Do KA, Kuhnert P, Pillay SP, Papadimos D, Conrad R, Jass JR. Diagnostic value of p53 immunohistochemistry in Barrett's esophagus: an endoscopic study. Pathology. 1998;30(2):136–40.

81. Murray L, Sedo A, Scott M, McManus D, Sloan JM, Hardie LJ, Forman D, Wild CP. TP53 and progression from Barrett's metaplasia to oesophageal adenocarcinoma in a UK population cohort. Gut. 2006;55(10):1390–7. https://doi.org/10.1136/gut.2005.083295.

82. Bani-Hani K, Martin IG, Hardie LJ, Mapstone N, Briggs JA, Forman D, Wild CP. Prospective study of cyclin D1 overexpression in Barrett's esophagus: association with increased risk of adenocarcinoma. J Natl Cancer Inst. 2000;92(16):1316–21.

83. Sikkema M, Kerkhof M, Steyerberg EW, Kusters JG, van Strien PM, Looman CW, van Dekken H, Siersema PD, Kuipers EJ. Aneuploidy and overexpression of Ki67 and p53 as markers for neoplastic progression in Barrett's esophagus: a case-control study. Am J Gastroenterol. 2009;104(11):2673–80. https://doi.org/10.1038/ajg.2009.437.

84. Shaheen NJ, Falk GW, Iyer PG, Gerson LB, American College of G. ACG clinical guideline: diagnosis and management of Barrett's esophagus. Am J Gastroenterol. 2016;111(1):30–50.; quiz 51. https://doi.org/10.1038/ajg.2015.322.

85. Sturm MB, Wang TD. Emerging optical methods for surveillance of Barrett's oesophagus. Gut. 2015;64(11):1816–23. https://doi.org/10.1136/gutjnl-2013-306706.

86. Coletta M, Sami SS, Nachiappan A, Fraquelli M, Casazza G, Ragunath K. Acetic acid chromoendoscopy for the diagnosis of early neoplasia and specialized intestinal metaplasia in Barrett's esophagus: a meta-analysis. Gastrointest Endosc. 2016;83(1):57–67e51. https://doi.org/10.1016/j.gie.2015.07.023.

87. Sharma P, Hawes RH, Bansal A, Gupta N, Curvers W, Rastogi A, Singh M, Hall M, Mathur SC, Wani SB, Hoffman B, Gaddam S, Fockens P, Bergman JJ. Standard endoscopy with random biopsies versus narrow band imaging targeted biopsies in Barrett's oesophagus: a prospective, international, randomised controlled trial. Gut. 2013;62(1):15–21. https://doi.org/10.1136/gutjnl-2011-300962.

88. Qumseya BJ, Wang H, Badie N, Uzomba RN, Parasa S, White DL, Wolfsen H, Sharma P, Wallace MB. Advanced imaging technologies increase detection of dysplasia and neoplasia in patients with Barrett's esophagus: a meta-analysis and systematic review. Clin Gastroenterol Hepatol. 2013;11(12):1562–70e1561-1562. https://doi.org/10.1016/j.cgh.2013.06.017.

89. Boerwinkel DF, Holz JA, Aalders MC, Visser M, Meijer SL, Van Berge Henegouwen MI, Weusten BL, Bergman JJ. Third-generation autofluorescence endoscopy for the detection of early neoplasia in Barrett's esophagus: a pilot study. Dis Esophagus. 2014;27(3):276–84. https://doi.org/10.1111/dote.12094.

90. Boerwinkel DF, Holz JA, Kara MA, Meijer SL, Wallace MB, Wong Kee Song LM, Ragunath K, Wolfsen HC, Iyer PG, Wang KK, Weusten BL, Aalders MC, Curvers WL, Bergman JJ. Effects of autofluorescence imaging on detection and treatment of early neoplasia in patients with Barrett's esophagus. Clin Gastroenterol Hepatol. 2014;12(5):774–81. https://doi.org/10.1016/j.cgh.2013.10.013.

91. Curvers WL, Alvarez Herrero L, Wallace MB, Wong Kee Song LM, Ragunath K, Wolfsen HC, Prasad GA, Wang KK, Subramanian V, Weusten BL, Ten Kate FJ, Bergman JJ. Endoscopic tri-modal imaging is more effective than standard endoscopy in identifying early-stage neoplasia in Barrett's esophagus. Gastroenterology. 2010;139(4):1106–14. https://doi.org/10.1053/j.gastro.2010.06.045.

92. Curvers WL, van Vilsteren FG, Baak LC, Bohmer C, Mallant-Hent RC, Naber AH, van Oijen A, Ponsioen CY, Scholten P, Schenk E, Schoon E, Seldenrijk CA, Meijer GA, ten Kate FJ, Bergman JJ. Endoscopic trimodal imaging versus standard video endoscopy for detection of early Barrett's neoplasia: a multicenter, randomized, crossover study in general practice. Gastrointest Endosc. 2011;73(2):195–203. https://doi.org/10.1016/j.gie.2010.10.014.

93. Li M, Anastassiades CP, Joshi B, Komarck CM, Piraka C, Elmunzer BJ, Turgeon DK, Johnson TD, Appelman H, Beer DG, Wang TD. Affinity peptide for targeted detection of dysplasia in Barrett's esophagus. Gastroenterology. 2010;139(5):1472–80. https://doi.org/10.1053/j.gastro.2010.07.007.

94. Bird-Lieberman EL, Neves AA, Lao-Sirieix P, O'Donovan M, Novelli M, Lovat LB, Eng WS, Mahal LK, Brindle KM, Fitzgerald RC. Molecular imaging using fluorescent lectins permits rapid endoscopic identification of dysplasia in Barrett's esophagus. Nat Med. 2012;18(2):315–21. https://doi.org/10.1038/nm.2616.

95. Sturm MB, Joshi BP, Lu S, Piraka C, Khondee S, Elmunzer BJ, Kwon RS, Beer DG, Appelman HD, Turgeon DK, Wang TD. Targeted imaging of esophageal neoplasia with a

fluorescently labeled peptide: first-in-human results. Sci Transl Med. 2013;5(184):184ra161. https://doi.org/10.1126/scitranslmed.3004733.

96. Neves AA, Di Pietro M, O'Donovan M, Waterhouse DJ, Bohndiek SE, Brindle KM, Fitzgerald RC. Detection of early neoplasia in Barrett's esophagus using lectin-based near-infrared imaging: an ex vivo study on human tissue. Endoscopy. 2018;50(6):618–25. https://doi.org/10.1055/s-0043-124080.

97. Kohli DR, Schubert ML, Zfass AM, Shah TU. Performance characteristics of optical coherence tomography in assessment of Barrett's esophagus and esophageal cancer: systematic review. Dis Esophagus. 2017;30(11):1–8. https://doi.org/10.1093/dote/dox049.

98. Wolfsen HC, Sharma P, Wallace MB, Leggett C, Tearney G, Wang KK. Safety and feasibility of volumetric laser endomicroscopy in patients with Barrett's esophagus (with videos). Gastrointest Endosc. 2015;82(4):631–40. https://doi.org/10.1016/j.gie.2015.03.1968.

99. Alshelleh M, Inamdar S, McKinley M, Stewart M, Novak JS, Greenberg RE, Sultan K, Devito B, Cheung M, Cerulli MA, Miller LS, Sejpal DV, Vegesna AK, Trindade AJ. Incremental yield of dysplasia detection in Barrett's esophagus using volumetric laser endomicroscopy with and without laser marking compared with a standardized random biopsy protocol. Gastrointest Endosc. 2018;88(1):35–42. https://doi.org/10.1016/j.gie.2018.01.032.

100. Leggett CL, Gorospe EC, Chan DK, Muppa P, Owens V, Smyrk TC, Anderson M, Lutzke LS, Tearney G, Wang KK. Comparative diagnostic performance of volumetric laser endomicroscopy and confocal laser endomicroscopy in the detection of dysplasia associated with Barrett's esophagus. Gastrointest Endosc. 2016;83(5):880–888.e2. https://doi.org/10.1016/j.gie.2015.08.050.

101. Xiong YQ, Ma SJ, Zhou JH, Zhong XS, Chen Q. A meta-analysis of confocal laser endomicroscopy for the detection of neoplasia in patients with Barrett's esophagus. J Gastroenterol Hepatol. 2016;31(6):1102–10. https://doi.org/10.1111/jgh.13267.

102. Peery AF, Hoppo T, Garman KS, Dellon ES, Daugherty N, Bream S, Sanz AF, Davison J, Spacek M, Connors D, Faulx AL, Chak A, Luketich JD, Shaheen NJ, Jobe BA, Barrett's Esophagus Risk C. Feasibility, safety, acceptability, and yield of office-based, screening transnasal esophagoscopy (with video). Gastrointest Endosc. 2012;75(5):945–53e942. https://doi.org/10.1016/j.gie.2012.01.021.

103. Shariff MK, Varghese S, O'Donovan M, Abdullahi Z, Liu X, Fitzgerald RC, di Pietro M. Pilot randomized crossover study comparing the efficacy of transnasal disposable endosheath with standard endoscopy to detect Barrett's esophagus. Endoscopy. 2016;48(2):110–6. https://doi.org/10.1055/s-0034-1393310.

104. Ross-Innes CS, Debiram-Beecham I, O'Donovan M, Walker E, Varghese S, Lao-Sirieix P, Lovat L, Griffin M, Ragunath K, Haidry R, Sami SS, Kaye P, Novelli M, Disep B, Ostler R, Aigret B, North BV, Bhandari P, Haycock A, Morris D, Attwood S, Dhar A, Rees C, Rutter MD, Sasieni PD, Fitzgerald RC, Group BS. Evaluation of a minimally invasive cell sampling device coupled with assessment of trefoil factor 3 expression for diagnosing Barrett's esophagus: a multi-center case-control study. PLoS Med. 2015;12(1):e1001780. https://doi.org/10.1371/journal.pmed.1001780.

105. Heberle CR, Omidvari AH, Ali A, Kroep S, Kong CY, Inadomi JM, Rubenstein JH, Tramontano AC, Dowling EC, Hazelton WD, Luebeck EG, Lansdorp-Vogelaar I, Hur C. Cost effectiveness of screening patients with gastroesophageal reflux disease for Barrett's esophagus with a minimally invasive cell sampling device. Clin Gastroenterol Hepatol. 2017;15(9):1397–404e1397. https://doi.org/10.1016/j.cgh.2017.02.017.

106. Ross-Innes CS, Chettouh H, Achilleos A, Galeano-Dalmau N, Debiram-Beecham I, MacRae S, Fessas P, Walker E, Varghese S, Evan T, Lao-Sirieix PS, O'Donovan M, Malhotra S, Novelli M, Disep B, Kaye PV, Lovat LB, Haidry R, Griffin M, Ragunath K, Bhandari P, Haycock A, Morris D, Attwood S, Dhar A, Rees C, Rutter MD, Ostler R, Aigret B, Sasieni PD, Fitzgerald RC, group Bs. Risk stratification of Barrett's oesophagus using a non-endoscopic sampling method coupled with a biomarker panel: a cohort study. Lancet Gastroenterol Hepatol. 2017;2(1):23–31. https://doi.org/10.1016/S2468-1253(16)30118-2.

107. Chettouh H, Mowforth O, Galeano-Dalmau N, Bezawada N, Ross-Innes C, MacRae S, Debiram-Beecham I, O'Donovan M, Fitzgerald RC. Methylation panel is a diagnostic biomarker for Barrett's oesophagus in endoscopic biopsies and non-endoscopic cytology specimens. Gut. 2018;67(11):1942–9. https://doi.org/10.1136/gutjnl-2017-314026.

108. Moinova HR, LaFramboise T, Lutterbaugh JD, Chandar AK, Dumot J, Faulx A, Brock W, De la Cruz CO, Guda K, Barnholtz-Sloan JS, Iyer PG, Canto MI, Wang JS, Shaheen NJ, Thota PN, Willis JE, Chak A, Markowitz SD. Identifying DNA methylation biomarkers for non-endoscopic detection of Barrett's esophagus. Sci Transl Med. 2018;10(424):eaao5848. https://doi.org/10.1126/scitranslmed.aao5848.

109. Matsuzaki J, Suzuki H. Circulating microRNAs as potential biomarkers to detect transformation of Barrett's oesophagus to oesophageal adenocarcinoma. BMJ Open Gastroenterol. 2017;4(1):e000160. https://doi.org/10.1136/bmjgast-2017-000160.

110. Buas MF, Gu H, Djukovic D, Zhu J, Onstad L, Reid BJ, Raftery D, Vaughan TL. Candidate serum metabolite biomarkers for differentiating gastroesophageal reflux disease, Barrett's esophagus, and high-grade dysplasia/esophageal adenocarcinoma. Metabolomics. 2017;13(3):23. https://doi.org/10.1007/s11306-016-1154-y.

111. Kelly P, Paulin F, Lamont D, Baker L, Clearly S, Exon D, Thompson A. Pre-treatment plasma proteomic markers associated with survival in oesophageal cancer. Br J Cancer. 2012;106(5):955–61. https://doi.org/10.1038/bjc.2012.15.

112. Chiam K, Wang T, Watson DI, Mayne GC, Irvine TS, Bright T, Smith L, White IA, Bowen JM, Keefe D, Thompson SK, Jones ME, Hussey DJ. Circulating serum Exosomal miRNAs as potential biomarkers for Esophageal adenocarcinoma. J Gastrointest Surg. 2015;19(7):1208–15. https://doi.org/10.1007/s11605-015-2829-9.

113. Paul S, Altorki N. Outcomes in the management of esophageal cancer. J Surg Oncol. 2014;110(5):599–610. https://doi.org/10.1002/jso.23759.

114. Gerson LB, Boparai V, Ullah N, Triadafilopoulos G. Oesophageal and gastric pH profiles in patients with gastro-oesophageal reflux disease and Barrett's oesophagus treated with proton pump inhibitors. Aliment Pharmacol Ther. 2004;20(6):637–43. https://doi.org/10.1111/j.1365-2036.2004.02127.x.

115. Kastelein F, Spaander MC, Steyerberg EW, Biermann K, Valkhoff VE, Kuipers EJ, Bruno MJ, ProBar Study G. Proton pump inhibitors reduce the risk of neoplastic progression in patients with Barrett's esophagus. Clin Gastroenterol Hepatol. 2013;11(4):382–8. https://doi.org/10.1016/j.cgh.2012.11.014.

116. Hvid-Jensen F, Pedersen L, Funch-Jensen P, Drewes AM. Proton pump inhibitor use may not prevent high-grade dysplasia and oesophageal adenocarcinoma in Barrett's oesophagus: a nationwide study of 9883 patients. Aliment Pharmacol Ther. 2014;39(9):984–91. https://doi.org/10.1111/apt.12693.

117. Roorda AK, Marcus SN, Triadafilopoulos G. Early experience with radiofrequency energy ablation therapy for Barrett's esophagus with and without dysplasia. Dis Esophagus. 2007;20(6):516–22.

118. Akiyama J, Marcus SN, Triadafilopoulos G. Effective intra-esophageal acid control is associated with improved radiofrequency ablation outcomes in Barrett's esophagus. Dig Dis Sci. 2012;57(10):2625–32. https://doi.org/10.1007/s10620-012-2313-2.

119. Jovov B, Shaheen NJ, Orlando GS, Djukic Z, Orlando RC. Defective barrier function in neosquamous epithelium. Am J Gastroenterol. 2013;108(3):386–91. https://doi.org/10.1038/ajg.2012.440.

120. Kastelein F, Spaander MC, Biermann K, Steyerberg EW, Kuipers EJ, Bruno MJ, Probar-study G. Nonsteroidal anti-inflammatory drugs and statins have chemopreventative effects in patients with Barrett's esophagus. Gastroenterology. 2011;141(6):2000–8;. quiz e2013-2004. https://doi.org/10.1053/j.gastro.2011.08.036.

121. Nguyen DM, Richardson P, El-Serag HB. Medications (NSAIDs, statins, proton pump inhibitors) and the risk of esophageal adenocarcinoma in patients with Barrett's esophagus. Gastroenterology. 2010;138(7):2260–6. https://doi.org/10.1053/j.gastro.2010.02.045.

122. Vaughan TL, Dong LM, Blount PL, Ayub K, Odze RD, Sanchez CA, Rabinovitch PS, Reid BJ. Non-steroidal anti-inflammatory drugs and risk of neoplastic progression in Barrett's oesophagus: a prospective study. Lancet Oncol. 2005;6(12):945–52.
123. Khalaf N, Nguyen T, Ramsey D, El-Serag HB. Nonsteroidal anti-inflammatory drugs and the Risk of Barrett's Esophagus. Clin Gastroenterol Hepatol. 2014;12(11):1832–9.e6. https://doi.org/10.1016/j.cgh.2014.04.027.
124. Spechler SJ, Lee E, Ahnen D, Goyal RK, Hirano I, Ramirez F, Raufman JP, Sampliner R, Schnell T, Sontag S, Vlahcevic ZR, Young R, Williford W. Long-term outcome of medical and surgical therapies for gastroesophageal reflux disease: follow-up of a randomized controlled trial. JAMA. 2001;285(18):2331–8.
125. Tran T, Spechler SJ, Richardson P, El-Serag HB. Fundoplication and the risk of esophageal cancer in gastroesophageal reflux disease: a veterans affairs cohort study. Am J Gastroenterol. 2005;100(5):1002–8.
126. Dunbar KB, Spechler SJ. The risk of lymph-node metastases in patients with high-grade dysplasia or intramucosal carcinoma in Barrett's esophagus: a systematic review. Am J Gastroenterol. 2012;107(6):850–62. quiz 863. https://doi.org/10.1038/ajg.2012.78.
127. Yang D, Zou F, Xiong S, Forde JJ, Wang Y, Draganov PV. Endoscopic submucosal dissection for early Barrett's neoplasia: a meta-analysis. Gastrointest Endosc. 2018;87(6):1383–93. https://doi.org/10.1016/j.gie.2017.09.038.
128. Konda VJ, Gonzalez Haba Ruiz M, Koons A, Hart J, Xiao SY, Siddiqui UD, Ferguson MK, Posner M, Patti MG, Waxman I. Complete endoscopic mucosal resection is effective and durable treatment for Barrett's-associated Neoplasia. Clin Gastroenterol Hepatol. 2014;12(12):2002–10.e1–2. https://doi.org/10.1016/j.cgh.2014.04.010.
129. Chung A, Bourke MJ, Hourigan LF, Lim G, Moss A, Williams SJ, McLeod D, Fanning S, Kariyawasam V, Byth K. Complete Barrett's excision by stepwise endoscopic resection in short-segment disease: long term outcomes and predictors of stricture. Endoscopy. 2011;43(12):1025–32. https://doi.org/10.1055/s-0030-1257049.
130. Desai M, Saligram S, Gupta N, Vennalaganti P, Bansal A, Choudhary A, Vennelaganti S, He J, Titi M, Maselli R, Qumseya B, Olyaee M, Waxman I, Repici A, Hassan C, Sharma P. Efficacy and safety outcomes of multimodal endoscopic eradication therapy in Barrett's esophagus-related neoplasia: a systematic review and pooled analysis. Gastrointest Endosc. 2017;85(3):482–95e484. https://doi.org/10.1016/j.gie.2016.09.022.
131. Orman ES, Li N, Shaheen NJ. Efficacy and durability of radiofrequency ablation for Barrett's Esophagus: systematic review and meta-analysis. Clin Gastroenterol Hepatol. 2013;11(10):1245–55. https://doi.org/10.1016/j.cgh.2013.03.039.
132. Shaheen NJ, Overholt BF, Sampliner RE, Wolfsen HC, Wang KK, Fleischer DE, Sharma VK, Eisen GM, Fennerty MB, Hunter JG, Bronner MP, Goldblum JR, Bennett AE, Mashimo H, Rothstein RI, Gordon SR, Edmundowicz SA, Madanick RD, Peery AF, Muthusamy VR, Chang KJ, Kimmey MB, Spechler SJ, Siddiqui AA, Souza RF, Infantolino A, Dumot JA, Falk GW, Galanko JA, Jobe BA, Hawes RH, Hoffman BJ, Sharma P, Chak A, Lightdale CJ. Durability of radiofrequency ablation in Barrett's esophagus with dysplasia. Gastroenterology. 2011;141(2):460–8. https://doi.org/10.1053/j.gastro.2011.04.061.
133. Cotton CC, Wolf WA, Overholt BF, Li N, Lightdale CJ, Wolfsen HC, Pasricha S, Wang KK, Shaheen NJ, Group AIMDT. Late recurrence of Barrett's Esophagus after complete eradication of intestinal metaplasia is rare: final report from ablation in intestinal metaplasia containing dysplasia trial. Gastroenterology. 2017;153(3):681–8e682. https://doi.org/10.1053/j.gastro.2017.05.044.
134. Qumseya BJ, Wani S, Desai M, Qumseya A, Bain P, Sharma P, Wolfsen H. Adverse events after radiofrequency ablation in patients with Barrett's esophagus: a systematic review and meta-analysis. Clin Gastroenterol Hepatol. 2016;14(8):1086–95e1086. https://doi.org/10.1016/j.cgh.2016.04.001.
135. Das KK, Falk GW. Long-term outcomes for cryotherapy in Barrett's esophagus with high-grade dysplasia: just cracking the ice. Gastrointest Endosc. 2017;86(4):633–5. https://doi.org/10.1016/j.gie.2017.03.1540.

136. Ramay FH, Cui Q, Greenwald BD. Outcomes after liquid nitrogen spray cryotherapy in Barrett's esophagus-associated high-grade dysplasia and intramucosal adenocarcinoma: 5-year follow-up. Gastrointest Endosc. 2017;86(4):626–32. https://doi.org/10.1016/j.gie.2017.02.006.
137. Phoa KN, van Vilsteren FG, Weusten BL, Bisschops R, Schoon EJ, Ragunath K, Fullarton G, Di Pietro M, Ravi N, Visser M, Offerhaus GJ, Seldenrijk CA, Meijer SL, ten Kate FJ, Tijssen JG, Bergman JJ. Radiofrequency ablation vs endoscopic surveillance for patients with Barrett esophagus and low-grade dysplasia: a randomized clinical trial. JAMA. 2014;311(12):1209–17. https://doi.org/10.1001/jama.2014.2511.
138. Duits LC, van der Wel MJ, Cotton CC, Phoa KN, Ten Kate FJW, Seldenrijk CA, Offerhaus GJA, Visser M, Meijer SL, Mallant-Hent RC, Krishnadath KK, Pouw RE, Tijssen JGP, Shaheen NJ, Bergman J. Patients with Barrett's esophagus and confirmed persistent low-grade dysplasia are at increased risk for progression to neoplasia. Gastroenterology. 2017;152(5):993–1001e1001. https://doi.org/10.1053/j.gastro.2016.12.008.
139. Hur C, Choi SE, Rubenstein JH, Kong CY, Nishioka NS, Provenzale DT, Inadomi JM. The cost effectiveness of radiofrequency ablation for Barrett's esophagus. Gastroenterology. 2012;143(3):567–75. https://doi.org/10.1053/j.gastro.2012.05.010.
140. Phoa KN, Rosmolen WD, Weusten B, Bisschops R, Schoon EJ, Das S, Ragunath K, Fullarton G, DiPietro M, Ravi N, Tijssen JGP, Dijkgraaf MGW, Bergman J, investigators S. The cost-effectiveness of radiofrequency ablation for Barrett's esophagus with low-grade dysplasia: results from a randomized controlled trial (SURF trial). Gastrointest Endosc. 2017;86(1):120–9e122. https://doi.org/10.1016/j.gie.2016.12.001.
141. Gordon LG, Mayne GC, Hirst NG, Bright T, Whiteman DC, Australian Cancer Study Clinical Follow-Up S, Watson DI. Cost-effectiveness of endoscopic surveillance of non-dysplastic Barrett's esophagus. Gastrointest Endosc. 2014;79(2):242–256.e246. https://doi.org/10.1016/j.gie.2013.07.046.
142. Guthikonda A, Cotton CC, Madanick RD, Spacek MB, Moist SE, Ferrell K, Dellon ES, Shaheen NJ. Clinical outcomes following recurrence of intestinal metaplasia after successful treatment of Barrett's esophagus with radiofrequency ablation. Am J Gastroenterol. 2017;112(1):87–94. https://doi.org/10.1038/ajg.2016.451.
143. Corley DA, Mehtani K, Quesenberry C, Zhao W, de Boer J, Weiss NS. Impact of endoscopic surveillance on mortality from Barrett's esophagus-associated esophageal adenocarcinomas. Gastroenterology. 2013;145(2):312–319.e311. https://doi.org/10.1053/j.gastro.2013.05.004.
144. Falk GW, Ours TM, Richter JE. Practice patterns for surveillance of Barrett's esophagus in the United States. Gastrointest Endosc. 2000;52(2):197–203.

Chemoprevention of Esophageal Cancer

5

Elizabeth G. Ratcliffe, Mohamed Shibeika,
Andrew D. Higham, and Janusz A. Jankowski

An emerging focus over the last few decades has been into cancer chemoprevention, using supplements or medication to avoid or delay the potential medical and psychological catastrophe of a cancer diagnosis. The idea is to take a safe, economically viable, well-tolerated, and well-understood medication which, given to a group in the population, could prevent carcinoma before invasion or at least delay the premalignant process to a later time point.

Esophageal cancer carries a huge burden of morbidity and mortality to patients around the world, with the UK having one of the worst rates of adenocarcinoma [1]. At diagnosis the disease is often at an advanced stage, surgery is extremely invasive, chemotherapy and radiotherapy treatments are aggressive, and endoscopic treatments limited to tertiary centers in areas of higher socioeconomic strength. Chemoprevention is an exciting prospect for this condition given the potential impact on patients and the potential relief to healthcare systems as populations age. Chemoprevention has been a key focus in other areas of medicine and has been extremely effective in reducing the burden of disease in cardiology, and many medications used in large populations for this purpose hold promise in cancer chemoprevention as will be described. The challenge going forward is narrowing down which

E. G. Ratcliffe (✉)
Wrightington Wigan and Leigh NHS Foundation Trust, Leigh, UK

M. Shibeika
East Lancashire Hospitals NHS Trust, Blackburn, UK

A. D. Higham
University Hospitals of Morecambe Bay NHS Foundation Trust, Lancaster, UK

J. A. Jankowski (✉)
Sherwood Forest Hospitals NHS Trust, Sutton in Ashfield, UK

National Institute for Health and Care Excellence, London, UK

University of Liverpool, Liverpool, UK
e-mail: JJankowski@rcsi.ie

© Springer Nature Switzerland AG 2020
N. F. Saba, B. F. El-Rayes (eds.), *Esophageal Cancer*,
https://doi.org/10.1007/978-3-030-29832-6_5

113

agents can be attractive to large populations of essentially healthy patients in the hope of preventing malignancy. Described below is an overview of the evidence for a few of the key areas of interest for esophageal chemoprevention, with an exploration of the associated side effects and some considerations for the future.

Proton Pump Inhibitors

Acid exposure plays an important role in the initiation of Barrett's esophagus (BE) and its progression to esophageal adenocarcinoma; therefore, proton pump inhibitors (PPIs) have been historically used as the backbone of medical treatment for the symptoms of gastroesophageal reflux disease (GERD). Several studies have investigated the role of proton pump inhibitors in the prevention of progression from BE to esophageal adenocarcinoma. In a large prospective cohort study, 75% of patients known to have BE and taking PPI had a reduction in the risk of neoplastic progression, independent of age, gender, BE length, esophagitis, histology, and use of other medications [2].

Other studies have shown that despite PPI use, 20% of BE patients experience pathological reflux, hence none of the PPIs have been proven to completely prevent neoplastic progression [3]. Maintenance of normal epithelial differentiation and cell proliferation is an important goal in cancer chemoprevention. Bearing in mind that intermittent esophageal acid exposure enhances cell proliferation, which is well correlated with the development of dysplasia, this may explain why BE patients remain at a certain risk for neoplastic progression during PPI use.

Several studies have hypothesized that effective intra-esophageal acid suppression may be beneficial in the long-term treatment of BE patients, due to the theoretical and logical concept that acid suppression should lead to well-differentiated BE epithelia while also minimizing cell proliferation, and thus should reduce the likelihood of progression to dysplasia or adenocarcinoma [4]. A systematic review that pooled the results of several trials investigating chemoprevention of esophageal adenocarcinoma reported mixed results [5]; some studies reported that PPIs cause regression of BE [6, 7], while others failed to reach statistical significance [8, 9]. These discrepancies in the literature at that stage resulted mainly from a lack of standardized method for measuring the length and distribution of Barrett's [10]. A lack of correlation between the acid suppression and symptom relief might also mean higher doses of PPI are required to achieve therapeutic acid suppression [11]. This concept has been investigated in a study which reported that standard doses of PPIs administered to BE patients could relieve symptoms of GERD after a 6-month period, but many participants continued to have pathological acid reflux as measured by 24-h pH monitoring, and remained, therefore, at risk of developing adenocarcinoma [4].

Peters et al. performed a randomized double-blind study, in which participants were given 40 mg omeprazole twice a day and underwent pH esophageal monitoring to confirm adequate acid suppression. After 2 years, there was a statistically significant regression of BE [12]. There is a paucity of data investigating the cellular effects of PPI treatment. Absolute suppression of acid reflux has been shown to reduce cell proliferation [4, 13] and increase expression of the cyclin-dependent kinase inhibitors p16 and p21 [14]. This therefore suggests that aggressive acid suppression may influence the alterations in cell cycle control that occur during carcinogenesis; reducing risk and therefore also supporting the findings reported by Peters et al. [12].

Whether aggressive acid-lowering treatment can modify the risk of cancer development is still unconfirmed due to a lack of robust clinical trials investigating this question. It may be that transformation of Barrett's to dysplasia is the most important step that should be focused upon rather than regression of Barrett's epithelium. A prospective analysis of over 200 patients over a 20-year period has shown that PPIs significantly reduced risk of dysplasia in Barrett's esophagus [15]. This study, unfortunately, remains in relative isolation; however, preliminary data is emerging from the Aspect trial, which is the largest randomized controlled trial looking at aspirin plus high or low dose omeprazole. Data presented at the ASCO annual conference at the time of writing showed high dose (40 mg BD) esomeprazole, in combination with aspirin, provided a significant effect on all-cause mortality in Barrett's patients versus 20 mg once daily if taken for at least 7 years. These data are encouraging but it is important to note that the study enrolled Barrett's confirmed cases and so this does not yet represent a course for all GERD cases, pending further information from the full dataset.

NSAIDs/Aspirin

Aspirin, a key agent in cardiovascular chemoprevention, has already been found to have a significant role in the prevention of colorectal cancer and is recommended for use in 50–59-year-olds with a significant cardiovascular risk profile (10% or more over 10 years) by the US Preventative Services Task Force [16]. Through evidence initially gathered in large cohort studies [17–19], this relationship was demonstrated in hereditary colorectal cancer patients in randomized controlled trials through the CAPP trial series [20]. The large cohorts also showed significant links with esophageal cancer and extensive work to define the biochemical process involved has been undertaken.

There are four main theories of why aspirin works in chemoprevention. Firstly, inflammation plays a significant role in the cancers that aspirin is considered to prevent and on one level it inhibits the release of inflammatory cytokines by immune cells, reducing downstream cellular changes, particularly through limiting release of TNF, INFy, WNT5A, IL-1, IL-6, and CXCL1 [21–23]. Platelet-mediated effects have also been described, linking reduced thromboxane production from platelets preventing cell proliferation that occurs as a reaction to neoplastic disruption to tissues [17].

However, the main causative pathways in esophageal cancer that appear to relate to aspirin and NSAIDs are the COX mediated pathways and the subsequent effects on β-catenin [24] (Fig. 5.1). Cell migration and proliferation are stimulated by the shift of β-catenin to the nucleus of the cell where it causes a gene expression sequence, hence it has pro-neoplastic effects at higher concentrations in the cell [21]. β-catenin is usually ubiquitylated after being flagged by T41 and S45 amino

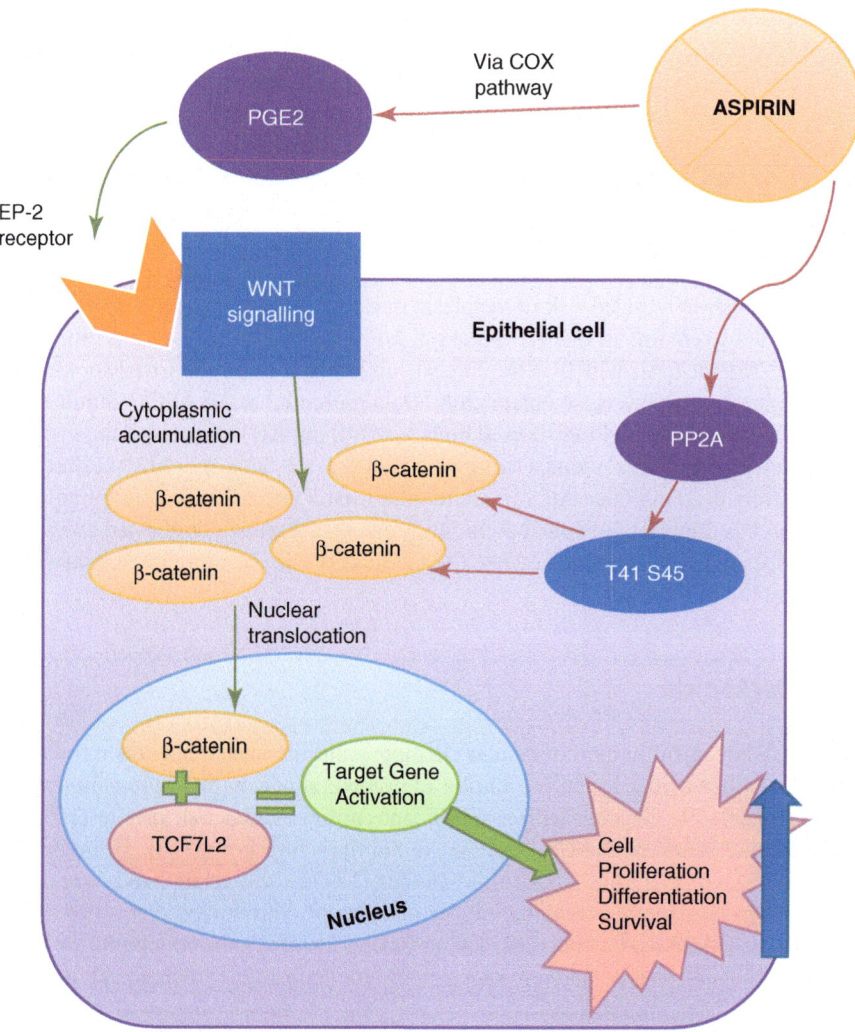

Fig. 5.1 A diagram showing the β-catenin pathways hypothesized to be affected by aspirin, modified from a diagram by Drew et al. in the 2016 paper "Aspirin and colorectal cancer: the promise of precision chemoprevention" Nature Reviews [21]. Green arrows represent stimulation pathways and red arrows inhibitory. Inhibiting the stabilization of β-catenin through inactivation of protein phosphatase 2A (PP2A)-promoting ubiquitylation; through inhibiting COX-2-mediated production of prostanoids by preventing COX-2 from converting arachidonic acid to prostaglandin E2 (PGE2) which in turn can stimulate the WNT signaling pathway

acid residues; however, in the context of aspirin this process is emphasized by inactivation of protein phosphatase 2A which is responsible for breaking down T41 and S45 [21]. PGE2 produced via the COX pathway stimulates the migration of β-catenin via stimulation of the EP-2 receptors in the epithelial cell and WNT-signaling.

In the COX pathway, arachidonic acid is metabolized through COX enzymes, resulting in the production of prostaglandins such as PGE2, PGF2, and PGD2. NSAIDs and aspirin disturb this process through interfering with the action of the COX enzyme [25]. There are two types of COX, denoted COX1 and COX2: high levels of COX2 have been implicated in neoplastic conditions [26]. It was also noted that metaplastic cell progression through to dysplasia and adenocarcinoma was associated with increased levels of COX2 mRNA and protein [27]. Barrett's esophagus and associated esophageal adenocarcinoma patients were found to have upregulation of COX2 mRNA expression, which occurs early in the neoplastic transformation process [28]. One of the studies carried out in the US concluded that inhibition of COX2 expression through using selective COX2 inhibitor has a chemopreventive effect in Barrett's esophagus [29]. This was supported further by another study which showed that food-borne natural flavonoid quercetin and selective COX2 inhibitors hinder cell proliferation and induce apoptosis in esophageal adenocarcinoma in vitro [30].

Clinical trials are encouraging. A meta-analysis by Rothwell et al. found a significant reduction in 20-year cancer-related mortality for patients with all solid cancers and particularly GI cancers taking daily aspirin versus control [31]. Evidence from Parkin et al. suggested an all-cancer reduction of 7–10% with 10 years of regular aspirin use in 50–65-year-olds, with most clear associations in GI cancers with esophageal, colorectal and gastric cancers all reduced by up to one-third [32]. A large population-based case-control study of UK and Netherlands populations by Masclee et al. looked at esophageal adenocarcinoma risk in Barrett's patients with concurrent use of PPI, NSAIDs, aspirin or statins and found no significantly significant associations [33]. However, a large case control study derived from Scotland-based general practice demonstrated decreased risk of upper aerodigestive tract cancer with usage of aspirin and not COX2 inhibitor [34]. Systematic review and meta-analysis supported the protective association between aspirin/NSAID and esophageal adenocarcinoma with more protection in patients with greater usage and longer duration [35].

The risks associated with long-term aspirin use are well understood, namely an increased risk of bleeding in general through unselective COX inhibition, which reduces thromboxane release, thus increasing the risk of platelet-mediated bleeding, and an increased risk of GI bleeding due to COX1 inhibition causing gastric ulceration through reduced production of prostaglandin E2 [17]. This creates concerns for many investigators regarding the use of aspirin in otherwise healthy populations; however encouraging data has come from Cuzick et al. suggesting a 10-year use of daily aspirin in 100 average > 55-year-olds would only produce 0.25 more GI bleeds in women and 0.49 in men for a benefit of 2.29 fewer cancers, strokes and MI in men and 1.32 in women over a 15-year period [36]. The use of combination therapy with PPI could ameliorate this risk further and we await data from the full publication of ASPECT [37]. Hur et al. assessed patient preferences for chemopreventive agents and found 76% of Barrett's patients would be open minded to the use of aspirin in this context [38]. The familiarity of aspirin to both patients and clinicians, and its extensive use in cardiovascular disease as a secondary effect strongly support its potential, and further studies are required prior to its widespread use for esophageal cancer prevention.

Statins

Statins, as a widely used cardiovascular risk reduction treatment, were also found in large cohort studies [39] to show potential for chemoprevention of cancer. Since then, statins have been linked with prevention in many different cancer types including colorectal [40], advanced prostate [41], hepatocellular [42, 43], and esophageal [39] cancers. The proposed mechanism for this relates to how statins affect the RAF-MAPK-ERK pathway resulting in an anti-inflammatory and proapoptotic state, and also prevent problems with normal cell survival and differentiation through inhibition of HMG CoA's conversion to mevalonate [44]. Activation of the mitogen-activated protein kinase (MAPK) signaling cascade was found to play a role in neoplastic progression of Barrett's esophagus [45] which creates a possible route for neoplasia suppression by statins, although overall the mechanism is not completely understood.

A recent meta-analysis of 39 cohort and two case-control studies were conducted to evaluate the role of statins in influencing mortality in esophageal cancer patients. This concluded that using statins prediagnosis and postdiagnosis has a positive impact on survival rate [46]. One of the population-based cohort studies showed that patients on statins prior to diagnosis of esophageal cancer had 19% reduction in their mortality [47]; however another cohort study in the UK concluded that although patients with esophageal adenocarcinoma experienced reduced risk of cancer related mortality, this effect was not observed in patients with esophageal squamous cell cancer [48].

Statins, like aspirin, have a crossover effect with cardiovascular disease prevention which gives them potential for secondary morbidity reduction and they are well known to clinicians and patients, allowing for ease of counseling. Unfortunately some major concerns have been raised about possible problems with the elderly including an increased risk of cancer [49, 50]. The numbers needed to treat coming out of trials are extremely high—for esophageal cancer they have been quoted as high as 1266 and are offset dramatically by numbers needed to harm of 91 for myopathy in men (moderate-severe myopathy) and 136 for severe liver derangement [51]. The link to esophageal cancer prevention at this stage is too weak to recommend use for chemoprevention, especially in the context of the concerns raised above. Large randomized controlled trials would help to assess the value of statins for esophageal cancer chemoprevention.

Metformin

Studies have looked at the antineoplastic and chemopreventative effects of metformin in esophageal squamous cell carcinoma in vivo and in vitro. It was found that metformin selectively inhibits human esophageal squamous cancer cell growth and induces apoptosis and autophagy through inactivating Stat3 and repressing Bcl-2 [52]. Associations have also been made with metformin triggering an AMPK-related stress response reducing cancer cell survival via the AMPK/LKB1 pathway [53].

Randomization has not been utilized to study the effects of metformin in esophageal cancer. However, metformin has been shown to improve radiological and pathological response in established esophageal adenocarcinoma patients when used as a neo-adjuvant to chemoradiation; this effect is dose-dependent [54]. Though it is not yet clear from the current evidence base if we can associate metformin with esophageal cancer reduction, certainly some risk factors for all cancers—obesity, sedentary lifestyle, and diabetes—relate to the metabolic state and there is evidence to suggest a link to metformin reducing the rate of all cancers by 31% in diabetic patients in long-term use [55]. GI upset in many patients can make metformin prohibitive in healthy patients and the evidence is not strong enough here either; there is possible stronger evidence in hepatocellular prevention [56], 31% overall risk reduction of all cancers and colonic adenoma rates [57] ($p = 0.034$, risk ratio 0·67 [95% CI 0·47–0·97]) in nondiabetic populations also. Increasing need for this medication in the general population due to rising obesity levels and early-onset type II diabetes may allow for more large-scale trials.

Conclusions

Chemoprevention is an extremely exciting prospect overall; however, moving this approach into widespread use is still a long way away (Table 5.1). There is strong evidence for the use of chemoprevention in a few cancer areas—aspirin for colorectal cancer and tamoxifen for estrogen-receptor positive breast cancers, and aspirin is recommended in high-risk groups [16, 58, 59]. If it would be possible to slow or halt the progression of Barrett's to dysplasia using a simple, cheap, readily available medication, combining this with improving our ability to perform targeted endoscopic assessment and build on the surveillance process could improve the

Table 5.1 Overview of agents discussed

Agent	Hypothesized pathway	Cancers prevented	Risks
PPI	Reduce inflammatory result of direct acid reaction with epithelial cells	Esophageal cancer	Increased gastric cancer in long-term cohort studies Electrolyte abnormalities Bone metabolism effects
Aspirin/ NSAIDS	β-Catenin, platelet mediated, COX inhibition, reducing inflammatory cytokines	Esophageal, CRC, hereditary CRC, breast, ovarian, pancreatic, prostate, lung	GI bleeding, intracranial hemorrhage, all bleeding
Statins	Proapotic via RAF-MAPK-ERK reducing cell survival via inhibition of HMG CoA to mevalonate	Esophageal, CRC, HCC, gastric, prostate	Liver injury, myopathy, renal derangement, increased cancer risk in the elderly
Metformin	Proapoptotic via inactivating Stat3 and repressing Bcl-2; AMPK stress response reducing survival	All cancers pancreatic, HCC	Diarrhea, nausea, abdominal discomfort

Table 5.2 An overview of current large-scale aspirin trials

Status	Trial name	Cancer target	Agent	Phase	Participants	Masking	Randomization	Completion date	Location
Completed	A study to assess the efficacy and safety of enteric-coated acetylsalicylic acid in patients at moderate risk of cardiovascular disease (ARRIVE)	Colorectal cancer (secondary end point)	Aspirin	3	12,546	Triple	Yes	Nov-16	Bayer, 673 international centers
Completed	The seAFOod (systematic evaluation of aspirin and fish oil) polyp prevention trial	Colorectal cancer	Aspirin	N/A	755	Double	Yes	Oct-17	University of Leeds, UK centers
Active	A phase III, randomized, study of aspirin and esomeprazole chemoprevention in Barrett's metaplasia (AspECT)	Esophageal	Omeprazole, aspirin	3	2513	Open label	Yes	May-17	Oxford
Active	Aspirin in reducing events in the elderly (ASPREE)	Colorectal cancer	Aspirin	4	19,000	Quadruple	Yes	Jan-18	Berman centre for outcomes and clinical research
Recruiting	A trial looking at different doses of aspirin to prevent cancer in people who have Lynch syndrome (CaPP3)	Colorectal cancer	Aspirin	3	Aim 2000	Double	Yes	2023	CRUK and international

Recruiting	Assessment of the effect of a daily chemoprevention by low-dose aspirin of new or recurrent colorectal adenomas in patients with lynch syndrome	Colorectal cancer	Aspirin	3	Aim 852	Quadruple	Yes	Dec-24	Hospital Avicenne France
Recruiting	Add-aspirin: A trial assessing the effects of aspirin on disease recurrence and survival after primary therapy in common nonmetastatic solid tumors	Breast, gastric, colorectal, esophageal, prostate	Aspirin	3	11,000	Triple	Yes	Oct-26	University College London
Recruiting	ASPirin intervention for the REDuction of colorectal cancer risk (ASPiRED)	Colorectal cancer	Aspirin	N/a	Aim 180	Double	Yes	Jul-28	Massachusetts General Hospital

incidence rates of esophageal cancer. The concern has been raised that preventing a curable malignancy by pushing the time to progression forward may result in patients being diagnosed too late for alternative modalities such as surgery, especially as many develop esophageal cancer in older age. Although some data support the concept of widespread aspirin or PPI chemoprevention, before the evidence is stronger, we would risk delaying a few cases while placing a healthy population at risk of adverse drug reactions. Further studies will help stratify these difficult decisions (Table 5.2). Genetic profiling trials are also underway looking for gene targets to risk stratify patients into chemoprevention programs. Certainly, until these genes can be defined, demographic risk stratification is likely to shape chemoprevention practice for esophageal cancer, as already occurs in cardiology.

Acknowledgement
Funding: Cancer Research UK, Royal College of Surgeons Ireland.
Declaration of Interests: Prof. Jankowski is the Chief Investigator for the Aspect trial.

References

1. Pennathur A, Gibson MK, Jobe BA, Luketich JD. Oesophageal carcinoma. Lancet. 2013;381:400–12. https://doi.org/10.1016/S0140-6736(12)60643-6.
2. Kastelein F, Spaander MC, Steyerberg EW, et al. Proton pump inhibitors reduce the risk of neoplastic progression in patients with Barrett's esophagus. Clin Gastroenterol Hepatol. 2013;11(4):382–8. https://doi.org/10.1016/j.cgh.2012.11.014.
3. Spechler SJ, Lee E, Ahnen D, et al. Long-term outcome of medical and surgical therapies for gastroesophageal reflux disease: follow-up of a randomized controlled trial. JAMA. 2001;285(18):2331–8. https://doi.org/10.1001/JAMA.285.18.2331.
4. Ouatu-Lascar R, Fitzgerald RC, Triadafilopoulos G. Differentiation and proliferation in Barrett's esophagus and the effects of acid suppression. Gastroenterology. 1999;117(2):327–35. https://doi.org/10.1053/gast.1999.0029900327.
5. Mehta S, Johnson IT, Rhodes M. Systematic review: the chemoprevention of oesophageal adenocarcinoma. Aliment Pharmacol Ther. 2005;22(9):759–68. https://doi.org/10.1111/j.1365-2036.2005.02667.x.
6. GORE S, HEALEY CJ, SUTTON R, et al. Regression of columnar lined (Barrett's) oesophagus with continuous omeprazole therapy. Aliment Pharmacol Ther. 1993;7(6):623–8. https://doi.org/10.1111/j.1365-2036.1993.tb00143.x.
7. El-Serag HB, Aguirre T, Kuebeler M, Sampliner RE. The length of newly diagnosed Barrett's oesophagus and prior use of acid suppressive therapy. Aliment Pharmacol Ther. 2004;19(12):1255–60. https://doi.org/10.1111/j.1365-2036.2004.02006.x.
8. Sharma P, Sampliner RE, Camargo E. Normalization of esophageal pH with high-dose proton pump inhibitor therapy does not result in regression of Barrett's esophagus. Am J Gastroenterol. 1997;92(4):582–5. http://www.ncbi.nlm.nih.gov/pubmed/9128303
9. Neumann CS, Iqbal TH, Cooper BT. Long term continuous omeprazole treatment of patients with Barrett's oesophagus. Aliment Pharmacol Ther. 1995;9(4):451–4. http://www.ncbi.nlm.nih.gov/entrez/query.fcgi?cmd=Retrieve&db=PubMed&dopt=Citation&list_uids=8527623
10. Armstrong D. Review article: towards consistency in the endoscopic diagnosis of Barrett's oesophagus and columnar metaplasia. Aliment Pharmacol Ther. 2004;20(Suppl 5):40–7.; discussion 61-2. https://doi.org/10.1111/j.1365-2036.2004.02132.x.

11. Yeh RW, Gerson LB, Triadafilopoulos G. Efficacy of esomeprazole in controlling reflux symptoms, intraesophageal, and intragastric pH in patients with Barrett's esophagus. Dis Esophagus. 2003;16(3):193–8. https://doi.org/10.1046/j.1442-2050.2003.00327.x.

12. Peters FTM, Ganesh S, Kuipers EJ, et al. Endoscopic regression of Barrett's oesophagus during omeprazole treatment; a randomised double blind study. Gut. 1999;45(4):489–94. https://doi.org/10.1136/gut.45.4.489.

13. Peters FT, Ganesh S, Kuipers EJ, et al. Effect of elimination of acid reflux on epithelial cell proliferative activity of Barrett esophagus. Scand J Gastroenterol. 2000;35(12):1238–44. http://www.ncbi.nlm.nih.gov/pubmed/11199360

14. Umansky M, Yasui W, Hallak A, et al. Proton pump inhibitors reduce cell cycle abnormalities in Barrett's esophagus. Oncogene. 2001;20(55):7987–91. https://doi.org/10.1038/sj.onc.1204947.

15. El-Serag HB, Aguirre TV, Davis S, Kuebeler M, Bhattacharyya A, Sampliner RE. Proton pump inhibitors are associated with reduced incidence of dysplasia in Barrett's esophagus. Am J Gastroenterol. 2004;99(10):1877–83. https://doi.org/10.1111/j.1572-0241.2004.30228.x.

16. U.S. Preventive Services Task force. Recommendation Statement: Aspirin to prevent cardiovascular disease and cancer U.S. Preventive Services Task Force. U.S. Preventative Task Force Online. https://www.uspreventiveservicestaskforce.org/Page/Document/UpdateSummaryFinal/aspirin-to-prevent-cardiovascular-disease-and-cancer?ds=1&s=aspirin. Accessed May 6, 2018.

17. Chan AT, Arber N, Burn J, et al. Aspirin in the chemoprevention of colorectal neoplasia: an overview. Cancer Prev Res. 2012;5(2):164–78. https://doi.org/10.1158/1940-6207.CAPR-11-0391.

18. Vaughan LE, Prizment A, Blair CK, Thomas W, Anderson KE. Aspirin use and the incidence of breast, colon, ovarian, and pancreatic cancers in elderly women in the Iowa Women's health study. Cancer Causes Control. 2016;27(11):1395–402. https://doi.org/10.1007/s10552-016-0804-8.

19. Cao Y, Nishihara R, Wu K, et al. Population-wide impact of long-term use of aspirin and the risk for Cancer. JAMA Oncol. 2016;2(6):762–9. https://doi.org/10.1001/jamaoncol.2015.6396.

20. Burn J, Gerdes AM, MacRae F, et al. Long-term effect of aspirin on cancer risk in carriers of hereditary colorectal cancer: an analysis from the CAPP2 randomised controlled trial. Lancet. 2011;378(9809):2081–7. https://doi.org/10.1016/S0140-6736(11)61049-0.

21. Drew DA, Cao Y, Chan AT. Aspirin and colorectal cancer: the promise of precision chemoprevention. Nat Rev Cancer. 2016;16(3):173–86. https://doi.org/10.1038/nrc.2016.4.

22. Cuzick J, Otto F, Baron JA, et al. Aspirin and non-steroidal anti-inflammatory drugs for cancer prevention: an international consensus statement. Lancet Oncol. 2009;10(5):501–7. https://doi.org/10.1016/S1470-2045(09)70035-X.

23. Jankowski JA, Hawk ET. A methodologic analysis of chemoprevention and cancer prevention strategies for gastrointestinal cancer. Nat Clin Pract Gastroenterol Hepatol. 2006;3(2):101–11. https://doi.org/10.1038/ncpgasthep0412.

24. Jankowski JA, Anderson M. Review article: management of oesophageal adenocarcinoma –control of acid, bile and inflammation in intervention strategies for Barrett's oesophagus. Aliment Pharmacol Ther. 2004;20(s5):71–80. https://doi.org/10.1111/j.1365-2036.2004.02143.x.

25. Vane JR, Botting RM. Anti-inflammatory drugs and their mechanism of action. Inflamm Res. 1998;47:78–87. https://doi.org/10.1007/s000110050284.

26. Tucker ON, Dannenberg AJ, Yang EK, et al. Cyclooxygenase-2 expression is up-regulated in human pancreatic cancer. Cancer Res. 1999;59(5):987–90. http://eutils.ncbi.nlm.nih.gov/entrez/eutils/elink.fcgi?dbfrom=pubmed&id=10070951&retmode=ref&cmd=prlinks%5Cnpapers3://publication/uuid/B59E91AA-82A7-40F0-BFA6-7F772463C3C5

27. Lagorce C, Paraf F, Vidaud D, et al. Cyclooxygenase-2 is expressed frequently and early in Barrett's oesophagus and associated adenocarcinoma. Histopathology. 2003;42(5):457–65. https://doi.org/10.1046/j.1365-2559.2003.01627.x.

28. Wilson KT, Fu S, Ramanujam KS, Meltzer SJ. Increased expression of inducible nitric oxide synthase and cyclooxygenase-2 in Barrett's esophagus and associated adenocarcinomas. Cancer Res. 1998;58(14):2929–34.

29. Buttar NS, Wang KK, Anderson MA, et al. The effect of selective cyclooxygenase-2 inhibition in Barrett's esophagus epithelium: an in vitro study. J Natl Cancer Inst. 2002;94(6):422–9. http://www.ncbi.nlm.nih.gov/entrez/query.fcgi?cmd=Retrieve&db=PubMed&dopt=Citation &list_uids=11904314

30. Cheong E, Ivory K, Doleman J, Parker ML, Rhodes M, Johnson IT. Synthetic and naturally occurring COX-2 inhibitors suppress proliferation in a human oesophageal adenocarcinoma cell line (OE33) by inducing apoptosis and cell cycle arrest. Carcinogenesis. 2004;25(10):1945–52. https://doi.org/10.1093/carcin/bgh184.

31. Rothwell PM, Fowkes FGR, Belch JF, Ogawa H, Warlow CP, Meade TW. Effect of daily aspirin on long-term risk of death due to cancer: Analysis of individual patient data from randomised trials. Lancet 2011.

32. Parkin DM, Boyd L, Walker LC. The fraction of cancer attributable to lifestyle and environmental factors in the UK in 2010. Br J Cancer. 2011;105:S77–81. https://doi.org/10.1038/bjc.2011.489.

33. Masclee GMC, Coloma PM, Spaander MCW, et al. NSAIDs, statins, low-dose aspirin and PPIs, and the risk of oesophageal adenocarcinoma among patients with Barrett's oesophagus: a population-based case–control study. BMJ Open. 2015;5:e006640. https://doi.org/10.1136/bmjopen-2014-006640.

34. Macfarlane TV, Lefevre K, Watson MC. Aspirin and non-steroidal anti-inflammatory drug use and the risk of upper aerodigestive tract cancer. Br J Cancer. 2014;111(9):1852–9. https://doi.org/10.1038/bjc.2014.473.

35. Corley DA, Kerlikowske K, Verma R, Buffler P. Protective association of aspirin/NSAIDs and esophageal cancer: a systematic review and meta-analysis. Gastroenterology. 2003;124(1):47–56. https://doi.org/10.1053/gast.2003.50008.

36. Cuzick J, Thorat MA, Bosetti C, et al. Estimates of benefits and harms of prophylactic use of aspirin in the general population. Ann Oncol. 2015;26(1):47–57. https://doi.org/10.1093/annonc/mdu225.

37. Jankowski JA. Aspirin chemoprevention for Barrett's and esophageal cancer: the AspECT trial. Cancer Prev Res. 2011;4(10). http://www.embase.com/search/result s?subaction=viewrecord&from=export&id=L71294276%5Cn;http://cancerprevention research.aacrjournals.org/cgi/content/meeting_abstract/4/10_MeetingAbstracts/ED04-03?sid=3a6f865f-6a2d-447b-ab11-801a2038933a%5Cn

38. Hur C, Broughton DE, Ozanne E, Yachimski P, Nishioka NS, Gazelle GS. Patient preferences for the chemoprevention of esophageal adenocarcinoma in Barrett's esophagus. Am J Gastroenterol. 2008;103(10):2432–42. https://doi.org/10.1111/j.1572-0241.2008.02117.x.

39. Hippisley-Cox J, Coupland C. Unintended effects of statins in men and women in England and Wales: population based cohort study using the QResearch database. BMJ. 2010;340:c2197. https://doi.org/10.1136/bmj.c2197.

40. Lytras T, Nikolopoulos G, Bonovas S. Statins and the risk of colorectal cancer: an updated systematic review and meta-analysis of 40 studies. World J Gastroenterol. 2014;20(7):1858–70. https://doi.org/10.3748/wjg.v20.i7.1858.

41. Platz EA, Leitzmann MF, Visvanathan K, et al. Statin drugs and risk of advanced prostate cancer. J Natl Cancer Inst. 2006;98(24):1819–25. https://doi.org/10.1093/jnci/djj499.

42. Singh S, Singh PP, Singh AG, Murad MH, Sanchez W. Statins are associated with a reduced risk of hepatocellular cancer: a systematic review and meta-analysis. Gastroenterology. 2013;144(2):323–32. https://doi.org/10.1053/j.gastro.2012.10.005.

43. Tsan Y-T, Lee C-H, Wang J-D, Chen P-C. Statins and the risk of hepatocellular carcinoma in patients with hepatitis B virus infection. J Clin Oncol. 2012;30(6):623–30. https://doi.org/10.1200/JCO.2011.36.0917.

44. Demierre MF, Higgins PDR, Gruber SB, Hawk E, Lippman SM. Statins and cancer prevention. Nat Rev Cancer. 2005;5(12):930–42. https://doi.org/10.1038/nrc1751.

45. Souza RF, Shewmake K, Pearson S, et al. Acid increases proliferation via ERK and p38 MAPK-mediated increases in cyclooxygenase-2 in Barrett's adenocarcinoma cells. Am J Physiol Gastrointest Liver Physiol. 2004;287(4):G743–8. https://doi.org/10.1152/ajpgi.00144.2004.
46. Zhong S, Zhang X, Chen L, Ma T, Tang J, Zhao J. Statin use and mortality in cancer patients: systematic review and meta-analysis of observational studies. Cancer Treat Rev. 2015;41(6):554–67. https://doi.org/10.1016/j.ctrv.2015.04.005.
47. Nielsen SF, Nordestgaard BG, Bojesen SE. Statin use and reduced Cancer-related mortality. N Engl J Med. 2012;367(19):1792–802. https://doi.org/10.1056/NEJMoa1201735.
48. Alexandre L, Clark AB, Bhutta HY, Chan SSM, Lewis MPN, Hart AR. Association between statin use after diagnosis of Esophageal Cancer and survival: apopulation-based cohort study. Gastroenterology. 2016;150(4):854–865.e1. https://doi.org/10.1053/j.gastro.2015.12.039.
49. Bonovas S, Sitaras NM. Does pravastatin promote cancer in elderly patients? A meta-analysis. CMAJ. 2007;176(5):649–54. https://doi.org/10.1503/cmaj.060803.
50. Weverling-Rijnsburger AW, Blauw GJ, Lagaay a M, Knook DL, Meinders AE, Westendorp RG. Total cholesterol and risk of mortality in the oldest old. Lancet. 1997;350(9085):1119–23. https://doi.org/10.1016/S0140-6736(97)04430-9.
51. Treatment C, Ctt T. Efficacy and safety of more intensive lowering of LDL choles-terol: a meta-analysis of data from 170 000 participants in 26 randomised trials. Lancet. 2010;376(9753):1670–81. https://doi.org/10.1016/S0140-6736(10)61350-5.
52. Feng Y, Ke C, Tang Q, et al. Metformin promotes autophagy and apoptosis in esophageal squamous cell carcinoma by downregulating Stat3 signaling. Cell Death Dis. 2014;5(2):e1088. https://doi.org/10.1038/cddis.2014.59.
53. Zhou G, Myers R, Li Y, et al. Role of AMP-activated protein kinase in mechanism of metformin action. J Clin Invest. 2001;108(8):1167–74. https://doi.org/10.1172/JCI200113505.
54. Skinner HD, McCurdy MR, Echeverria AE, et al. Metformin use and improved response to therapy in esophageal adenocarcinoma. Acta Oncol. 2013;52(5):1002–9. https://doi.org/10.31 09/0284186X.2012.718096.
55. DeCensi A, Puntoni M, Goodwin P, et al. Metformin and cancer risk in diabetic patients: a systematic review and meta-analysis. Cancer Prev Res. 2010;3(11):1451–61. https://doi.org/10.1158/1940-6207.CAPR-10-0157.
56. Singh S, Singh PP, Roberts LR, Sanchez W. Chemopreventive strategies in hepatocellular carcinoma. Nat Rev Gastroenterol Hepatol. 2014;11(1):45–54. https://doi.org/10.1038/nrgastro.2013.143.
57. Higurashi T, Hosono K, Takahashi H, et al. Metformin for chemoprevention of metachronous colorectal adenoma or polyps in post-polypectomy patients without diabetes: a multicentre double-blind, placebo-controlled, randomised phase 3 trial. Lancet Oncol. 2016;17(4):475–83. https://doi.org/10.1016/S1470-2045(15)00565-3.
58. Cuzick J, DeCensi A, Arun B, et al. Preventive therapy for breast cancer: a consensus statement. Lancet Oncol. 2011;12(5):496–503. https://doi.org/10.1016/S1470-2045(11)70030-4.
59. National Collaborating Centre for Cancer. Familial breast cancer: classification, care and managing breast cancer and related risks in people with a family history of breast cancer. National Institute for Health and Clinical Excellence: Guidance, Clinical guideline [CG164]. Cardiff: NCC-C; 2013. p. 253.

Staging of Cancer of the Esophagus and Esophagogastric Junction

6

Thomas W. Rice and Eugene H. Blackstone

Staging of cancer of the esophagus and esophagogastric junction for the eighth edition of the AJCC and UICC cancer staging manuals [1, 2] was constructed on a strong foundation of seventh edition data and analysis [3, 4]. A greatly expanded eighth edition Worldwide Esophageal Cancer Collaboration (WECC) database, with a substantial increase in both numbers of patients entered and variables collected [5–7], facilitated a more robust and reliable Random Forest-based machine learning analysis. Random Forest techniques provided risk-adjusted survival estimates for all patients from which distinctive and homogeneous stage groups with monotonically decreasing survival were identified.

Key to eighth edition staging is stage groupings by classifications. There are three separate classifications each with separate recommendations for both adenocarcinoma and squamous cell carcinoma: the classic reference pathologic (pTNM) stage groupings, the newly introduced neoadjuvant pathologic (ypTNM) stage groupings, and clinical (cTNM) stage groupings [8–10].

Cancer Classifications

Published in 1977, the AJCC "first edition" Manual for Staging of Cancer introduced AJCC designated TNM definitions and, where possible, stage groupings for 18 disease sites, including the esophagus. Importantly, "general rules and the relationship between time and the staging of cancer" were introduced. These "Rules for Classification" included pretreatment information, which was designated clinical diagnostic staging (cTNM); information obtained at surgical exploration, designated surgical-evaluation staging (sTNM); information from gross and histologic examination of the resection specimen, designated posttreatment pathologic staging

T. W. Rice (✉) · E. H. Blackstone
Department of Thoracic and Cardiovascular Surgery, Cleveland Clinic, Cleveland, OH, USA
e-mail: ricet@ccf.org

© Springer Nature Switzerland AG 2020
N. F. Saba, B. F. El-Rayes (eds.), *Esophageal Cancer*,
https://doi.org/10.1007/978-3-030-29832-6_6

127

(pTNM); information obtained at treatment failure and before additional treatment, designated retreatment staging (rTNM); and information found at autopsy, designated autopsy staging (aTNM) [11]. These have evolved primarily into clinical (cTNM), pathological (pTNM), and postneoadjuvant (ypTNM) stage groups.

Inconsistent and ineffective clinical staging modalities and newness of neoadjuvant therapy, compared to the conclusiveness of pathologic assessment of resection specimens, have led to sharing of pathologic stage grouping (pTNM) with corresponding cTNM or ypTNM groups. However, this sharing implies more than a common TNM language. The dual purpose of staging as outlined in the "first edition" UICC Cancer Staging Manual states "(TNM) classification is a means of recording facts observed by the clinician [about the cancer] whereas staging implies interpretation of these facts regarding prognosis" [12]. Therefore both terminology and prognosis need to be shared. This sharing of stage groups among classifications was examined by the AJCC Upper GI Task Force in preparing the eighth edition cancer staging manual. The need for separate stage groups based on category (TNM) was identified, although the need to harmonize with prognosis was not. As a consequence, a given clinical stage group does not carry the same prognosis as the identical pathologic stage group or the identical postneoadjuvant stage group.

Cancer Categories

Another consequence of sharing among classifications was the sloppy use of the term "classification," to describe both the relationship of time to cancer staging (classification) and the cancer characteristics, now defined as categories [1]. Criteria define the elements of categories. Esophageal anatomic cancer categories include primary tumor (T), regional lymph node (N), and distant site (M) (Table 6.1; Fig. 6.1). Subcategorization of pT1 into pT1a and pT1b has refined and improved Stage I grouping. Regional lymph nodes (N), which are found in the periesophageal tissue from the upper esophageal sphincter to the celiac artery, are clarified in a new map (Fig. 6.2). The non-anatomic cancer category Grade (G) is important for pathologic stage grouping (pTNM) of early-stage cancers (Table 6.1). Undifferentiated cancers require additional analyses to expose a histopathologic cell type. If glandular origin can be determined, the cancer is staged as a Grade 3 adenocarcinoma, if a squamous origin can be determined or if the cancer remains undifferentiated after full analysis, it is staged as a Grade 3 squamous cell carcinoma (Table 6.1). Cancer location is not important for adenocarcinoma stage grouping but in conjunction with Grade is necessary to subgroup pT3N0M0 squamous cell carcinoma. The definition of the esophogastric junction is revised such that cancers involving the esophogastric junction with epicenters no more than 2 cm into the gastric cardia are staged as adenocarcinomas of the esophagus, and those with more than 2 cm involvement of the gastric cardia are staged as stomach cancers (Fig. 6.3). Location was considered by the AJCC Upper Gastrointestinal Expert Panel as a placeholder until comprehensive genomic analysis could identify cell of origin rather than arbitrary measurement locations [13].

Table 6.1 Cancer staging categories for cancer of the esophagus and esophagogastric junction

T Category	Criteria
Tx	Tumor cannot be assessed
T0	No evidence of primary tumor
Tis	High-grade dysplasia, malignant cells confined by the basement membrane
T1	Tumor invades the lamina propria, muscularis mucosa, or submucosa
T1a[a]	Tumor invades the lamina propria or muscularis mucosa
T1b[a]	Tumor invades the submucosa
T2	Tumor invades the muscularis propria
T3	Tumor invades adventitia
T4	Tumor invades adjacent structures
T4a[a]	Tumor invading pleura, pericardium, azygos vein, diaphragm, or peritoneum
T4b[a]	Tumor invading other adjacent structures, such as aorta, vertebral body, and airway.
N category	*Criteria*
NX	Regional lymph nodes cannot be accessed
N0	No regional lymph node metastasis
N1	Metastasis in 1–2 regional lymph nodes
N2	Metastasis in 3–6 regional lymph nodes
N3	Metastasis in 7 or more regional lymph nodes
M category	*Criteria*
M0	No distant metastasis
M1	Distant metastasis
Adenocarcinoma G category	*Criteria*
G1	Well differentiated, > 95% of tumor is composed by well-formed glands
G2	Moderately differentiated, 50% to 95% of tumor shows gland formation
G3	Poorly differentiated, tumors composed of nest and sheets of cells with <50% of tumor demonstrating glandular formation. Undifferentiated, if glandular origin can be identified
Squamous cell carcinoma G category	*Criteria*
G1	Well-differentiated, prominent keratinization with pearl formation and a minor component of nonkeratinizing basal-like cells. Tumor cells are arranged in sheets, and mitotic counts are low
G2	Moderately differentiated, variable histologic features, ranging from parakeratotic to poorly keratinizing lesions. Generally, pearl formation is absent
G3	Poorly differentiated, consists predominantly of basal-like cells forming large and small nests with frequent central necrosis. The nests consist of sheets or pavement-like arrangements of tumor cells, and occasionally are punctuated by small numbers of parakeratotic or keratinizing cells

[a]Subcategories

Cancer Stage Groupings

Pathologic Stage Grouping (pTNM)

Historically, pathologic stage groupings after esophagectomy alone have been the sole basis for all cancer staging. Today pathologic staging is losing its clinical relevance for advanced stage cancer as neoadjuvant therapy replaces esophagectomy

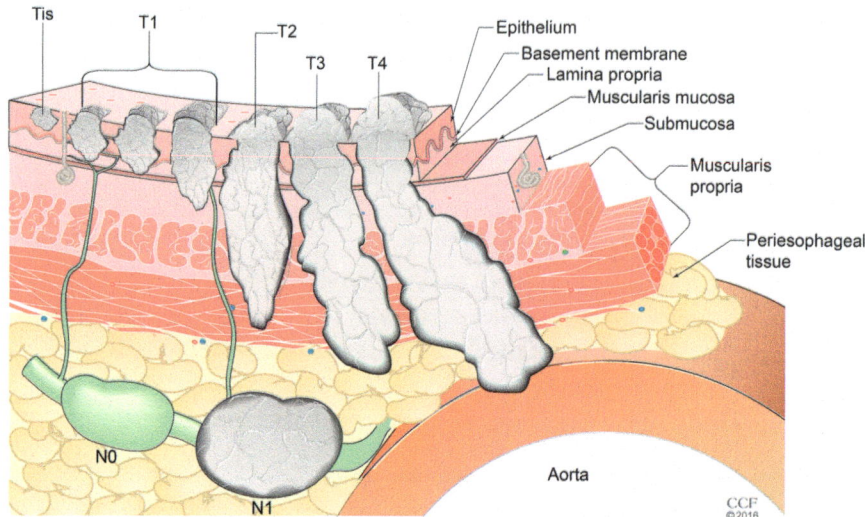

Fig. 6.1 Eighth edition TNM categories. T is categorized as Tis: high-grade dysplasia; T1: cancer invade lamina propria, muscularis mucosae, or submucosa and are subcategorized into T1a (cancer invades lamina propria or muscularis mucosae) and T1b (cancer invades submucosa); T2: cancer invades muscularis propria; T3: cancer invades periesophageal tissue; T4: cancer invades local structures and are subcategorized as T4a (cancer invades adjacent structures such as pleura, pericardium, azygos vein, diaphragm, or pericardium; and T4b (cancer invades major adjacent structures, such as aorta, vertebral body, or trachea). N is categorized as N0: no regional lymph node metastasis; N1: regional lymph node metastases involving 1–2 nodes; N2: regional lymph node metastases involving 3–6 nodes; and N3: regional lymph node metastases involving 7 or more nodes. M is categorized as M0: no distant metastasis; and M1: distant metastasis

alone. However, it remains relevant for early-stage cancers and as an important staging and survival reference point.

Squamous Cell Carcinoma

In the eighth edition, there is no net change in the number of staging subgroups; however, there is significant rearrangement and renaming (Table 6.2a). pStage 0 is restricted to high-grade glandular dysplasia, pTis. Subcategorization of T1 combined with Grade requires 2 pStage I subgroups: pStage IA (pT1aN0M0G1) and pStage IB (pT1aN0M0G2-3, pT1bN0M0, and pT2N0M0G1). pT2N0M0G2-3 cancers, pT3N0M0 cancers of the lower thoracic esophagus, and pT3N0M0G1 cancers of the upper thoracic esophagus comprise pStage IIA. pStage IIB is comprised of T3N0M0G2-3 cancers of the upper thoracic esophagus and pT1N1M0 cancers. pStage III and pStage IV are identical for both adenocarcinoma and squamous cell carcinoma.

Adenocarcinoma

Staging subgroups increased from 9 in the seventh edition to 10 in the eighth (Table 6.2b). pStage 0 is restricted to high-grade glandular dysplasia, pTis.

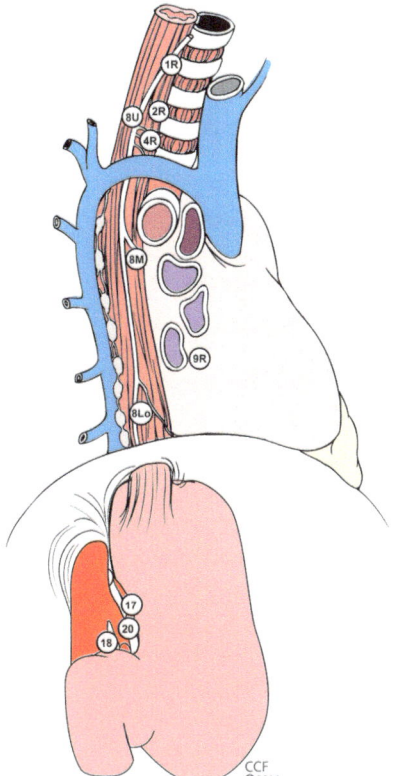

Fig. 6.2 (**a–c**): Lymph node maps for esophageal cancer regional lymph nodes, from left (**a**), right (**b**), and anterior (**c**). The regional lymph nodes are as follows: 1R: Right lower cervical paratracheal nodes: between the supraclavicular paratracheal space and apex of the lung, 1L: Left lower cervical paratracheal nodes: between the supraclavicular paratracheal space and apex of the lung, 2R: Right upper paratracheal nodes: between the intersection of the caudal margin of the innominate artery with the trachea and the apex of the lung, 2L: Left upper paratracheal nodes: between the top of the aortic arch and apex of the lung, R4: Right lower paratracheal nodes: between the intersection of the caudal margin of the innominate artery with the trachea and cephalic border of the azygos vein, L4: Left lower paratracheal nodes: between the top of the aortic arch and the carina, 7: Subcarinal nodes: caudal to the carina of the trachea, 8U: Upper thoracic paraesophageal lymph nodes: from the apex of the lung to the tracheal bifurcation, 8M Middle thoracic paraesophageal lymph nodes: from the tracheal bifurcation to the caudal margin of the inferior pulmonary vein, 8Lo: Lower thoracic paraesophageal lymph nodes: from the caudal margin of the inferior pulmonary vein to the EGJ, 9R: Pulmonary ligament nodes: within the right inferior pulmonary ligament, 9L: Pulmonary ligament nodes: within the left inferior pulmonary ligament, 15: Diaphragmatic nodes: lying on the dome of the diaphragm and adjacent to or behind its crura, 16: Paracardial nodes: immediately adjacent to the gastroesophageal junction, 17: Left gastric nodes: along the course of the left gastric artery, 18: Common hepatic nodes: immediately on the proximal common hepatic artery, 19: Splenic nodes: immediately on the proximal splenic artery, 20: Celiac nodes: at the base of the celiac artery, Cervical periesophageal level VI and level VII lymph nodes are named as per the head and neck map

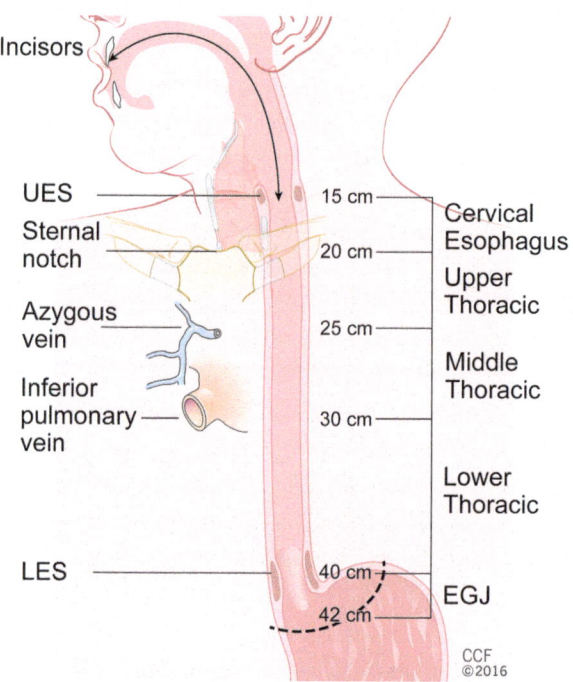

Fig. 6.3 Location of esophageal cancer primary site, including typical endoscopic measurements of each region measured from the incisors. Exact measurements depend on body size and height. Location of cancer primary site is defined by cancer epicenter. Cancers involving the EGJ that have their epicenter within the proximal 2 cm of the cardia (Siewert types I/II) are to be staged as esophageal cancers. Cancers whose epicenter is more than 2 cm distal from the EGJ, even if the EGJ is involved, will be staged using the stomach cancer TNM and stage groupings. EGJ esophagogastric junction, LES lower esophageal sphincter, UES upper esophageal sphincter

Subcategorization of T1 combined with Grade requires 3 pStage I subgroups: pStage IA (pT1aN0M0G1), pStage IB (pT1aN0M0G2 and pT1bN0M0G1-2), and pStage IC (pT1N0M0G3 and pT2N0M0G1-2). pT2N0M0G3 remains the sole cancer in pStage IIA. T3N0M0 and pT1N1M0 comprise pStage IIB. pStage III is reserved for advanced cancers with relatively good survival. pT2N1M0 and pT1N2M0 form pStage IIIA, while pT2N2M0, pT3N1-2M0, and pT4aN0-1M0 form pStage IIIB. pStage IV was subcategorized with the realization that the most locally advanced cancers have survival similar to cancers with metastasis to distant sites (M1). pT4aN2M0, pT4bN0-2M0, and pTanyN3M0 are pStage IVA. Cancers with metastasis to distant sites (M1) are restricted to pStage IVB.

Neoadjuvant Pathologic Stage Grouping (ypTNM)

New to the eighth edition is stage grouping of patients with esophageal cancers that have undergone neoadjuvant therapy and pathologic review of the resection specimen. Drivers of this addition include absence of equivalent pathologic (pTNM)

Table 6.2 (**a**) Pathologic Stage Groupings (pTNM)—squamous cell carcinoma. (**b**) Pathologic Stage Groupings (pTNM)—adenocarcinoma

a

		N0		N1	N2	N3	M1
		L	U/M				
Tis		O					
T1a	G1	IA	IA	IIB	IIIA	IVA	IVB
	G2-3	IB	IB				
T1b		IB		IIB	IIIA	IVA	IVB
T2	G1	IB	IB	IIIA	IIIB	IVA	IVB
	G2-3	IIA	IIA				
T3	G1	IIA	IIA	IIIB	IIIB	IVA	IVB
	G2-3	IIA	IIB				
T4a		IIIB		IIIB	IVA	IVA	IVB
T4b		IVA		IVA	IVA	IVA	IVB

b

		N0	N1	N2	N3	M1
Tis		O				
T1a	G1	IA	IIB	IIIA	IVA	IVB
	G2	IB				
	G3	IC				
T1b	G1	IB	IIB	IIIA	IVA	IVB
	G2	IB				
	G3	IC				
T2	G1	IC	IIIA	IIIB	IVA	IVB
	G2	IC				
	G3	IIA				
T3		IIB	IIIB	IIIB	IVA	IVB
T4a		IIIB	IIIB	IVA	IVA	IVB
T4b		IVA	IVA	IVA	IVA	IVB

categories for the peculiar neoadjuvant pathologic categories (ypT0N0-3M0 and ypTisN0-3M0), dissimilar stage group compositions, and markedly different survival profiles.

The groupings are identical for both histopathologic cell types (Table 6.3). Grade plays no role in neoadjuvant pathologic stage grouping. ypStage I is comprised of ypT0-2N0M0 cancers. ypStage II is the single entity ypT3N0M0. ypStage IIIA is comprised of cancers confined to the esophageal wall with ypN1 regional nodal

Table 6.3 Neoadjuvant pathologic stage groupings (ypTNM)—adenocarcinoma and squamous cell carcinoma

	N0	N1	N2	N3	M1
T0	I	IIIA	IIIB	IVA	IVB
Tis	I	IIIA	IIIB	IVA	IVB
T1	I	IIIA	IIIB	IVA	IVB
T2	I	IIIA	IIIB	IVA	IVB
T3	II	IIIB	IIIB	IVA	IVB
T4a	IIIB	IVA	IVA	IVA	IVB
T4b	IVA	IVA	IVA	IVA	IVB

category (ypT0-2N1M1). ypStage IIIB is comprised of ypT1-3N2M0, ypT3N1M0, and ypT4aN0M0 cancers. ypStage IVA includes ypT4aN1-2M0, ypT4bN0-2M0, and yp TanyN3M0. ypStage IVB is comprised of ypM1 cancers.

Clinical Stage Grouping (cTNM)

Also new to the eighth edition is clinical stage grouping (cTNM) prior to treatment decision (Table 6.4). Clinical staging is done largely in the absence of histologic cancer data in that the TNM categories are typically defined by imaging and not by microscopic examination of a resection specimen. Dissimilar stage group composition (Tables 6.2 and 6.4) and survival profiles necessitated clinical stage grouping (cTNM) separate from pathologic stage grouping (pTNM).

Squamous Cell Carcinoma
cStage 0 is comprised of cTis (Table 6.3a). cStage I is exclusivelycT1N0-1M0. cStage II is comprised of cT2N0-1M0 and cT3N0M0 cancers. cStage III is comprised of cT3N1M0 and cT1-3N2M0 cancers. cT4a-bN0-2M0 and all cN2-N3M0 cancers are placed in cStage IVA. cStage IVB is reserved for cM1 cancers.

Adenocarcinoma
cStage 0 is comprised of cTis (Table 6.3b). cStage I is exclusively cT1N0M0. cStage IIA is cT1N1M0 and cStage IIB is cT2N0M0. cStage III is cT2N1, cT3-4aN0-1M0. T4bN0-1M0, and all cN2-N3M0 comprise cStage IVA. cStage IVB is comprised of all cM1 cancers.

Table 6.4 (a) Clinical stage groupings (cTNM)—squamous cell carcinoma. (b) Clinical stage groupings (cTNM)—adenocarcinoma

a

	N0	N1	N2	N3	M1
Tis	O				
T1	I	I	III	IVA	IVB
T2	II	II	III	IVA	IVB
T3	II	III	III	IVA	IVB
T4a	IVA	IVA	IVA	IVA	IVB
T4b	IVA	IVA	IVA	IVA	IVB

b

	N0	N1	N2	N3	M1
Tis	O				
T1	I	IIA	IVA	IVA	IVB
T2	IIB	III	IVA	IVA	IVB
T3	III	III	IVA	IVA	IVB
T4a	III	III	IVA	IVA	IVB
T4b	IVA	IVA	IVA	IVA	IVB

Changes Between Seventh and Eighth Edition Cancer Staging

The changes in classifications and categories between the seventh and eighth edition are listed in Table 6.5.

Table 6.5 8th edition: changes from the seventh edition

pTNM		
Categories	T	T1 subcategorized as T1a and T1b, producing stage subgroups IA and IB for squamous cell carcinoma and IA and IC for adenocarcinoma T2 squamous cell carcinoma: Location removed as staging category T4a includes direct invasion of peritoneum
	G	G4 was eliminated, and additional testing is required to uncover glandular (G3 adenocarcinoma) or squamous (G3 squamous) differentiation. If the cancer remains undifferentiated, it is categorized as G3 squamous cell carcinoma
	L	Cancers of the esophagogastric junction that have their epicenters within the proximal 2 cm of the gastric cardia are staged as esophageal cancers. Those with epicenters >2 cm distal to the esophagogastric junction, staged in the seventh edition as esophageal cancers, even if the esophagus is involved, are staged as stomach cancers
Stage groups	pStage III	Subgroup IIIC in seventh edition removed
	pStage IV	Subgrouped as IVA and IVB
ypTNM		
Stage groups		No longer shared with pTNM, separate groupings identical for squamous cell carcinoma and adenocarcinoma
cTNM		
Stage groups		No longer shared with pTNM, separate groupings for squamous cell carcinoma and adenocarcinoma

Conclusions

Eighth edition staging for cancer of the esophagus and esophagogastric junction are data-driven and expanded from pathologic stage grouping (pTNM) to pathologic stage grouping after neoadjuvant therapy (ypTNM) and clinical staging (cTNM) before treatment decision.

References

1. Rice TW, Kelsen DP, Blackstone EH, et al. Esophagus and esophagogastric junction. In: Amin MB, Edge SB, Greene FL, et al., editors. AJCC cancer staging manual. 8th ed. New York, NY: Springer; 2017. p. 185–202.
2. International Union Against Cancer. Oesphagus including oesophagogastric junction. In: Brierley JD, Gospodarowicz MK, Wittekind C, editors. TNM classification of malignant Tumors. 8th ed. Oxford, England: Wiley; 2017. p. 57–62.
3. Edge SB, Byrd DR, Compton CC, Fritz AG, Greene FL, Trotti A, editors. American Joint Committee on Cancer Staging Manual. 7th ed. New York: Springer-Verlag; 2010.
4. Sobin LH, Gospodarrowicz MK, Wittekind C, editors. TNM classifications of malignant tumors. International Union against Cancer. 7th ed. Oxford, England: Wiley-Blackwell; 2009.
5. Rice TW, Chen L-Q, Hofstetter WL, et al. Worldwide Esophageal cancer collaboration: pathologic staging data. Dis Esophagus. 2016;29:724–33.
6. Rice TW, Lerut TEMR, Orringer MB, et al. Worldwide Esophageal cancer collaboration: neoadjuvant pathologic staging data. Dis Esophagus. 2016;29:715–23.

7. Rice TW, Apperson-Hansen C, DiPaola LM, et al. Worldwide Esophageal Cancer Collaboration: clinical staging data. Dis Esophagus. 2016;29:707–14.
8. Rice TW, Ishwaran H, Hofstetter WL, Kelsen D, Blackstone EH. Recommendations for pathologic stage grouping (pTNM) of cancer of the esophagus and esophagogastric junction for the 8th edition AJCC/UICC staging manuals. Dis Esophagus. 2016;29:897–905.
9. Rice TW, Ishwaran H, Kelsen D, Hofstetter WL, Blackstone EH. Recommendations for neoadjuvant pathologic stage grouping (ypTNM) of cancer of the esophagus and esophagogastric junction for the 8th edition AJCC/UICC staging manuals. Dis Esophagus. 2016;29:906–12.
10. Rice TW, Ishwaran H, Blackstone EH, Hofstetter WL, Kelsen D. Recommendations for clinical stage grouping (cTNM) of cancer of the esophagus and esophagogastric junction for the 8th edition AJCC/UICC staging manuals. Dis Esophagus. 2016;29:913–9.
11. Manual for Staging of Cancer 1977. American Joint Committee for Cancer Staging and End-Results Reporting. Chicago; 1977.
12. International Union Against Cancer (UICC). TNM Classification of Malignant Tumors. Geneva; 1968.
13. Hayakawa Y, Sethi N, Sepulveda AR, Bass AJ, Wang TC. Oesophageal adenocarcinoma and gastric cancer: should we mind the gap? Nat Rev Cancer. 2016;16:305–18.

Radiologic Assessment of Esophageal Cancer

7

Valeria M. Moncayo, A. Tuba Kendi, and David M. Schuster

Introduction

Esophageal cancer represents the third most common gastrointestinal tract malignancy and sixth most common cause of cancer death worldwide [1, 2]. About 17,290 new cases of esophageal cancer will be diagnosed in the United States in 2018 (13,480 in men and 3810 in women) and about 15,850 deaths from esophageal cancer are estimated by the American Cancer Society [3]. The majority of esophageal cancers are either squamous cell carcinoma (SCC) or adenocarcinomas [1, 2]. SCC is the most common pathologic subtype with a higher incidence in developing countries [1, 2, 4]. Esophageal adenocarcinomas comprise 15% of all esophageal cancers [4]. Other malignant tumors such as sarcomas, lymphoma, and small cell carcinoma (neuroendocrine tumor) are rather rare [4]. Accurate initial staging of esophageal cancer is required to guide treatment protocols and to estimate prognosis [1, 2, 4–6].

Diagnosis

For many developing countries, barium esophagogram remains the primary diagnostic test for esophageal cancer [5]. The most common radiographic appearance is the presence of an abrupt irregular narrowing with an ulcerated surface in a stricture [5, 7] (Fig. 7.1). Modern barium esophagogram detects a lesion in 98% of studies of patients

V. M. Moncayo (✉) · D. M. Schuster
Division of Nuclear Medicine and Molecular Imaging,
Department of Radiology and Imaging Sciences, Emory University,
Atlanta, GA, USA
e-mail: vmoncay@emory.edu; dschust@emory.edu

A. T. Kendi
Department of Radiology, Mayo Clinic, Rochester, MN, USA
e-mail: kendi.ayse@mayo.edu

© Springer Nature Switzerland AG 2020
N. F. Saba, B. F. El-Rayes (eds.), *Esophageal Cancer*,
https://doi.org/10.1007/978-3-030-29832-6_7

Fig. 7.1 Barium esophagogram of a patient with esophageal cancer shows abrupt narrowing of esophagus and focal areas of ulceration (arrow) with stricture

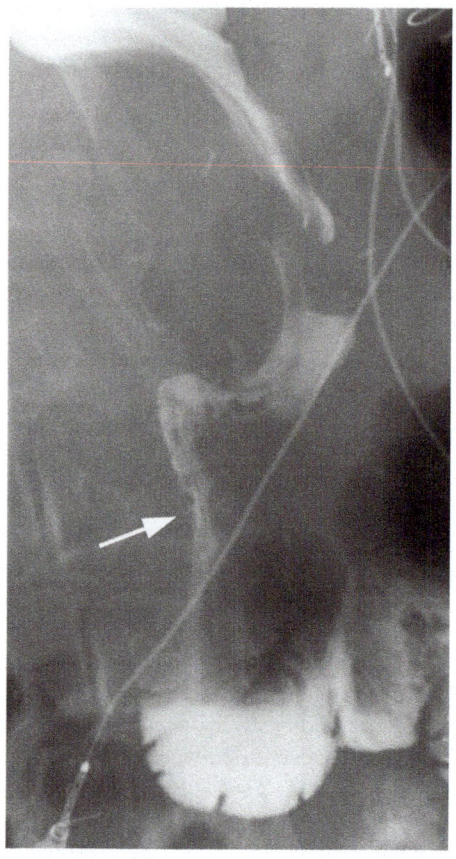

with esophageal cancer and is suggestive of esophageal cancer in 96%, with an estimated positive predictive value of 42% [5, 8]. As clinical diagnosis of esophageal cancer requires tissue confirmation, most centers in developed countries perform esophagoscopy with tissue sampling instead of esophagogram. Although the flexible fiberoptic system is most commonly utilized, in cases with severe stricture, esophagoscopy may not be possible. In these circumstances, endoscopic esophageal ultrasound (EUS) and EUS fine-needle aspiration (EUS FNA) are the procedures of choice. FNA with biopsy of suspicious findings is an important step during the staging process [5].

Staging

Clinical staging tools include esophagoscopy with biopsy, EUS, EUS-FNA, CT, and FDG positron emission tomography/computed tomography (PET/CT). Bronchoscopy, cervical lymph node biopsy, endoscopic bronchial ultrasound (EBUS) and EBUS-FNA, ultrasound, or CT-directed biopsies can be used in specific cases [1, 2, 4, 5, 7].

CT [9] and EUS have been the mainstay imaging modalities for initial staging; however, these modalities may over- or understage as many as 30–40% of cases [10]. PET/CT demonstrates superiority to other modalities especially given its effectiveness in the detection of distant metastatic disease [10]. Wallace et al. examined multiple imaging modalities for staging and concluded that the preferred staging procedure was PET/CT followed by EUS in cases where no evidence of metastasis was observed by PET/CT [10, 11].

Staging of esophageal cancer has been updated in the eighth edition of the American Joint Committee on Cancer (AJCC)/Union for International Cancer Control (UICC) cancer staging manuals [12]. This new edition includes separate clinical (CTNM), pathologic (pTNM), and postneoadjuvant therapy (ypTNM) staging groupings [12]. It is relevant to acknowledge that clinical staging is in general limited by the resolution of the imaging methods used for such staging. The limitations and strengths of each modality should, therefore, be taken into consideration.

Depth of invasion defines the T staging of primary cancer. T *is* (in situ) tumors are intra-epithelial without invasion of the basal membrane, currently termed high-grade dysplasia. T1 cancers extend beyond the basal membrane and invade the lamina propria, muscularis mucosa, or submucosa. T1 cancers can be classified as mucosal (T1a) or submucosal (T1b). T2 cancers breach into but not beyond the muscularis propria. T3 cancers invade beyond the esophageal wall without invading adjacent structures. T4 cancers invade structures adjacent to the esophagus. T4a cancers are still resectable, invading adjacent structures like the pleura, pericardium, and diaphragm. T4b tumors are unresectable due to invasion of other adjacent structures like the aorta, vertebral bodies, or trachea [2, 4, 5, 13].

A regional lymph node is defined as any paraesophageal lymph node extending from cervical nodes to celiac nodes. N classification includes N0 (no cancer-positive nodes), N1 (1 or 2 nodes), N2 (3–6 nodes), and N3 (7 or more) [2, 4, 5].

Distant metastasis is classified as either M0, no distant metastasis, or M1, distant metastasis. Histopathologic cell type is either squamous cell carcinoma or adenocarcinoma as AJCC/UICC staging is based on cancers arising from the esophageal epithelium. Histologic grade is categorized as G1 well differentiated, G2 moderately differentiated, G3 poorly differentiated, and G4 undifferentiated [4, 5, 13]. The histologic grade has been eliminated from the AJCC/UICC eighth edition, with the expectation for it to be considered for the ninth edition.

In this new edition, cancer location is expressed as the distance of the epicenter of the cancer from the incisors. Upper and lower border of the tumor and cancer length are needed to provide the epicenter. This is new compared to the prior determination of tumor location in the seventh edition, which was the proximal end of the cancer from the incisors. This location can be correlated with anatomic imaging. If the tumor is above the sternal notch, the esophageal cancer is located in the cervical esophagus. An upper thoracic location on CT corresponds to the region between the sternal notch and lower border of the azygos vein. Middle thoracic tumors are located between the azygos vein and inferior pulmonary vein. The lower thoracic region is below the inferior pulmonary vein to the stomach or gastroesophageal junction (Fig. 7.2) [4, 5, 11]. Adenocarcinomas with epicenter no more than 2 cm

Fig. 7.2 Anatomic localization of esophageal cancer

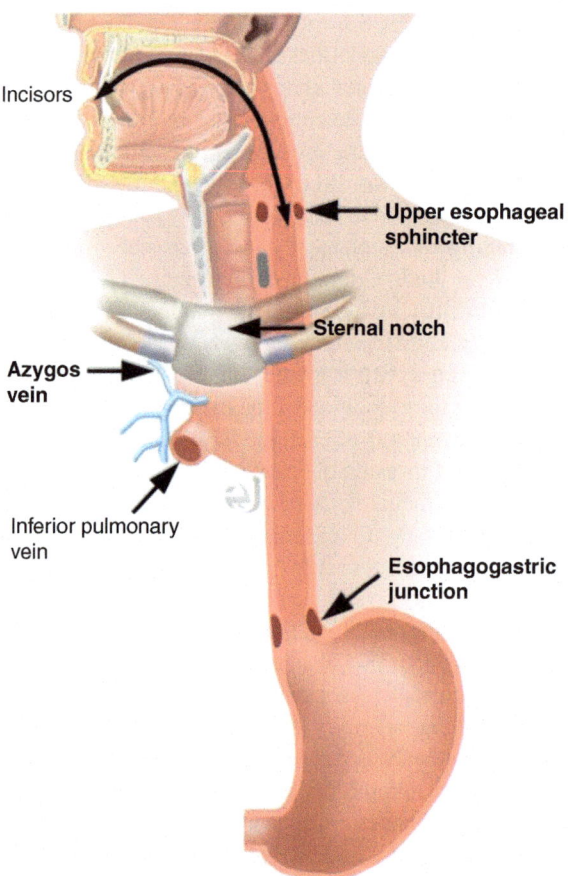

into the gastric cardia are staged as esophageal adenocarcinomas, and those extending further are staged as stomach cancers.

T Staging

T1 and T2 tumors are generally treated with surgery, whereas patients with T3 and T4 tumors are frequently offered preoperative chemotherapy and/or radiation therapy. Hence, the detection of depth of invasion for proper T staging becomes crucial [1, 2, 4, 5, 7].

EUS

EUS is the most accurate imaging tool that provides information about involvement of the esophageal wall that is necessary to define T stage. EUS may detect the involvement of adjacent structures, specifically the invasion through the muscularis propria layer, so that it may upstage a cancer to T4 in the presence of invasion [6]. The performance of EUS has been shown to improve as the T stage increases [2, 7]. The distinction between T1 or T2 and T2 or T3 cancers is essential for decision making because the former are typically N0, requiring resection alone, while T3–4 cancers have a higher probability of N1 disease requiring neoadjuvant therapy [12, 14].

EUS is not accurate in differentiating T *is* from T1. However, US performed with high-frequency probes showed very good results in distinguishing mucosal versus submucosal invasion [1]. In comparison to CT, EUS is more accurate in differentiating between T1, T2, and T3 tumors [2]. However, there are shortcomings of EUS. Like any other sonographic examination, it is operator dependent, and in cases where the esophageal lumen is narrowed, it may be impossible to pass the endoscope through the stricture [2, 4]. In these cases, mechanical dilatation can be performed; however, there is increased risk of esophageal perforation [1, 4].

The appropriate therapy for esophageal cancer partly relies on the accurate assessment of disease extent. This information is often acquired from PET/CT and EUS. The length of disease (LoD) is an important measurement that can influence therapy decisions. The results from a recent study showed that PET/CT tends to under-measure LoD compared to EUS [15].

Evaluation of depth of invasion for superficial esophageal cancer is generally performed by white light imaging (WLI) and EUS. Recent advances in magnifying endoscopy and narrow band imaging (M-NBI) enabled the assessment of the pattern of intra-epithelial papillary capillary loops and avascular area to predict the histology and cancer invasion depth. As the classification method for M-NBI is complicated, it is not widely used in clinical practice. Recently, a simplified method of classification was suggested by the Japanese Esophageal Society. A study by Wang et al. confirmed that a training program for this new simplified method improved the diagnostic accuracy of cancer invasion depth [16].

CT and MRI

Assessment of the esophagus by CT can be challenging especially for T1 and T2 esophageal cancers, as the detection of a small tumor in a poorly distended tubular structure is quite difficult. Usually, the esophageal wall measures less than 3 mm on CT of a distended esophagus [2, 4]. A wall thickness more than 5 mm is considered abnormal [4]. Asymmetric thickening of the esophageal wall is a primary but nonspecific finding [4] for esophageal cancer. CT assessment is less accurate for the detection and staging of esophageal cancer compared to EUS [1, 2, 4] (Fig. 7.3).

In circumstances when esophagoscopy is not possible, mostly due to the presence of a marked stricture, CT may provide information about the location of the tumor.

The most useful aspect of CT in T staging is to evaluate for the presence of invasion of adjacent soft tissues. Direct invasion or obliteration of the fat plane between the tumor and the anatomic structure may indicate local invasion [1, 2, 4, 7]. However caution is advised in cachectic patients and in patients with prior history of radiation therapy or surgery as fat planes on CT may not be clearly depicted [1, 2, 7].

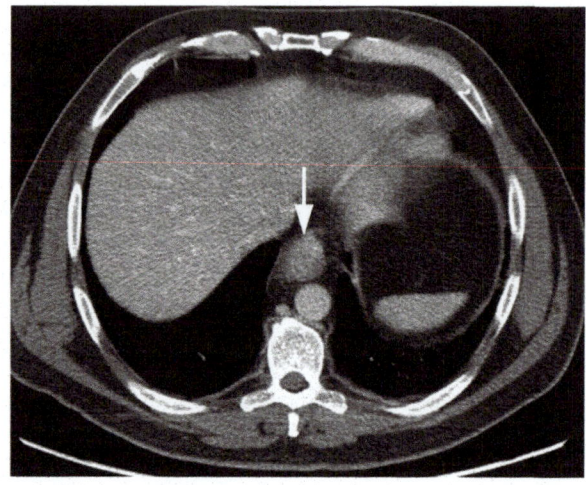

Fig. 7.3 Axial contrast-enhanced CT of the upper abdomen shows marked circumferential thickening of the distal esophagus (arrow), consistent with known esophageal cancer. Unfortunately, CT was not able to properly determine T staging as the assessment of esophageal wall layers was limited with this imaging technique

In addition, local invasion is suggested by a contact angle of more than 90° between the cancer and the aorta or thickening and displacement or indentation of the posterior membrane of the trachea or left mainstem bronchus, yet neither of these findings is definitive [1, 4, 6]. Finally, tumor extension in the airway or a fistula between the esophagus and airway may be visualized; still bronchoscopic confirmation is necessary. Pleural effusion and pleural wall thickening are suspicious findings on CT for tumoral invasion. Direct extension of tumor to the heart or loss of pericardial fat plane can also be detected by CT.

With recent advances in CT technology, it is possible to provide higher quality images with isotropic voxels as well as CT esophagography or virtual endoscopy [4].

Multi-planar reformatted images (MPRs) are useful to estimate tumor length and assessment of the exact location of esophageal cancer is more accurate compared to that achieved with axial images only [1, 4]. MPRs are also useful in evaluating esophageal cancers at the esophagogastric junction (EGJ) [1]. Pneumo-CT is a technique developed to image stenotic lesions, optimizing tumor visualization at the esophageal wall [17]. Administration of effervescent granules, air insufflations, or ingestion of large amounts of water is another method to better visualize the esophageal wall by CT [4].

Magnetic resonance imaging (MRI) has a limited role in imaging of esophageal cancer due to technical shortcomings. Early studies with MRI demonstrated poor quality especially due to motion artifacts and cardiac/respiratory-related artifacts. Recent developments in cardiac respiratory gating, availability of high field magnets (1.5 and 3 T) for imaging, and the development of new and faster imaging sequences have resulted in better-quality images. The addition of sequences such as diffusion-weighted imaging and dynamic contrast enhancement has improved esophageal cancer imaging. Preliminary studies with high-resolution MR imaging report high accuracies for T staging, close to that of EUS [18–20].

FDG PET

The first report in the literature of the use of FDG PET in a patient with esophageal cancer was described in 1995, by Yasuda [10, 21]. Given that FDG PET provides mostly metabolic information about the tumor, determination of T stage is not one of its strengths. Though 92–100% of esophageal cancers are FDG avid, lack of visualization of esophageal wall layers, even with combined FDG PET/CT limits accurate assessment of T stage. Some authors, such as Kato, report that T1 tumors lack FDG uptake, likely due to their size below the resolution for PET (0.7–1 cm) [22]. In the study by Kato, it was found that T2, T3, and T4 tumors have similar levels of FDG uptake [23]. Advanced T staging could be seen with combined PET/CT, when the metabolic activity extends to adjacent soft tissues in the mediastinum, and the fat planes are lost suggesting invasion [1].

Increasing data exist to support the use of quantitative measures or metabolic parameters of the primary tumor as prognostic predictors. These include standardized uptake value (SUV), metabolic tumor volume (MTV) and total tumor glycolysis (TLG), among others [23–25]. A meta-analysis of ten studies with 542 patients by Pan reports that high SUVs are associated with a significantly poorer overall survival and disease free survival. Foley studied these independent predictors of survival, and the most significant was TLG (defined by the product of metabolic volume of primary tumor times SUVmean). In Foley's study, another significant predictive factor was the "Metastatic Length of Disease" defined as the total length of disease including nonregional lymph node metastases and distant metastases measured in mm. The total count of involved local lymph node metastases on PET/CT was also a significant predictor of survival [24].

Finally, FDG uptake secondary to inflammation from esophagitis may confound accurate T staging, although the pattern of FDG uptake is usually linear and diffuse compared to focal for malignancies [26].

N Stage

Lymphatic involvement can occur at very early stages of esophageal cancer due to the unique bidirectional lymphatic drainage system of the esophagus. The intramural (mucosal) drainage system is located in the lamina propria. Unlike other parts of the gastrointestinal system, this location can result in early dissemination of tumor cells. The second, longitudinal system is localized in the submucosa, within the muscular layer [4].

EUS

EUS and EUS FNA are primary tools to identify regional nodal involvement. EUS has an accuracy of 72–80% [2]. CT has an accuracy ranging between 46 and 58% [1]. Although EUS is superior to CT in detecting lymph node metastasis, the sensitivity and specificity vary depending on location; for example, detection of celiac axis lymph nodes is better than that of mediastinal lymph nodes with EUS [1].

Combined use of EUS with FNA improves accuracy [1, 2, 4]. However, EUS FNA can only be performed in lymph nodes that are approachable [4]. Metastatic lymph nodes can appear as well-defined (clear border), round, homogeneous, and low-echoic lesions measuring more than 10 mm in diameter [4]. According to Rice et al. [7], the accuracy of detecting nodal metastasis in lymph nodes with all five of these features is 100% [7]. However, very few metastatic lymph nodes present with all of these findings, especially in a peri-esophageal location.

Recent study by Goense et al. showed that cervical ultrasonography has no additional value over PET/CT in assessment of cervical lymph node metastases. PET/CT provides a better diagnostic confidence compared to cervical ultrasonography. However, FNA can be still needed for cervical lesions that are identified on PET/CT [27].

CT and MRI

CT provides information about nonregional lymph nodes, mainly supraclavicular, abdominal, retrocrural lymph nodes. A short axis of more than 1 cm of a lymph node on CT is the most widely used criterion for suspicious lymph node involvement (Fig. 7.4). The cut offs for retrocrural and supraclavicular nodes are 0.6 cm and 0.5 cm, respectively. However, normal-sized lymph nodes may contain tumor deposits, resulting in false negative examination. Also an enlarged lymph node may not be malignant but could be inflammatory, resulting in false positive results with CT [2, 4]. Therefore, sensitivity and specificity of detection of nodal metastasis with CT are low, with reported accuracy of 46–58% [2, 4].

MRI in its current state has moderate-to-poor diagnostic value for N staging. There are studies showing markedly improved diagnostic accuracy of MRI for N staging by using fast sequences and SPIO contrast agent [28, 29].

Fig. 7.4 Axial contrast-enhanced CT of the lower thoracic/upper abdomen region shows periesophageal lymphadenopathy, most consistent with malignant lymphadenopathy (arrow) as well as abnormal thickening of adjacent esophageal wall consistent with known esophageal cancer

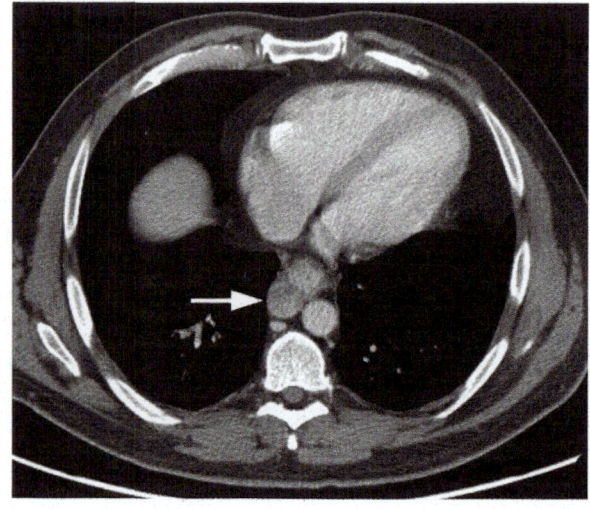

FDG PET

FDG PET/CT combines the anatomic delineation of CT with PET, which can also identify tumoral deposits by the presence of FDG activity. FDG PET is limited in the detection of locoregional lymph nodes in close proximity to the primary tumor in which intense FDG activity may obscure FDG uptake in small adjacent lymph nodes [1, 4, 19]. The reported sensitivity and specificity for detection of locoregional lymph nodes by PET/CT is 59% and 81%, respectively, from a meta-analysis of 12 publications [5]. The sensitivity of EUS compared with PET/CT is superior for the detection of lymph nodes, although specificity is lower [9, 30]. The presence of locoregional lymph nodes does not preclude surgery; yet, if lymph nodes are seen beyond these boundaries, such as in the retroperitoneum or upper/mid-neck, the patient would be considered to have distant metastatic disease where surgery is contraindicated [31].

Compared to the detection of lymph node metastasis from lung cancer and other cancers, FDG PET/CT is less accurate in esophageal cancer [5]. The addition of FDG PET to EUS FNA does not change N classification significantly [5]. The sensitivity of PET/CT for the detection of distant nodal metastasis is 90% [2]. The combined use of PET and CT improves the detection rate of nodal disease (Fig. 7.5). Still, false-positive findings due to chronic inflammation may be a limitation [1].

Metabolic parameters have also been used in the evaluation of N staging. A study by Moon evaluated patients with clinically N0 disease, and reported that combined use of T classification and SUVmax were strong predictors of occult metastatic disease [32]. Other metabolic parameters such as TLG and MTV have been also studied by different groups. Hsu found a significant correlation between extratumoral maximum SUV and N classification [33].

Fig. 7.5 Sagittal fused PET/CT image of the thoracic level shows the hypermetabolic esophageal cancer (arrow) and more cranially located hypermetabolic periesophageal lymph node (arrowhead)

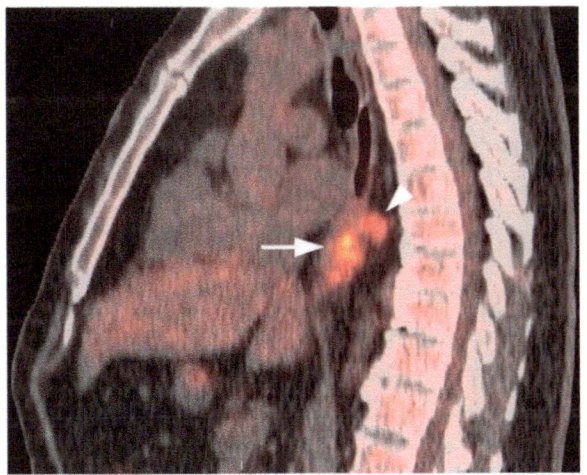

M Stage

In patients with recent diagnosis of esophageal cancer, 20–30% will have distant metastasis at the time of diagnosis [1, 2]. Metastases are mostly found in the liver, lung, adrenals, and bones [1, 2, 4, 7]. Except for the brain, contrast-enhanced CT of the chest, abdomen, and pelvis will cover most of the areas that may have metastatic deposits. The most updated National Comprehensive Cancer Network (NCCN) guidelines propose the use of PET/CT in initial staging when upper gastrointestinal endoscopy, biopsy, and CT scan with and without contrast of the chest and abdomen fail to reveal M1 disease [34].

EUS

EUS has limited value in the assessment of distant metastasis. EUS can only detect distant metastasis if there is direct contact between the involved organ and the EUS probe, as in the retroperitoneum, left lateral segment of the liver, or celiac axis lymph nodes [1, 4, 7].

CT and MRI

Although CT is only 63–74% sensitive, it remains the mainstay for imaging of distant metastasis [4]. Hepatic metastases are visualized as low-density ill-defined lesions. Contrast-enhanced CT imaging during portal venous phase is mostly used for hepatic metastasis [1]. Lesions less than 1 cm are difficult to detect with CT, which may result in false-negative results [5]. Adrenal metastases usually appear as focal adrenal enlargement or an adrenal nodule. Optimized CT, MR imaging, percutaneous FNA, or laparoscopy may be required to confirm the etiology of these lesions [7, 35].

Solitary pulmonary metastases are rare at initial presentation. Solitary pulmonary nodules are more likely to be either benign or synchronous lung malignancies [5]. Therefore, tissue confirmation of solitary pulmonary nodules detected during staging should be considered [4]. Multiple pulmonary metastatic nodules are uncommon at initial presentation, though are seen more at late stages. CT is very sensitive at detecting pulmonary metastasis. Most pulmonary metastases are round, well defined, and noncalcified [1].

Brain metastases are reported in 2–4% of patients presenting with esophageal cancer. They tend to occur in patients with large EGJ adenocarcinomas, which have local invasion or lymph node metastasis [5, 36], and are best detected with optimized CT or brain MRI.

FDG PET

The most common sites for distant metastasis from esophageal cancer are liver, lung, bones, and adrenal glands. Less commonly seen are metastases to the brain, subcutaneous tissues, thyroid gland, skeletal muscles, and pancreas [37]. The pivotal role of FDG PET in esophageal cancer is the detection of distant metastases (Figs. 7.6 and 7.7). As M stage is a major determinant of treatment planning, PET/CT performed at initial workup is becoming the standard of care [1].

Fig. 7.6 Axial fused PET/CT images of the lower thoracic region show the large markedly hypermetabolic esophageal mass, two metastatic pulmonary nodules (one is hypermetabolic marked with arrow), and periesophageal metastatic adenopathy

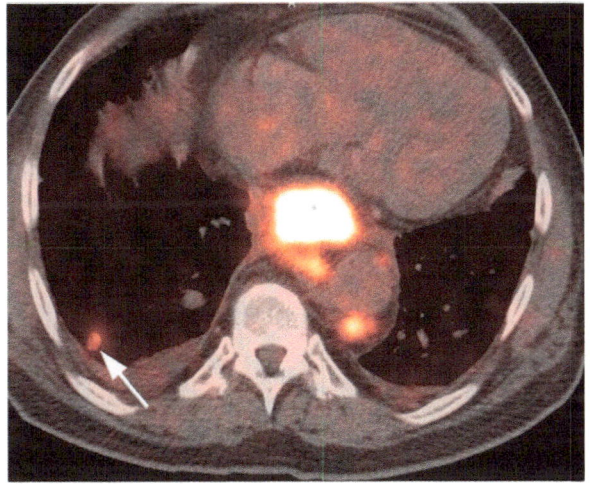

Fig. 7.7 Coronal fused PET/CT image shows hypermetabolic esophageal cancer with multiple periesophageal metastatic adenopathy. There is also left supraclavicular and celiac axis hypermetabolic metastatic lymph nodes (arrows). There is also curvilinear hypermetabolic activity at the right perihepatic region, consistent with subdiaphragmatic metastatic implants

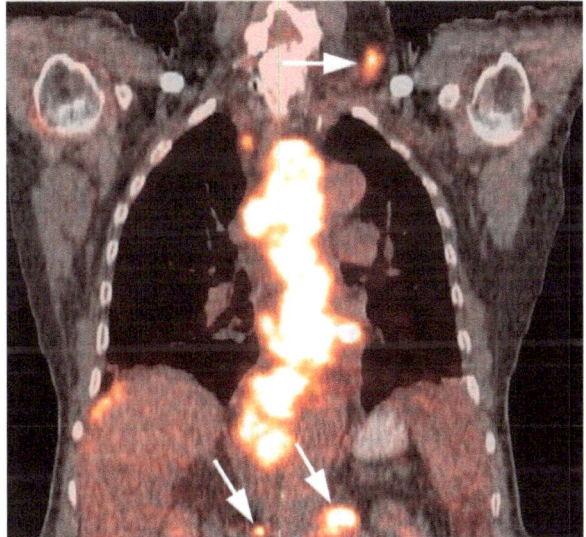

In comparison with other modalities, PET alone is superior to CT in detecting metastatic cancer [1, 2, 5], yet combined PET/CT has lower sensitivity for lesions less than 1 cm. PET/CT detects radiologically occult distant metastases in 10–20% of cases [1, 7, 22]. FDG PET can be cost effective in preventing noncurative surgery by the detection of metastasis that are not identified with conventional imaging [1]. A meta-analysis reported that PET has 71% sensitivity and 93% specificity in the detection of distant metastases in comparison to 52% and 91% for CT, respectively [7, 38]. Disease management strategies may change in up to 38% of cases, by using PET/CT [39, 40].

Co-registered PET/CT has greater sensitivity, specificity, and overall accuracy than PET alone [1]. The combination of PET with CT has diagnostic accuracy of 80–92%. A relative limitation of PET/CT is lower sensitivity for liver metastases, secondary to the use of noncontrast CT by most centers [1]. Magnetic resonance is now considered the most sensitive noninvasive imaging modality for the detection of liver metastasis from gastrointestinal tract malignancies, followed closely by PET/CT in comparison with ultrasonography and CT [41]. Distant lymph node metastases without involvement of locoregional lymph nodes have been reported to occur in 25% of cases [37, 42, 43] (Fig. 7.7).

Therapeutic Response

The same staging modalities used for clinical staging can be used during assessment of therapeutic response.

EUS

EUS is inaccurate in determining T stage after therapy as it cannot distinguish inflammation/fibrosis from cancer; hence overstaging is the most common error [1]. Understaging can also occur secondary to difficulty in detection of residual microscopic disease [1]. Accuracy of EUS for detection of pathologic lymph nodes is also reduced by alterations in the appearance of pathological lymph nodes after therapy and possibly smaller metastatic deposits within the lymph nodes that are difficult to detect by ultrasound [7]. Use of EUS is also limited in some post-therapy conditions, including luminal stenosis and post-radiation esophagitis [1].

CT

Although CT is widely used during staging of esophageal cancer, it has very limited value in the assessment of therapy response as both viable tumor and post-therapy inflammatory changes have similar appearance on CT [1].

FDG PET

The prediction of tumor response early, during the neoadjuvant regimen, is of crucial importance. FDG PET is very useful in this regard. Decrease in FDG uptake early in the process, compared with initial metabolic activity in the primary tumor has been validated as a potential prognostic predictor in several studies [44] (Fig. 7.8).

It is important to remember that patients who have had radiation therapy may demonstrate higher levels of FDG uptake compared to patients receiving only chemotherapy [44]. Metabolic parameters may aid in assessing response to neoadjuvant therapy. Hatt studied SUV and TLG and found that the latter had better sensitivity and specificity for tumor response [45]. A prospective, multicenter study by Palie found that tumor volume, TLG, and maximum SUV are good predictors of poor response to neoadjuvant therapy. Other studies have found that a decrease in

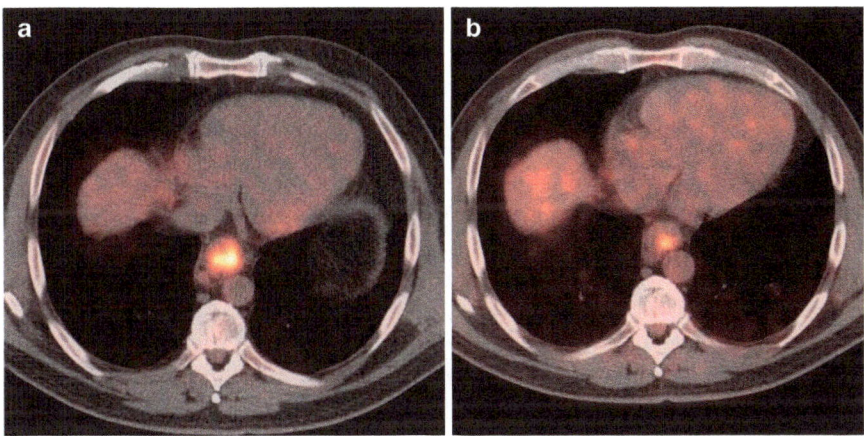

Fig. 7.8 Axial fused PET/CT images before (**a**) and after (**b**) therapy show the marked improvement of FDG activity of the tumor, most consistent with good therapy response

SUVmax of 35–60% between initial staging and after therapy PET/CT correlates with pathologic response [37, 46–49]. PET/CT has been found useful and superior to other modalities in the detection of new interval metastasis after neoadjuvant chemotherapy in 8–17% of cases [37]. Further studies are still needed to define the role of FDG PET in measuring response to therapy.

The NCCN guidelines recommend the use of PET/CT for the assessment of disease response at 5–8 weeks after preoperative or definite chemoradiation before surgery or initiation of postoperative treatment. PET alone is no longer offered in clinical practice. Also, these guidelines emphasize that ulceration caused by radiation therapy is a common false positive finding on PET/CT, therefore its combination with endoscopy may be useful to identify patients with high risk of residual tumor after preoperative chemoradiation [34].

Surveillance and Restaging

CT
The presence of new regional adenopathy or new soft tissue thickening is a CT finding concerning for recurrence [31].

FDG PET
FDG PET has a very good detection rate of recurrence or metastatic disease. It has been shown that FDG PET can provide additional information in up to 27% of cases [31]. One of the shortcomings of FDG PET is the presence of FDG activity with infection or inflammation. Hence, tissue sampling is required when an FDG avid focus is noted that is concerning for recurrence [31].

Treatment Complications

Patients undergoing multimodality therapy are at risk for more acute toxicities. Nonhematologic toxicities including esophagitis, infection, aspiration, and gastro-intestinal or cardiac events can be diagnosed with the combination of clinical/labo-ratory and imaging information (Fig. 7.9) [31].

Anastomotic leakage is the most common surgical complication, with cervical anastomosis having higher risk than distal anastomosis [31]. Fluoroscopic esopha-gography with water-soluble contrast agents is the study of choice [31]. CT evalua-tion by an initial noncontrast study followed with oral administration of a low-osmolar IV contrast material is also used [31]. A recent study by Lantos con-cluded that esophagography had slightly lower sensitivity and substantially higher specificity compared to CT. Combined use of both modalities had 100% sensitivity. Hence, both studies can confidently exclude postoperative leaks [50]. Shoji et al. suggested a positive air bubble sign on CT as an objective and a noninvasive screen-ing method for esophageal leaks [51].

A major surgical challenge is to have an adequate resection without compromis-ing the blood supply for the esophageal conduit. Esophageal conduit necrosis is a rare but a life-threatening complication. A recent study by Lainas et al. suggested that esophageal conduit necrosis after esophagectomy may be due to preexisting celiac axis stenosis, either extrinsic stenosis by the median arcuate artery or intrinsic stenosis by atherosclerosis. Both of these findings can be evaluated by preoperative CT [52].

Late complications include esophageal stricture and perforation, which may be assessed with esophagography. Pulmonary toxicities such as pneumonitis may also be diagnosed with cross-sectional imaging, including CT or PET/CT [31].

Fig. 7.9 Axial CT at lower thoracic level of a patient after esophageal cancer resection and gastric pull through. There are foci of ground glass opacities (arrow), and focal areas of pulmonary nodules (arrow) secondary to aspiration

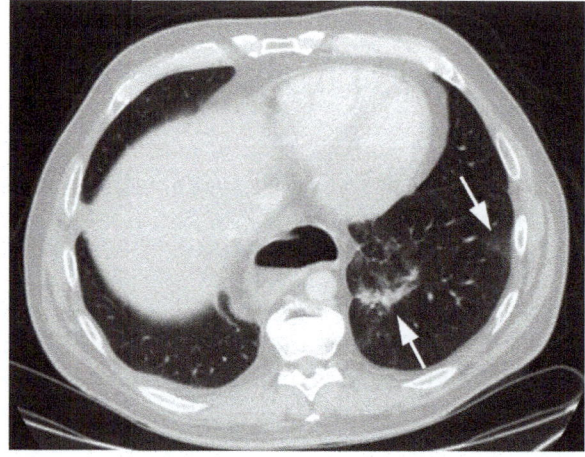

Novel Imaging Modalities for Esophageal Cancer

A recently available hybrid modality (PET/MR) imaging allows the combination of both anatomic and functional information [35]. Lee investigated the role of PET/MR imaging in preoperative staging of esophageal cancer patients and compared MRI with FDG PET, EUS, and CT. In this study, PET/MR showed T staging accuracy comparable to EUS, and higher accuracy than EUS and PET in the prediction of N staging. PET/MR may have substantial potential in the imaging of esophageal cancer [35].

There is ongoing research in nuclear oncology with the development of novel radiotracers. 18F-fluorothymidine (FLT), a nucleoside analogue which is a marker of cell proliferation, has been evaluated as a potential relevant radiotracer in esophageal cancer. Early studies testing the capabilities of 18F-FLT PET for initial T and N staging were not encouraging, as 18F-FLT PET/CT scans showed less uptake in the tumors and more false negative findings [53, 54]. However, several more recent studies have evaluated 18F-FLT for the prediction of tumor response after chemotherapy, suggesting that this radiotracer could perform superiorly to F18-FDG, although more studies are needed to further validate its use [55–57].

Other novel PET radiotracers include 18F-FAMT, which accumulates in tumor cells via the L-type amino-acid transporter 1 (LAT1), which has been found to be associated with cell proliferation and angiogenesis. Suzuki correlated PET parameters with the development of lymph node metastasis in clinically N0 esophageal SCC cancer patients and it was found that elevated uptake correlated with advanced stage and lymph node metastasis. Although more studies are needed to determine the clinical use of F18-FAMT, it represents a potential target for guided therapeutic interventions [58].

CT texture analysis assessing components of the tumor and intratumoral heterogeneity has been studied in preoperative evaluation of esophageal cancer. A recent texture analysis study by Liu et al. showed that texture analysis has great potential in differentiating different T and N stages of esophageal cancer [59].

Machine learning methods have gained use to predict complex biological problems. One of the machine learning models is support vector models (SVMs). A recent study showed that assessment of CT images by using SVMs performed better than CT size criteria in diagnosing lymph node metastases in esophageal cancer before chemotherapy [60].

References

1. Kim TJ, Kim HY, Lee KW, Kim MS. Multimodality assessment of esophageal cancer: preoperative staging and monitoring of response to therapy. Radiographics. 2009;29(2):403–21.
2. Napier KJ, Scheerer M, Misra S. Esophageal cancer: a review of epidemiology, pathogenesis, staging workup and treatment modalities. World J Gastrointest Oncol. 2014;6(5):112–20.
3. American Cancer Socity. Esophageal Cancer Key Statistics; 2017. https://www.cancer.org/cancer/esophagus-cancer/about/key-statistics.html.

4. Shin KE, Lee KS, Choi JY, Kim HK, Shim YM. Esophageal malignancy and staging. Semin Roentgenol. 2013;48(4):344–53.
5. Li Z, Rice TW. Diagnosis and staging of cancer of the esophagus and esophagogastric junction. Surg Clin North Am. 2012;92(5):1105–26.
6. Sonavane S, Watts J Jr, Terry N, Singh SP. Expected and unexpected imaging features after oesophageal cancer treatment. Clin Radiol. 2014;69(8):e358–66.
7. Rice TW. Clinical staging of esophageal carcinoma. CT, EUS, and PET. Chest Surg Clin N Am. 2000;10(3):471–85.
8. Levine MS, Chu P, Furth EE, Rubesin SE, Laufer I, Herlinger H. Carcinoma of the esophagus and esophagogastric junction: sensitivity of radiographic diagnosis. AJR Am J Roentgenol. 1997;168(6):1423–6.
9. Flamen P, Lerut A, Van Cutsem E, De Wever W, Peeters M, Stroobants S, et al. Utility of positron emission tomography for the staging of patients with potentially operable esophageal carcinoma. J Clin Oncol. 2000;18(18):3202–10.
10. Esteves FP, Schuster DM, Halkar RK. Gastrointestinal tract malignancies and positron emission tomography: an overview. Semin Nucl Med. 2006;36(2):169–81.
11. Wallace MB, Nietert PJ, Earle C, Krasna MJ, Hawes RH, Hoffman BJ, et al. An analysis of multiple staging management strategies for carcinoma of the esophagus: computed tomography, endoscopic ultrasound, positron emission tomography, and thoracoscopy/laparoscopy. Ann Thorac Surg. 2002;74(4):1026–32.
12. Rice TW, Patil DT, Blackstone EH. 8th edition AJCC/UICC staging of cancers of the esophagus and esophagogastric junction: application to clinical practice. Ann Cardiothorac Surg. 2017;6(2):119–30.
13. Rice TW, Blackstone EH, Rusch VW. 7th edition of the AJCC cancer staging manual: esophagus and esophagogastric junction. Ann Surg Oncol. 2010;17(7):1721–4.
14. Kelly S, Harris KM, Berry E, Hutton J, Roderick P, Cullingworth J, et al. A systematic review of the staging performance of endoscopic ultrasound in gastro-oesophageal carcinoma. Gut. 2001;49(4):534–9.
15. Foley KG, Morgan C, Roberts SA, Crosby T. Impact of positron emission tomography and endoscopic ultrasound length of disease difference on treatment planning in patients with oesophageal cancer. Clin Oncol. 2017;29(11):760–6.
16. Wang WL, Chiu SY, Lee CT, Tseng CH, Chen CC, Han ML, et al. A training program of a new simplified classification of magnified narrow band imaging for superficial esophageal squamous cell carcinoma. J Gastroenterol Hepatol. 2018;33(6):1248–55.
17. Ulla M, Gentile E, Yeyati EL, Diez ML, Cavadas D, Garcia-Monaco RD, et al. Pneumo-CT assessing response to neoadjuvant therapy in esophageal cancer: imaging-pathological correlation. World J Gastrointest Oncol. 2013;5(12):222–9.
18. Puli SR, Reddy JB, Bechtold ML, Antillon D, Ibdah JA, Antillon MR. Staging accuracy of esophageal cancer by endoscopic ultrasound: a meta-analysis and systematic review. World J Gastroenterol. 2008;14(10):1479–90.
19. Riddell AM, Allum WH, Thompson JN, Wotherspoon AC, Richardson C, Brown G. The appearances of oesophageal carcinoma demonstrated on high-resolution, T2-weighted MRI, with histopathological correlation. Eur Radiol. 2007;17(2):391–9.
20. van Rossum PS, van Hillegersberg R, Lever FM, Lips IM, van Lier AL, Meijer GJ, et al. Imaging strategies in the management of oesophageal cancer: what's the role of MRI? Eur Radiol. 2013;23(7):1753–65.
21. Yasuda S, Raja S, Hubner KF. Application of whole-body positron emission tomography in the imaging of esophageal cancer: report of a case. Surg Today. 1995;25(3):261–4.
22. Karaosmanoglu AD, Blake MA. Applications of PET-CT in patients with esophageal cancer. Diagn Interv Radiol. 2012;18(2):171–82.
23. Kato H, Kuwano H, Nakajima M, Miyazaki T, Yoshikawa M, Ojima H, et al. Comparison between positron emission tomography and computed tomography in the use of the assessment of esophageal carcinoma. Cancer. 2002;94(4):921–8.

24. Foley KG, Fielding P, Lewis WG, Karran A, Chan D, Blake P, et al. Prognostic significance of novel (1)(8)F-FDG PET/CT defined tumour variables in patients with oesophageal cancer. Eur J Radiol. 2014;83(7):1069–73.
25. Pan L, Gu P, Huang G, Xue H, Wu S. Prognostic significance of SUV on PET/CT in patients with esophageal cancer: a systematic review and meta-analysis. Eur J Gastroenterol Hepatol. 2009;21(9):1008–15.
26. Goerres GW, Von Schulthess GK, Hany TF. Positron emission tomography and PET CT of the head and neck: FDG uptake in normal anatomy, in benign lesions, and in changes resulting from treatment. AJR Am J Roentgenol. 2002;179(5):1337–43.
27. Goense L, Meziani J, van Rossum PSN, Wessels FJ, Lam M, van Hillegersberg R, et al. Cervical ultrasonography has no additional value over negative ^{18}F-FDG PET/CT scans for diagnosing cervical lymph node metastases in patients with oesophageal cancer. Eur Radiol. 2018;28(5): 2031–37.
28. Nishimura H, Tanigawa N, Hiramatsu M, Tatsumi Y, Matsuki M, Narabayashi I. Preoperative esophageal cancer staging: magnetic resonance imaging of lymph node with ferumoxtran-10, an ultrasmall superparamagnetic iron oxide. J Am Coll Surg. 2006;202(4):604–11.
29. Alper F, Turkyilmaz A, Kurtcan S, Aydin Y, Onbas O, Acemoglu H, et al. Effectiveness of the STIR turbo spin-echo sequence MR imaging in evaluation of lymphadenopathy in esophageal cancer. Eur J Radiol. 2011;80(3):625–8.
30. Rasanen JV, Sihvo EI, Knuuti MJ, Minn HR, Luostarinen ME, Laippala P, et al. Prospective analysis of accuracy of positron emission tomography, computed tomography, and endoscopic ultrasonography in staging of adenocarcinoma of the esophagus and the esophagogastric junction. Ann Surg Oncol. 2003;10(8):954–60.
31. Godoy MC, Bruzzi JF, Viswanathan C, Truong MT, Guimaraes MD, Hofstetter WL, et al. Multimodality imaging evaluation of esophageal cancer: staging, therapy assessment, and complications. Abdom Imaging. 2013;38(5):974–93.
32. Moon SH, Kim HS, Hyun SH, Choi YS, Zo JI, Shim YM, et al. Prediction of occult lymph node metastasis by metabolic parameters in patients with clinically N0 esophageal squamous cell carcinoma. J Nucl Med. 2014;55(5):743–8.
33. Hsu PK, Lin KH, Wang SJ, Huang CS, Wu YC, Hsu WH. Preoperative positron emission tomography/computed tomography predicts advanced lymph node metastasis in esophageal squamous cell carcinoma patients. World J Surg. 2011;35(6):1321–6.
34. National Comprehensive Cancer Network Guidelines. Esophageal and Esophagogastric Junction Cancers (Version 4.2017); 2017. http://www.nccn.org/professionals/physician_gls/pdf/esophageal.pdf.
35. Lee G, I H, Kim SJ, Jeong YJ, Kim IJ, Pak K, et al. Clinical implication of PET/MR imaging in preoperative esophageal cancer staging: comparison with PET/CT, endoscopic ultrasonography, and CT. J Nucl Med. 2014;55(8):1242–7.
36. Quint LE, Hepburn LM, Francis IR, Whyte RI, Orringer MB. Incidence and distribution of distant metastases from newly diagnosed esophageal carcinoma. Cancer. 1995;76(7):1120–5.
37. Bruzzi JF, Munden RF, Truong MT, Marom EM, Sabloff BS, Gladish GW, et al. PET/CT of esophageal cancer: its role in clinical management. Radiographics. 2007;27(6):1635–52.
38. van Vliet EP, Heijenbrok-Kal MH, Hunink MG, Kuipers EJ, Siersema PD. Staging investigations for oesophageal cancer: a meta-analysis. Br J Cancer. 2008;98(3):547–57.
39. Barber TW, Duong CP, Leong T, Bressel M, Drummond EG, Hicks RJ. 18F-FDG PET/CT has a high impact on patient management and provides powerful prognostic stratification in the primary staging of esophageal cancer: a prospective study with mature survival data. J Nucl Med. 2012;53(6):864–71.
40. Chatterton BE, Ho Shon I, Baldey A, Lenzo N, Patrikeos A, Kelley B, et al. Positron emission tomography changes management and prognostic stratification in patients with oesophageal cancer: results of a multicentre prospective study. Eur J Nucl Med Mol Imaging. 2009;36(3):354–61.

41. Mainenti PP, Mancini M, Mainolfi C, Camera L, Maurea S, Manchia A, et al. Detection of Colo-rectal liver metastases: prospective comparison of contrast enhanced US, multidetector CT, PET/CT, and 1.5 Tesla MR with extracellular and reticulo-endothelial cell specific contrast agents. Abdom Imaging. 2010;35(5):511–21.
42. Akiyama H, Tsurumaru M, Kawamura T, Ono Y. Principles of surgical treatment for carcinoma of the esophagus: analysis of lymph node involvement. Ann Surg. 1981;194(4):438–46.
43. Clark GW, Peters JH, Ireland AP, Ehsan A, Hagen JA, Kiyabu MT, et al. Nodal metastasis and sites of recurrence after en bloc esophagectomy for adenocarcinoma. Ann Thorac Surg. 1994;58(3):646–53; discussion 53-4
44. Omloo JM, van Heijl M, Hoekstra OS, van Berge Henegouwen MI, van Lanschot JJ, Sloof GW. FDG-PET parameters as prognostic factor in esophageal cancer patients: a review. Ann Surg Oncol. 2011;18(12):3338–52.
45. Hatt M, Visvikis D, Pradier O, Cheze-le Rest C. Baseline (1)(8)F-FDG PET image-derived parameters for therapy response prediction in oesophageal cancer. Eur J Nucl Med Mol Imaging. 2011;38(9):1595–606.
46. Brucher BL, Weber W, Bauer M, Fink U, Avril N, Stein HJ, et al. Neoadjuvant therapy of esophageal squamous cell carcinoma: response evaluation by positron emission tomography. Ann Surg. 2001;233(3):300–9.
47. Kato H, Kuwano H, Nakajima M, Miyazaki T, Yoshikawa M, Masuda N, et al. Usefulness of positron emission tomography for assessing the response of neoadjuvant chemoradiotherapy in patients with esophageal cancer. Am J Surg. 2002;184(3):279–83.
48. Kroep JR, Van Groeningen CJ, Cuesta MA, Craanen ME, Hoekstra OS, Comans EF, et al. Positron emission tomography using 2-deoxy-2-[18F]-fluoro-D-glucose for response monitoring in locally advanced gastroesophageal cancer; a comparison of different analytical methods. Mol Imaging Biol. 2003;5(5):337–46.
49. Smith JW, Moreira J, Abood G, Aranha GV, Nagda S, Wagner RH, et al. The influence of (18) flourodeoxyglucose positron emission tomography on the management of gastroesophageal junction carcinoma. Am J Surg. 2009;197(3):308–12.
50. Lantos JE, Levine MS, Rubesin SE, Lau CT, Torigian DA. Comparison between esophagography and chest computed tomography for evaluation of leaks after esophagectomy and gastric pull-through. J Thorac Imaging. 2013;28(2):121–8.
51. Shoji Y, Takeuchi H, Fukuda K, Nakamura R, Wada N, Kawakubo H, et al. Air bubble sign: a new screening method for anastomotic leakage after esophagectomy for esophageal cancer. Ann Surg Oncol. 2018;25(4):1061–8.
52. Lainas P, Fuks D, Gaujoux S, Machroub Z, Fregeville A, Perniceni T, et al. Preoperative imaging and prediction of oesophageal conduit necrosis after oesophagectomy for cancer. Br J Surg. 2017;104(10):1346–54.
53. van Westreenen HL, Cobben DC, Jager PL, van Dullemen HM, Wesseling J, Elsinga PH, et al. Comparison of 18F-FLT PET and 18F-FDG PET in esophageal cancer. J Nucl Med. 2005;46(3):400–4.
54. Han D, Yu J, Zhong X, Fu Z, Mu D, Zhang B, et al. Comparison of the diagnostic value of 3-deoxy-3-18F-fluorothymidine and 18F-fluorodeoxyglucose positron emission tomography/computed tomography in the assessment of regional lymph node in thoracic esophageal squamous cell carcinoma: a pilot study. Dis Esophagus. 2012;25(5):416–26.
55. Park SH, Ryu JS, Oh SJ, Park SI, Kim YH, Jung HY, et al. The feasibility of (18) F-fluorothymidine PET for prediction of tumor response after induction chemotherapy followed by chemoradiotherapy with S-1/oxaliplatin in patients with resectable esophageal cancer. Nucl Med Mol Imaging. 2012;46(1):57–64.
56. Chen H, Li Y, Wu H, Sun L, Lin Q, Zhao L, et al. 3′-Deoxy-3′-[F]-fluorothymidine PET/CT in early determination of prognosis in patients with esophageal squamous cell cancer: comparison with [F]-FDG PET/CT. Strahlenther Onkol. 2015;191(2):141–52.
57. Chao KS. Functional imaging for early prediction of response to chemoradiotherapy: 3′-deoxy-3′-18F-fluorothymidine positron emission tomography--a clinical application model of esophageal cancer. Semin Oncol. 2006;33(6 Suppl 11):S59–63.

58. Suzuki S, Kaira K, Ohshima Y, Ishioka NS, Sohda M, Yokobori T, et al. Biological significance of fluorine-18-alpha-methyltyrosine (FAMT) uptake on PET in patients with oesophageal cancer. Br J Cancer. 2014;110(8):1985–91.
59. Liu S, Zheng H, Pan X, Chen L, Shi M, Guan Y, et al. Texture analysis of CT imaging for assessment of esophageal squamous cancer aggressiveness. J Thorac Dis. 2017;9(11):4724–32.
60. Wang ZL, Zhou ZG, Chen Y, Li XT, Sun YS. Support vector machines model of computed tomography for assessing lymph node metastasis in esophageal cancer with neoadjuvant chemotherapy. J Comput Assist Tomogr. 2017;41(3):455–60.

Role of Endoscopy in the Diagnosis, Staging, and Management of Esophageal Cancer

8

Michelle P. Clermont and Field F. Willingham

Introduction

The incidence of esophageal adenocarcinoma (EAC) has increased approximately 700% since the late 1970s, outpacing the rate of growth of other major epithelial malignancies [1]. Over 10,000 cases are now diagnosed annually in the USA and most patients do not live more than 5 years after diagnosis [2, 3]. Meanwhile, the incidence of esophageal squamous cell carcinoma (SCC) has declined over several decades [1]. While SCC has no known premalignant condition amenable to screening, EAC is preceded by Barrett's esophagus (BE) in a metaplasia-dysplasia-carcinoma sequence. Barrett's esophagus has been a target for screening efforts and eradication via endoscopic approaches in order to detect and prevent progression to EAC. The risk of developing EAC among patients with untreated Barrett's esophagus is approximately 0.4–0.5% per year [4]. Multiple risk factors such as male gender and long-segment Barrett's esophagus increase the risk of progression [5]. The relatively good 5-year prognosis in early-stage disease compared with advanced stages has led to efforts aimed at the early detection of esophageal cancer in Barrett's esophagus [6, 7]. The use of endoscopy for the prevention, diagnosis, and treatment of esophageal cancer continues to evolve.

M. P. Clermont
Department of Medicine, Division of Gastroenterology, University of Pennsylvania Perelman School of Medicine, Philadelphia, PA, USA

F. F. Willingham (✉)
Department of Medicine, Division of Digestive Diseases,
Emory University School of Medicine, Atlanta, GA, USA
e-mail: field.willingham@emoryhealthcare.org

© Springer Nature Switzerland AG 2020
N. F. Saba, B. F. El-Rayes (eds.), *Esophageal Cancer*,
https://doi.org/10.1007/978-3-030-29832-6_8

Screening for Barrett's Esophagus

The relatively low prevalence of Barrett's esophagus among patients with gastro-esophageal reflux disease (GERD), the current lack of reliable methods for identifying high-risk individuals, and the risk and cost associated with upper endoscopy make population-based screening for Barrett's with upper endoscopy imperfect. The American Gastroenterological Association (AGA) in 2011 recommended endoscopic screening for Barrett's esophagus in patients with multiple risk factors for esophageal adenocarcinoma. These risk factors include age greater than or equal to 50 years, male sex, Caucasian race, chronic GERD, presence of a hiatal hernia, elevated body mass index (BMI), and intra-abdominal distribution of body fat (Table 8.1). This recommendation was graded as weak with moderate-quality evidence, underscoring the lack of consensus in this area.

The British Society of Gastroenterology (BSG) in 2014 recommended screening patients with chronic GERD symptoms plus three of the following: age 50 years or greater, Caucasian race, male gender, and obesity (Table 8.1). They suggest that the threshold to screen for BE should be lowered if there is a family history with one first-degree relative with BE or esophageal adenocarcinoma (grade C recommendation) [8]. While current screening efforts focus on patients with GERD symptoms, BE is known to be present in patients without GERD, and up to 57% of patients with esophageal adenocarcinoma never report typical symptoms of GERD [9, 10]. Some studies have shown that the current practice of using endoscopy after 5 years of GERD symptoms may detect only a limited number of patients who are actually at risk for progression to esophageal adenocarcinoma [4, 11]. The American College of Gastroenterology (ACG) in 2016 continues to recommend against screening for Barrett's esophagus in the general population as noted in the 2008 guidelines but has added a focus on screening men with ≥ 5 years of GERD symptoms with two additional risk factors [12]. Screening is less emphasized in women with chronic GERD in the absence of multiple risk factors due to a lower risk of EAC.

A case-control study of 63 patients with esophageal adenocarcinoma found that laryngopharyngeal reflux symptoms, such as asthma, aspiration, and hoarseness, might be more prevalent in those with EAC than typical GERD symptoms. Chronic cough was found to be an independent risk factor for EAC, and some have suggested that it may be helpful for screening purposes in identifying people at risk [13].

The low overall incidence of high-grade dysplasia (HGD) and intramucosal carcinoma (IMC) disfavors population-based screening with conventional endoscopy [4, 14–16]. Efforts are underway to identify screening methods that may be more broadly applicable. Unsedated examinations and non-endoscopic options utilizing cytology or capsule esophagoscopy are being evaluated [17, 18]. A veteran population with or without GERD symptoms was randomized to unsedated transnasal esophagoscopy (TNE) or capsule esophagoscopy (ECE) to evaluate BE screening and 12.6% of those randomized to TNE crossed the minimal clinically important threshold for overall procedure tolerability as opposed to none randomized to ECE ($p = 0.001$) [19]. A study involving 96 patients assessing the accuracy and feasibility of unsedated exams with disposable endoscopes compared to conventional upper

Table 8.1 Screening and surveillance endoscopy

	AGA 2011 [5]	ASGE 2012 [119]	BSG 2014 [8]	ACG 2016 [12]	ESGE 2017 [33]
Screening endoscopy	White male, age >50 years, GERD, hiatal hernia, obesity	GERD >5 years, white, male, age >50 years, family history of BE or EAC	Chronic GERD symptoms +3: (50 years or older, white, male, obese). Screening threshold lower for family history of BE or EAC in first degree relative	Men with >5 years and/or frequent (weekly or more) symptoms of GERD (heartburn or acid regurgitation) and two or more risk factors for BE or EAC. RF: age >50 years, Caucasian race, central obesity (waist circumference >102 cm or waist-hip ratio >0.9), current or past history of smoking, confirmed family history of BE or EAC (in first-degree relative)	>5 years GERD, multiple risk factors (age ≥50 years, white race, male sex, obesity, first-degree relative with BE or EAC
Surveillance endoscopy					
No dysplasia on 2 exams	3–5-year interval	3-year interval	2–3 years if max segment length ≥3 cm; 3–5 years if max length <3 cm	3–5-year interval Repeat in 1–2 years if suspected BE but no dysplasia detected	≥1 cm < 3 cm: 5-year interval - ≥3 and <10 cm 3-year interval ≥10 cm: Refer to BE expert center
LGD	Every 6–12 months	Repeat within 6 months, then every 12 months. Consider ablation	Every 6 months	Every 12 months	Every 6 months until no dysplasia and then every 1 year
HGD surveillance	Every 3 months if no eradication therapy	Endoscopic ablation	Multidisciplinary team discussion. Typically endoscopic ablation	Endoscopic management	Every 3 months if repeat biopsy is negative for dysplasia. Treat with RFA if HGD on repeat

ACG American College of Gastroenterology, AGA American Gastroenterological Association, BSG British Society of Gastroenterology, ASGE American Society for Gastrointestinal Endoscopy, ESGE European Society of Gastrointestinal Endoscopy, GERD gastroesophageal reflux disease, BE Barrett's esophagus, EAC esophageal adenocarcinoma, LGD low-grade dysplasia, HGD high-grade dysplasia, EMR esophageal mucosal resection, APC argon plasma coagulation, PDT photo-dynamic therapy, RF radiofrequency ablation endoscopy found a moderate level of diagnostic agreement between the two modalities, with Kappa coefficients of 0.409 for erosive GERD and 0.617 for Barrett's esophagus [20]. The procedure was well tolerated, fast, and considered safe. In a study of 121 patients undergoing conventional endoscopy and unsedated small-caliber endoscopy, 71% indicated that they would prefer to have unsedated small-caliber endoscopy performed [17]. In this study, BE was found in 26% of the population undergoing conventional endoscopy and in 30% of those undergoing unsedated endoscopy. The level of diagnostic agreement was moderate with a Kappa of 0.591. An ingestible esophageal sampling device coupled with immuno-cytochemistry for trefoil factor 3 is being studied as a non-endoscopic screening modality for BE. A study with 504 patients found a sensitivity of 90% and specificity of 93.5% for identifying Barrett's 2 cm or longer when compared to conventional upper endoscopy [21]. A study in 2015 attempted to determine whether a minimally invasive cell sampling device, the Cytosponge, coupled with immunohistochemical staining for the biomarker Trefoil Factor 3 (TFF3), may be able to select patients who need endoscopy for BE screening. The study involved 11 UK hospitals with 1110 patients and found that 93.9% successfully swallowed the Cytosponge without any serious adverse events. The Cytosponge was also favorably rated compared to upper endoscopy ($p < 0.001$). The test sensitivity was found to be 79.9% (95% CI 76.4%–83.0%) which increased to 87.2% (95% CI 83.0%–90.6%) in patients with ≥3 cm of circumferential BE. The specificity for diagnosing BE was 92.4% (95% CI 89.5%–94.7%) [22].

Surveillance

The rate of progression to cancer in non-dysplastic BE was initially thought to be close to 1% per year in small studies [23]; however, subsequent studies have suggested a rate of progression to cancer as low as 0.12% per year [24]. The ACG and AGA estimate the likely rate of progression to cancer to be around 0.2–0.5% per year [5, 12].

The goal of endoscopic surveillance in Barrett's esophagus is to detect dysplasia, especially HGD and IMC, which can be treated through endoscopic measures before progression to invasive adenocarcinoma or metastatic disease occurs. The AGA recommends using high-resolution endoscopes (>850,000 pixels) when examining BE. The availability of this technology has allowed endoscopists to better identify areas of concern within the Barrett's epithelium and to improve biopsy targeting of suspicious lesions. After obtaining targeted biopsies, 4-quadrant biopsies are taken every 1–2 cm for patients with non-dysplastic BE and every 1 cm for patients with dysplastic BE (whether high grade or low grade). This protocol has become the standard of care though questions arise regarding the time and cost involved with the extensive sampling and subsequent interpretation. Some research has suggested that large-capacity or jumbo biopsy forceps may also increase the amount of tissue acquired and the detection of dysplasia [25]. Use of a systematic protocol for biopsies has been shown to be more effective in detecting BE and dysplasia in BE [26]. The presence of dysplasia should be confirmed by two expert pathologists [5]. Surveillance endoscopy for BE is performed based on the highest degree of dysplasia present. If no dysplasia is identified initially, a second endoscopy with protocol-based biopsies as above should be performed within 1 year. Subsequent surveillance endoscopy should be performed every 3 years for non-dysplastic Barrett's esophagus (Table 8.1) [27].

When BE is identified, control of acid reflux is indicated. Reduction of inflammation with a proton pump inhibitor (PPI) may improve visual recognition of a lesion or nodule on surveillance endoscopy and could theoretically interfere with carcinogenesis [27]. Biopsies from each segment of BE should be submitted to pathology in separate containers to better focus future treatment in areas of concern if dysplasia is discovered.

BE is classified endoscopically according to the Prague classification, using C for the circumferential segment and M for the maximal length of involvement [28]. The length of circumferential Barrett's from the gastroesophageal (GE) junction is recorded, as is the length of the maximal extent of Barrett's extending proximally from the lower esophageal sphincter. There is good interobserver agreement in using these criteria [12, 28], and the approach provides a clear method of communicating the extent of the Barrett's involvement.

If low-grade dysplasia (LGD) is identified, another endoscopy should be performed within 6 months to confirm the degree of dysplasia. Surveillance endoscopy should then be performed every year until no dysplasia is identified on two consecutive exams (Table 8.1) [27]. Recent data have suggested a benefit with radiofrequency ablation (RFA) for low-grade BE, and this practice is becoming more established [29, 30]. The current approach for BE with high-grade dysplasia is to treat with RFA for flat Barrett's esophagus with high-grade dysplasia. Other options including esophagectomy and continued surveillance with upper endoscopy every 3 months may be considered in some circumstances. Endoscopic mucosal resection should be performed for areas of nodularity and mucosal irregularity prior to initiating RFA [31, 32].

The BSG has several similarities in its surveillance guidelines compared to those of the AGA and ACG (Table 8.1). They recommend surveillance every 2–3 years for non-dysplastic BE (ND-BE) if the maximum segment length is greater than or equal to 3 cm and 3–5 years if the maximum segment length is less than 3 cm. They also recommend surveillance with endoscopy every 6 months if LGD is discovered until two consecutive exams show non-dysplastic BE. When HGD or carcinoma is discovered, they recommend discussion with the patient and a multidisciplinary team (MDT) determination for surveillance intervals and treatment. The MDT should include an interventional endoscopist, gastrointestinal pathologist, radiologist, and surgeon. This team should consider factors such as comorbidities, nutritional status, patient preference, and staging. They suggest an outpatient discussion regarding the morbidity and mortality related to the potential treatment options, long-term survival, and quality of life [8].

The European Society of Gastrointestinal Endoscopy (ESGE) in 2017 recommends surveillance depending on the size of non-dysplastic BE lesion discovered:

5-year interval for ≥1 cm <3 cm disease, 3-year interval for ≥3 and <10 cm disease, and disease ≥10 cm requiring referral to a BE expert center. For LGD they recommend surveillance every 6 months until no more dysplasia is found and then every 1 year thereafter. For HGD they recommend surveillance every 3 months if repeat biopsy is negative for dysplasia and to treat with RFA if HGD is found on repeat endoscopy [33].

A study from the Netherlands Cancer Registry compared patients participating in a surveillance program for BE before EAC diagnosis with those not participating in such a program between 1999 and 2009 [1]. Two-year and five-year mortality rates were lower in patients undergoing adequate surveillance (adjusted hazard ratio (HR) = 0.79, 95% confidence interval (CI) = 0.64–0.92) when compared with patients with a prior BE diagnosis who were not participating. This study suggested that there is a mortality reduction from EAC if adequate surveillance for BE is performed.

There are many novel and advanced imaging modalities being incorporated into surveillance endoscopy, including narrow band imaging, confocal laser endomicroscopy, and optical coherence tomography. The technologies might improve targeting and detection. While early studies suggest utility, these advanced imaging modalities are currently being studied primarily in specialty centers and academic institutions. Broader adoption may await standardized diagnostic criteria for differentiating ND-BE, LGD, and HGD [34].

Endoscopic Treatment of Gastroesophageal Reflux Disease

Gastroesophageal reflux disease (GERD) has been implicated in the development of BE, and multiple endoscopic approaches have been studied to control GERD. Some trials have been disappointing and thus far no one endoscopic modality has emerged as a standard. One device involves the use of radiofrequency energy delivered through a catheter equipped with a flexible balloon-basket assembly with four electrode needle sheaths [35]. Radiofrequency energy is delivered at varying levels from the lower esophageal sphincter to the gastric cardia. This procedure was approved by the FDA in 2000 [36]. The endoscopic treatment is performed with sedation and is typically an outpatient procedure [37]. The procedure may lead to collagen deposition at the gastroesophageal junction (GEJ) and may increase lower esophageal sphincter (LES) pressure. It is thought that the procedure also has neuromodulatory effects from selective neurolysis of vagal afferents leading to reduced transient LES relaxations. The ablation may also decrease the perception of heartburn pain due to the influence on sensory nerves as well as reduce reflux [38–40].

Another device involves an endoluminal gastroplication with suture placement at the LES for reduction of symptoms. It was also approved by the FDA in 2000 [41]. Its function is to mechanically restore a barrier against reflux. There is some data suggesting that there is a decrease in esophageal sensitivity to acid after placement of the sutures [37, 42, 43]. Other endoscopic gastroplication devices creating layered full thickness plications of the wall of the cardia have been described [44].

Another endoscopic anti-reflux device creates a transoral incisionless esophago-gastric fundoplication (TIF). It creates an anterior partial fundoplication by attaching the fundus of the stomach to the anterior and left lateral wall of the distal esophagus. Patients with moderate to severe GERD or those who are partially responsive to PPIs may benefit from treatment. Contraindications include BMI greater than 35 kg/m^2, Barrett's esophagus, esophageal varices, hiatal hernia greater than 2 cm, and major connective tissue disorders [45, 46].

A non-absorbable ethylene-vinyl-alcohol polymer which was injected into the musculature or deep submucosa of the LES where it solidified into a sponge-like implant to increase the LES pressure was previously described [47–49]. The device was voluntarily recalled in 2005 due to major reported side effects.

In summary, some data suggest that radiofrequency energy produces an improvement in GERD symptoms and quality of life with negligible morbidity [50–52], and that this approach has a good safety profile and low complication rate (<0.07% by 2006) [53]. There continues to be active development in plicating devices for the endoscopic treatment of GERD. Other systematic reviews have reviewed endoluminal therapies for the treatment of gastroesophageal reflux [54]. Especially in the presence of a large hiatal hernia, laparoscopic nissen fundoplication remains a very effective approach.

Diagnosis of Barrett's Esophagus and Esophageal Adenocarcinoma

Upper Endoscopy for Tissue Diagnosis

The standard approach for the diagnosis of esophageal adenocarcinoma and Barrett's esophagus involves visually directed biopsied obtained at an upper endoscopy. For Barrett's esophagus, the Seattle protocol involves 4-quadrant biopsies every 1–2 cm under white light endoscopy with a goal of detecting dysplasia [55]. The BSG Guidelines published in 2014 recommend a 2 cm biopsy interval protocol in addition to the sampling of any visible lesions (BSG Grade B). They state that adherence to this method is variable (10–79%), with lower adherence for longer segments. Lower adherence may contribute to less dysplasia detection [56–58].

To establish the diagnosis of BE, endoscopic and histologic criteria must be met. Endoscopic criteria include displacement of the Z-line (the squamocolumnar junction) proximal to the GEJ, identified by the pinch of the lower esophageal sphincter. In BE, salmon-colored Barrett's mucosa extends proximally and is distinguished from the pale, glossy appearing squamous mucosa [59]. Pathologic criteria include the presence of intestinal metaplasia with goblet cells in the mucosa. Because of the implications for management, the diagnosis of dysplasia or adenocarcinoma should be confirmed by two expert histopathologists [8]. However, even experienced gastrointestinal pathologists may disagree on a diagnosis of HGD and intramucosal adenocarcinoma [60]. Nodularity and mucosal irregularity within the Barrett's epithelium are more likely to contain dysplasia or carcinoma and should be targeted with focal biopsy or removed with endoscopic mucosal resection (EMR). Flat and occult lesions may be easier to detect with specialized modalities such as narrow band imaging [55].

Advanced Modalities to Improve Detection

Narrow Band Imaging

Narrow band imaging (NBI) is a high-resolution endoscopic technique that enhances the imaging of the fine structure of the mucosal surface without requiring the instillation of staining agents. It involves the use of selective wavelengths of light [55]. The depth of penetration of light directly correlates to its wavelength, and increased depth of light penetration leads to a similar increase in wavelength of visible light. For instance, the blue light used in NBI allows optimal superficial imaging [61], while red light has longer wavelengths and penetrates deeper. The blue light (415 nm) and green light (540 nm) of NBI are absorbed by hemoglobin and demonstrate superficial vasculature [62]. NBI may be preferred in some settings to chromoendoscopy, which involves instillation of a dye such as methylene blue to stain the mucosa in the gastrointestinal tract for enhanced visualization. The dye in chromoendoscopy requires formulation and attention to application and may not distribute evenly over the mucosa.

A meta-analysis of eight studies including 446 patients and 2194 lesions demonstrated that the sensitivity and specificity for detecting HGD with NBI with magnification were 96% and 94%, respectively. The sensitivity for IMC was 95% and the specificity was 65% [63]. A randomized crossover trial of 123 patients showed that NBI without magnification identified a higher proportion of patients with dysplasia compared to white light (30% vs. 21% with $p = 0.0001$) [64]. A similar number of patients found to have IMC were discovered with the use of fewer biopsies using NBI compared to white light (3.6 vs. 7.6 with $p = 0.0001$). However, interobserver agreement regarding interpretation of NBI images of IMC and dysplasia between expert and nonexpert endoscopists may be low [65–67]. NBI does not increase cost or add any significant risk and requires a negligible amount of time and is therefore often considered a standard part of the endoscopic examination in Barrett's esophagus.

Confocal Laser Endomicroscopy

Confocal laser endomicroscopy (CLE) uses a low-power laser to illuminate tissue and detects the reflected fluorescent light. The laser is directed at a certain depth and light is reflected back through a very thin focal plane, refocused, and passed through the confocal aperture which enhances spatial resolution. Scanning is performed in both the horizontal and vertical planes and an in vivo microscopic image of biological tissue is produced. White-light endoscopy and CLE are performed together with images displaying simultaneously. It provides gray-scale imaging of tissue microstructures at or near the level of histopathology. These images may be at 1000-fold magnification [68]. An endoscope-based system (eCLE) (Optiscan Pty., Ltd.,

Notting Hill, Australia; Pentax) for CLE is no longer on the market. The probe-based system (pCLE) passed through the working channel of the endoscope is in use (Cellvizio; Mauna Kea Technologies, Paris, France) [55].

One study using the Mainz criteria (confocal Barrett's classification system) demonstrated a sensitivity and specificity of 98% and 94% for BE and 93% and 94% for BE-associated dysplasia, respectively, in predicting in vivo histology [69]. Strong inter-observer and intra-observer agreement was reported using this classification system (kappa 0.84 and 0.89, respectively). A randomized controlled study involving 192 patients with BE compared high-definition white-light endoscopy (HD-WLE) with random biopsies to endoscopy plus eCLE with targeted biopsies. In this study, the combination of HD-WLE and eCLE increased the diagnostic yield of biopsies for neoplasia (22% vs. 6%) and significantly lowered the number of biopsies required [70]. A multicenter study of 101 patients suggested that adding pCLE to HD-WLE significantly improved the detection of neoplasia; sensitivity and specificity with HD-WLE alone were 34.2% and 92.7%, respectively, compared to 68.3% and 87.8% with combined pCLE and HD-WLE ($p = 0.002$ and $p < 0.001$) [71]. Another smaller study did not show as promising results with 68 patients in three centers when assessing pCLE vs. WLE. Specificity and negative predictive value were low at 12% and 18%, respectively [72]. A recent meta-analysis comparing NBI and CLE for detecting neoplasia in BE suggested that CLE significantly increased the per-lesion detection rate for esophageal neoplasia, HGD, and EAC in BE patients. Of the five studies including 251 patients, the pooled additional detection rate (ADR) of CLE for per-lesion detection of neoplasia was 19.3% (95% CI: 0.05–0.33, $I^2 = 74.6\%$). The pooled sensitivity of NBI was not significantly lower than that of CLE and the pooled specificities were similar [73]. While CLE offers the promise of real-time histology, caveats include the fluorescein administration, cost, small field of view, and learning curve. Further investigation may better define the role for the technology [55].

Optical Coherence Tomography

Optical coherence tomography (OCT) is similar to ultrasound technology but uses light waves in place of sound. It creates a cross-sectional image of tissue using infrared light by penetrating up to 3 mm in depth using a catheter through a standard endoscope. It does not require the administration of fluorescein. The intensity of the back-scattering of light creates cross-sectional and 3-dimensional images of tissue microstructures. The images are similar to coarse black and white histopathology. OCT does not require contact with esophageal tissue and can visualize the epithelium, basement membrane, vasculature, and lamina propria. Nuclear dysplasia cannot be observed [74]. A prospective study involving 33 patients with BE demonstrated the accuracy in the detection of dysplasia in BE. The sensitivity and specificity of OCT for detecting dysplasia were 68% and 82% [75], respectively, and the diagnostic accuracy for the four endoscopists involved ranged from 56 to 98%. Computer-aided diagnosis (CAD) algorithms might increase accuracy of detection of dysplasia and metaplasia. A recent study used histology as a reference standard and developed a CAD algorithm with a sensitivity of 82%, specificity of 74%, and accuracy of 83% for detecting dysplasia in BE [76]. OCT is not currently widely available [77].

A study assessing the presence of dysplasia in BE looked at 177 biopsy-correlated images to evaluate a novel dysplasia index using OCT image characteristics of IMC and HGD in Barrett's esophagus. The sensitivity and specificity rates for diagnosing HGD/adenocarcinoma were 83% and 75%, respectively. There was significant correlation between diagnoses of IMC/HGD by histopathology and scores for the image features including dysplasia, surface maturation, and gland architecture [78].

Endoscopic Mucosal Resection for Diagnosis

Endoscopic mucosal resection (EMR) is recommended for patients with Barrett's esophagus with nodules, raised lesions, or mucosal irregularity. With EMR, a specialized cap is affixed to the end of an endoscope, and tissue is suctioned into the cap. A band is deployed at the base to create a pseudopolyp of tissue. The tissue is then removed using snare electrocautery. This technique allows the removal of an approximately 1 cm area of mucosa and a portion of the underlying submucosa for histologic examination. Repeated contiguous EMR may be performed to resect a larger area of tissue (piecemeal EMR). EMR provides a much larger tissue specimen for examination by pathologists than traditional forceps biopsy. It is more likely to detect cancer or dysplasia, and it allows pathologists to define the precise depth of invasion in early cancers for staging [59]. The technology was originally developed as a diagnostic procedure in the 1980s and has now evolved into an effective therapeutic modality as well [6].

In a retrospective analysis involving 35 patients with BE undergoing both EMR and mucosal tissue biopsy, 63% of specimens were discordant [79]. Fifty-three percent of biopsy results were upstaged with EMR, and the most common change was an upstaging to invasive adenocarcinoma. Approximately 10% of biopsy specimens were downstaged via examination of EMR specimens. Of the 13 cases of invasive adenocarcinoma discovered through EMR, 92% were upstaged, leading to management change in 34% of cases. Another study demonstrated that EMR changed the grade or T-stage in 48% of patients when compared to traditional biopsies. EMR has also been employed in eliminating the affected Barrett's segment in 94% of cases and has been shown to reduce the need for esophagectomy [80]. EMR is a critical component in the accurate staging and proper management of BE-related lesions (Figs. 8.1 and 8.2).

EMR may also help to diagnose invasive squamous cell carcinoma. In one study, 51 patients diagnosed with high-grade intraepithelial squamous neoplasia upon biopsy after endoscopic iodine staining were evaluated with EMR for comparison of results [81]. Histologic examination of EMR specimens showed that 23.5% (12/51) had tumor invasion of the lamina propria and 7.8% (4/51) had muscularis mucosa invasion. The other 68.6% (35/51) had confirmed high-grade intraepithelial squamous neoplasia. Follow-up was a median of 23 months with two recurrences both needing a second EMR. Per 2016 ACG guidelines, patients with LGD and HGD should have EMR performed if mucosal abnormalities are present [12].

Staging

Endoscopic Ultrasound for Locoregional Staging

Endoscopic ultrasound (EUS) is the procedure of choice to establish the depth of invasion and lymph node (LN) status and is the most accurate tool for the TNM staging of esophageal neoplasia [82]. EUS is preceded by a careful upper endoscopic examination which provides information about the location of the disease, the extent of the background Barrett's epithelium, and also may reveal features such as gastric extension and the presence of a hiatal hernia. EUS establishes the T-stage by visualizing the wall layers and defining the depth of invasion. EUS does not visualize nuclear and cellular changes [83], and with early-stage N0 disease, an EMR may be performed for pathologic examination to establish the precise T-stage, grade, and histopathologic features such as lymphovascular invasion. EUS may not be required for HGD and small intramucosal tumors before endoscopic or surgical treatment [55].

The main use of EUS in Barrett's-related disease has been the detection of invasive tumors and the presence of lymph node metastases (LNM). This can allow ablative therapy in those with disease limited to the mucosa and select submucosal

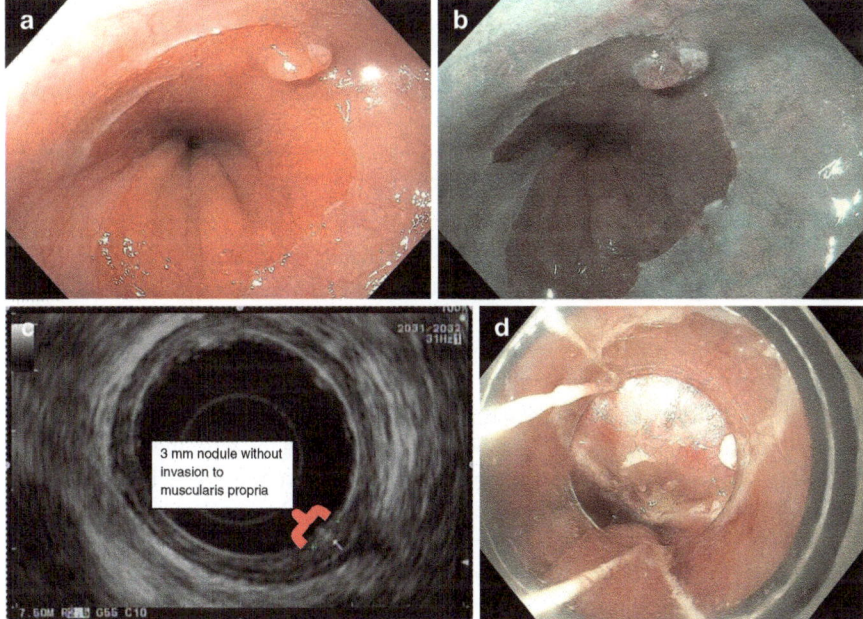

Fig. 8.1 Endoscopic staging of T1a esophageal adenocarcinoma. (**a**) 3 mm nodule at Z-line. (**b**) The same lesion visualized under narrow band imaging. (**c**) Endoscopic ultrasound showing the lesion limited to the mucosa. (**d**) Endoscopic mucosal resection (EMR) of the lesion. The pathology results revealed intramucosal adenocarcinoma with 4 mm negative margins. In this case the EMR was therapeutic as well as diagnostic

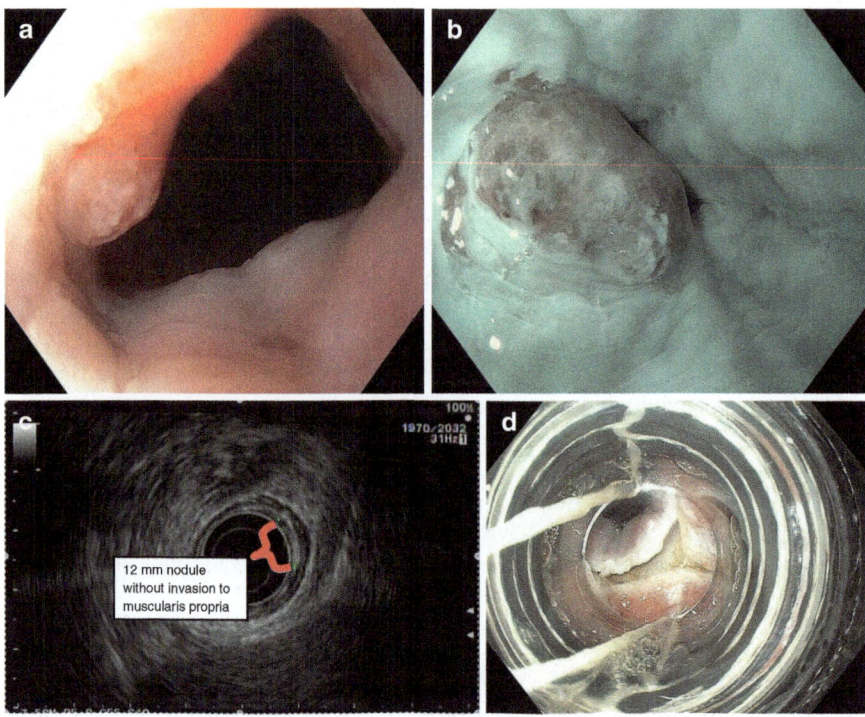

Fig. 8.2 Endoscopic staging of T1b esophageal adenocarcinoma. (**a**) 12 mm nodular mass at Z-line. (**b**) The same lesion visualized under narrow band imaging. (**c**) Endoscopic ultrasound showing the lesion not invading the muscularis propria. For this reason, endoscopic mucosal resection was indicated for staging. (**d**) Endoscopic mucosal resection of the lesion

tumors without malignant-appearing LNs [83]. Many studies show that when EUS is inaccurate it tends to overstage more often than understage, especially in superficial Barrett's neoplasms [84, 85]. In a study involving 125 patients with esophageal carcinoma (86% with adenocarcinoma), EUS was 80% sensitive for determining nodal metastasis compared to 40% for CT ($p < 0.001$). The diagnostic accuracy was 81% with EUS compared to 61% with CT ($p = <0.001$) [86].

Miniprobe EUS utilizes a slim catheter introduced via the working channel of an endoscope to provide high-resolution radial echoendosonographic images over a shorter depth of penetration. It can be used to examine the esophageal wall even in situations of stenosis. In a study involving 143 patients with esophageal carcinoma, 112 having EAC, 78% of patients were accurately staged and would have been assigned to the appropriate therapy group, while 11% were overstaged and would have been overtreated, and 11% were understaged and would have been undertreated using miniprobe EUS to differentiate locally advanced from limited cancer [87].

EUS is accurate in differentiating T1 and T2 lesions and superior to CT for lymph node staging according to a prospective trial with 100 patients with early Barrett's-related carcinoma [87]. The T-stage diagnosed with CT was T1 or less in every patient. Using EUS, the T-stage was T1 in 92% of cases and >T1 in 8%. Significantly more LNs were found with EUS compared to CT (28 vs. 19), and the sensitivity of CT for N-staging was low compared with EUS (38% vs. 7%) [87]. In another study involving 48 patients with 8 having submucosal invasion, EUS provided accurate staging in 41/48 patients (85%) with only one patient overstaged and 6 patients understaged compared to the histologic diagnosis [88].

In another study involving 33 patients with adenocarcinoma, 21 with squamous cell carcinoma, and 1 with lymphoepithelial-like carcinoma, 86% of the 40 T1 m lesions on EUS were confirmed on pathology. Of the 33 T1sm lesions diagnosed on EUS, 66% were confirmed as T1sm. The accuracy of EUS in evaluation of LNM was 71% with negative predictive value of 84%. The accuracy by histological type was 70% for adenocarcinoma and 81% for squamous cell carcinoma, which was not found to be statistically significant [89].

Early detection of SCC is also very important as finding and treating these lesions can lead to a 5-year survival rate of more than 90% after endoscopic or surgical management [90]. EUS is considered to be the best option for staging esophageal SCC. A study showed that the accuracy of EUS for staging T1a lesions (mucosal lamina propria and muscularis mucosa infiltration) and T1b (submucosal infiltration) lesions was 70.8% (51/72) with a sensitivity of 74.3%. Multivariate analysis suggested that the accuracy of EUS was related to the length of the lesion ($p = 0.029$) [91].

A more recent study investigated the use of EUS and computed tomography-positron emission tomography (CT-PET) in relation to survival in esophageal cancer. In Kaplan-Meier analyses, patients who had EUS or EUS + CT-PET had improved survival for all stages compared with no EUS or CT-PET except in stage 0 disease. EUS increased the likelihood of receiving endoscopic therapies, esophagectomy, and chemoradiation. Multivariable Cox proportional hazards models demonstrated that receiving EUS was a predictor for improved 1-year (HR 0.49, 95% CI 0.39–0.59, $p < 0.0001$), 3-year (HR 0.57, 95% CI 0.48–0.66, $p < 0.0001$), and 5-year (HR 0.59, 95% CI 0.50–0.68) survival [92].

Endoscopic Treatment of Early Esophageal Cancer

Traditional therapy for early-stage esophageal cancer and BE with HGD had been esophagectomy with lymph node dissection. However, esophagectomy carries significant morbidity, ranging from 20 to 50% [93], and may have lifelong quality of life implications. In addition, the mortality from esophagectomy ranges from 2 to 9% [93–95]. Definitive endoscopic therapy with EMR of malignancy followed by subsequent RFA of residual BE has been increasingly utilized in BE with HGD as well as early-stage esophageal cancer, defined as Tis, T1a, and T1b tumors.

Endoscopic Mucosal Resection as Therapy for Intramucosal Adenocarcinoma

As discussed above, endoscopic mucosal resection (EMR) should be performed for diagnostic purposes in areas within BE with concerning features such as nodularity or mucosal irregularity. In these cases, it may provide diagnostic information (precise T-stage, degree of differentiation, margins, presence or absence of lymphovascular invasion). The precise depth of tumor invasion may further refine treatment allocation. EMR may also be therapeutic in select cases of HGD, Tis, T1a, and certain T1b tumors, as it allows resection of the superficial layers from the submucosa (Fig. 8.1).

The efficacy and safety of endoscopic therapy with EMR in Tis and T1a lesions has been demonstrated [96]. Longer-term mortality outcomes for early-stage cancers have been similar between endoscopic therapy and esophagectomy [97–100]. Prospective studies have demonstrated complete oncologic eradication and low mortality with endoscopic therapy for Tis and T1a lesions [101–105]. The National Comprehensive Cancer Network (NCCN) recommends endoscopic resection of Tis and T1a esophageal adenocarcinoma followed by RFA as the preferred therapy. A recent study also demonstrated excellent outcomes with endoscopic therapy in highly selected cases with T1b adenocarcinoma limited to the superficial-most third of the submucosa (T1b sm1 lesions), though this approach continues to be debated [106].

Patient selection remains the critical question when deciding between endoscopic resection and esophagectomy for early-stage tumors. Since a decision to pursue endoscopic therapy over esophagectomy implies foregoing lymph node dissection, patient selection must be aimed at identifying patients at low risk for nodal metastasis. The risk of nodal metastasis and thereby the risk of incomplete oncologic outcome can be weighed against the risk of surgical mortality in selecting a treatment modality [5, 106].

A 2012 review of 70 studies and 1874 patients with surgical pathology showed no nodal metastasis in 524 patients with HGD and 26 of 1350 patients with intramucosal carcinoma, representing a 1.93% incidence of nodal metastasis in this group. More recently, an analysis of 715 patients with early-stage esophageal adenocarcinoma undergoing esophagectomy in the Surveillance, Epidemiology and End Results (SEER) database of the National Cancer Institute helped to stratify patients by risk of nodal metastasis according to tumor size and degree of differentiation. There were no cases of nodal metastasis among Tis cases. Among 323 T1a cases, 6.8% had nodal metastasis. The incidence was 5.2% among low-grade tumors, 2.3% among tumors smaller than 2 cm in diameter, and 1.7% among tumors that were both low grade and smaller than 2 cm. Among 353 T1b cases, 18.1% had nodal metastasis, with an incidence of 8.6% for low-grade tumors smaller than 2 cm and 3.0% for low-grade tumors smaller than 1 cm [107].

Other than depth of invasion, size, and histologic grade, lymphovascular invasion has been identified as a risk factor for nodal metastasis. Tumors with lymphovascular invasion are typically considered for esophagectomy due to the higher risk of nodal metastasis.

In a retrospective study involving 62 patients with superficial esophageal adenocarcinoma, there was a local recurrence in 14 of 64 patients, 3–36 months after EMR. Larger diameters were most commonly associated with recurrence ($p = 0.01$) [108]. Typically, a local recurrence is managed with repeat EMR. A prospective study of EMR in patients with either early esophageal adenocarcinoma or HGD in Barrett's esophagus showed promising results for use of EMR in lower risk disease. Complete local remission was achieved in 97% of a group of 35 patients with "low-risk" disease, including macroscopic types I, IIa, IIB, IIc, lesion diameter up to 20 mm, mucosal lesion, histologic grades G1 and G2, and/or HGD. EMR may be a less invasive option for highly selected early cancers [96].

A study of 176 patients treated for mucosal EAC (T1a) with EMR or surgery had similar cumulative mortality (17%) with either method. Treatment modality was not a significant predictor of survival on multivariable analysis. Recurrent EAC was detected in 12% of patients treated endoscopically and all of the recurrences were successfully re-treated endoscopically [91]. In a study involving 114 patients with mucosal EAC treated surgically or endoscopically, complete remission (CR) was achieved in all patients except for one in the EMR group who died from other causes before CR could be achieved. Complications from surgery were found in 32% of patients with 0% major complications found in the EMR group ($p < 0.001$). There was a higher recurrence rate in patients who underwent EMR with one patient having local recurrence and four with metachronous neoplasia. Repeat endoscopic treatment was possible in all patients [109].

Another study involved the role of EMR in curing esophageal adenocarcinoma. The lesions had to meet low-risk criteria which included: lesion diameter <20 mm and macroscopically type I (polypoid), IIa (elevated), IIb (flat), or IIc (depressed) lesions that were <10 mm and well-differentiated or moderately differentiated adenocarcinoma (grade G1 (well differentiated)/G2 (moderately differentiated)) and lesions limited to mucosa (m type) without known nodal metastasis or lymphovascular invasion proven by histology. One hundred patients met these criteria and were treated with EMR. Results showed that complete local remission was achieved in 99 of 100 patients [103]. Median follow-up was 33 months, and during that time 11 patients developed metachronous lesions classified as high-grade dysplasia or mucosal cancer. After repeat endoscopic management all patients again achieved complete local remission. The authors calculated 1-, 2-, 3-, and 5-year survival rates as 99%, 99%, 98%, and 98%, respectively. No severe complications, such as bleeding or perforation occurred in the acute phase and no patients died. Common minor complications that occurred with EMR included hemorrhage after EMR successfully treated with epinephrine [103].

A study involving 107 patients with BE and suspected HGD or IMC had reassuring results for the eradication of neoplasia with EMR [110]. In 80.4% of patients, the BE was eradicated completely. Over the follow-up time of 40 months there was a 71.6% (53 of 74) complete remission rate from intestinal metaplasia and 100% complete remission rate from HGD (74 of 74) or cancer (74 of 74). HGD and IMC recurred in one patient each, and they were both treated to complete remission with EMR. Complications involved strictures in 41.1% and symptomatic dysphagia in 37.3% of patients requiring dilations. Perforations occurred in two patients after EMR and in one after dilation.

Some centers have reported good results with superficially invasive submucosal EAC treated endoscopically. One study showed no lymph node metastases in T1b sm1 lesions (tumor invasion limited to the superficial third of the submucosa) [111]. In another study of 120 patients with HGD or T1 adenocarcinoma, 1% showed LNM in T1m1–3/sm1 tumors compared with 44% of T1sm2 and 3 tumors [112].

EMR has also been used for small, localized esophageal squamous cell neoplasms as an alternative to surgical therapy. It has been shown to have similar efficacy when compared to esophagectomy [113]. EMR is limited by the size of the lesion due to the increased risk of piecemeal resection in larger lesions leading to more recurrence of disease and incorrect histological evaluation [114]. Endoscopic submucosal dissection (ESD) is common in Asia and allows removal of larger esophageal lesions en bloc. ESD may have a lower local recurrence rate than EMR [114–116].

Radiofrequency Ablation for Barrett's Esophagus with Dysplasia

The recommended management for BE with HGD without adenocarcinoma is EMR for any suspicious lesions followed by RFA [5]. In a landmark multicenter, sham-controlled trial, 127 patients with dysplastic BE underwent RFA or a sham procedure. Among patients with LGD, complete eradication occurred in 90.5% in the RFA group and 22.7% in the control group ($p < 0.001$). In the HGD group, there was an 81% eradication rate in the RFA group compared with 19% in the control group ($p < 0.001$). In the RFA group, 77.4% of patients had complete eradication of intestinal metaplasia compared with 2.3% in the control group ($p < 0.001$) [14]. Given the high rate of progression to adenocarcinoma typically observed among patients with HGD, this study established the utility of RFA for patients with HGD.

The use of RFA for LGD in BE is being evaluated. The rate of progression from LGD to adenocarcinoma is lower than in HGD. Reports of the use of RFA for treatment of low-grade dysplasia are heterogeneous with short follow-up periods as found in a meta-analysis of 37 studies and 521 patients with LGD [117]. Due to the lack of data on long-term follow up, the potential benefit of ablation in reducing carcinoma risk in those with LGD compared to the risks and cost of treatment with RFA is incompletely characterized [5, 118]. The American Society for Gastrointestinal Endoscopy (ASGE) recommended in 2011 that select patients with BE LGD be considered for ablation procedures [119]. In a study involving 68 patients with LGD randomized to RFA and 68 patients with LGD randomized to endoscopic surveillance, ablation reduced the risk of progression to HGD or adenocarcinoma by 25% (1.5% for ablation v. 26.5% for control, $p < 0.001$) [30]. The absolute risk of progression from LGD to adenocarcinoma was reduced by 7.4% ($p = 0.03$). Among patients receiving RFA, complete eradication occurred in 92.6% with dysplasia and 88.2% with intestinal metaplasia compared to 27.9% with dysplasia and 0% with intestinal metaplasia in the control group. Follow-up was over a 3-year period. In practice, due to the good safety profile of RFA and anxiety surrounding observational management for a premalignant lesion in the esophagus, RFA is frequently offered in the setting of LGD.

In 2013, a systematic review and meta-analysis of studies examined the rate of complete eradication of dysplasia and intestinal metaplasia and the rate of IMC recurrence after treatment. Complete eradication of metaplasia and dysplasia occurred in 78% and 91% of patients, respectively. IMC recurrence occurred in

13% of patients. Stage advancement to cancer occurred in 0.2% of patients during treatment and in 0.7% after complete eradication of metaplasia. Heterogeneity was a noted limitation [120].

A retrospective review involving 36 patients at two tertiary care facilities with biopsy-proven IMC were treated with RFA after or during treatment with EMR. Complete eradication of IMC/dysplasia was achieved in 89% with patients requiring a mean of 1–2 EMRs and 2–3 RFA sessions to achieve eradication. The mean follow-up period was 24 ± 19 months and complete eradication at that time was 81%. Treatment complications included bleeding in 3% and stricture formation in 19% [121].

HGD or carcinoma can develop in some patients even after previous successful eradication of neoplasia or intestinal metaplasia. There have been reports of patients developing subsquamous neoplasia at least 6 months after RFA and two patients who developed subsquamous neoplasia after EMR and before RFA. It is possible that anatomical characteristics could interfere with the energy delivery of RFA to lesions. While continued surveillance is indicated in patients who have undergone RFA, the proper intervals are unknown. One approach has been to perform surveillance endoscopy every 3 months for 1 year after ablation and then increase the interval to every 6 months for 1 year, subsequently increasing to annually [122]. EMR and RFA have been used in tandem to increase the rate of complete remission of Barrett's-related lesions. However, using RFA after EMR may increase the risk of complications such as esophageal scarring. This can lead to increased risk of tears, strictures, and perforations. However, several studies have shown that these risks are low and may be equal to using RFA alone [34, 123, 124].

A more recent study involving a large, multicenter registry investigated the safety and efficacy of RFA vs. RFA after preceding EMR for nodular BE with advanced neoplasia (HGD or IMC). Safety outcomes included stricture, bleeding, and hospitalization while efficacy outcomes included complete eradication of intestinal metaplasia (CEIM), complete eradication of dysplasia (CED), and number of RFA treatments needed to achieve CEIM. CEIM was achieved in 84% of patients treated with RFA alone or after EMR. CED was achieved in 94% of patients with combination therapy and 92% with RFA only ($p = 0.17$). Safety outcomes and durability of eradication were not different between groups [125].

Another study comparing RFA in BE with HGD and IMC using a UK registry showed that in 515 patients, those with IMC were more likely to have visible lesions requiring preceding EMR than those with HGD and these may carry a higher risk of cancer progression. Patients underwent RFA every 3 months until all visible BE mucosa was ablated or cancer developed. The 12-month complete response for dysplasia and IM were almost identical ($p = 0.7$) and progression to invasive cancer was not significantly different at 12 months ($p = 0.19$). In IMC, RFA with preceding EMR was associated with superior durability compared with RFA alone ($p = 0.01$) [32]. A 6-year follow-up study looking at 508 patients completing therapy with combined EMR and RFA for BE-related neoplasia showed that complete remission of dysplasia (CR-D) and complete remission of intestinal metaplasia (CR-IM) improved significantly from 77% and 56% to 92% and 83%, respectively

($p < 0.0001$). EMR for visible lesions before RFA increased from 48% to 60% ($p = 0.013$). Rescue EMR after RFA decreased from 13% to 2% ($p < 0.0001$). No difference was seen to be significant in terms of progression to OAC at 12 months ($p = 0.51$) [29].

The EURO-II study involved 13 European centers and looked at EMR followed by RFA to eradicate BE with HGD and/or IMC. There were 132 patients undergoing a median 3 RFA treatments with complete eradication of neoplasia achieved in 92% and CE-IM in 87%, per intention to treat analysis, and 98% and 93%, respectively, in the per-protocol analysis. Mild-to-moderate adverse events occurred in 19% of patients. This study showed that intensive multimodality endotherapy with EMR and RFA is safe and highly effective [31].

Conclusions

The incidence of esophageal adenocarcinoma is progressively increasing and its growth rate outpaces that of the other major epithelial malignancies. Endoscopy has a critical role in the evaluation, diagnosis, staging, and management of Barrett's esophagus and esophageal cancer. Screening may be considered for patients with GERD, especially in the presence of any red-flag symptoms such as weight loss, dysphagia, or bleeding. Surveillance is utilized in patients with Barrett's esophagus to detect progression to dysplasia and early cancer, when tumors are superficial and curable by endoscopic or surgical modalities. Endoscopic ultrasound is the modality of choice for the locoregional evaluation of esophageal tumors, establishing the T and the N stage. EMR provides very specific diagnostic and staging information with early tumors, further refining considerations for treatment allocation. EMR forms the cornerstone of endoscopic treatment for early cancers. EMR is also indicated for any nodularity or mucosal irregularity in patients with dysplasia. Radiofrequency ablation is the treatment of choice for flat Barrett's esophagus with high-grade dysplasia, and following EMR once all the nodularity has been resected. As technology continues to progress, endoscopic approaches stand to provide ever-greater detection, more accurate staging, and less invasive management options for the large population of patients with esophageal cancer.

References

1. Gamboa AM, et al. Mo1135 trends in the incidence of esophageal adenocarcinoma and early stage esophageal adenocarcinoma in the United States. Gastroenterology. 2014;146(5):S-566–7.
2. Siegel R, Naishadham D. Cancer statistics, 2013. CA A Cancer J. 2013;63(1):11–30. http://onlinelibrary.wiley.com/doi/10.3322/caac.21166/full?dmmsmid=68954&dmmspid=8282470&dmmsuid=1829598%5Cnpapers2://publication/uuid/1268646D-F787-441F-B50E-43B02A2D9FB3
3. Pohl H, Welch HG. The role of overdiagnosis and reclassification in the marked increase of esophageal adenocarcinoma incidence. J Natl Cancer Inst. 2005;97(2):142–6.

4. Sappati Biyyani RS, Chak A. Barrett's esophagus: review of diagnosis and treatment. Gastroenterol Rep. 2013;1(1):9–18. http://www.ncbi.nlm.nih.gov/pubmed/24759662%5Cnhttp://www.pubmedcentral.nih.gov/articlerender.fcgi?artid=PMC3941437

5. Association AG. American gastroenterological association medical position statement on the management of Barrett'S esophagus. Gastroenterology. 2011;140(3):1084–91. https://doi.org/10.1053/j.gastro.2011.01.030.

6. Mino-Kenudson M, Hull MJ, Brown I, Muzikansky A, Srivastava A, Glickman J, et al. EMR for Barrett's esophagus-related superficial neoplasms offers better diagnostic reproducibility than mucosal biopsy {a figure is presented}. Gastrointest Endosc. 2007;66(4):660–6.

7. Rice TW, Blackstone EH, Adelstein DJ, Zuccaro G, Vargo JJ, Goldblum JR, et al. Role of clinically determined depth of tumor invasion in the treatment of esophageal carcinoma. J Thorac Cardiovasc Surg. 2003;125(5):1091–102.

8. Fitzgerald RC, Di Pietro M, Ragunath K, Ang Y, Kang JY, Watson P, et al. British Society of Gastroenterology guidelines on the diagnosis and management of Barrett's oesophagus. Gut. 2014;63(1):7–42.

9. Green JA, Amaro R, Barkin JS. Symptomatic gastroesophageal reflux as a risk factor for esophageal adenocarcinoma. Dig Dis Sci. 2000;45:2367–8.

10. Lagergren J, Bergstromeinhold R, Lingren A, Nyren O. Symptomatic gastoroesophageal reflux as a risk factor for esophageal adenocarcinoma. NEJM. 1999;340:825–31.

11. Shaheen NJ, Weinberg DS, Denberg TD, Chou R, Qaseem A, Shekelle P. Upper endoscopy for gastroesophageal reflux disease: best practice advice from the clinical guidelines committee of the american college of physicians. Ann Intern Med. 2012;157:808–17.

12. Shaheen NJ, Falk GW, Iyer PG, Gerson LB. ACG clinical guideline: diagnosis and management of Barrett/'s esophagus [internet]. Am J Gastroenterol. 2016;111:30–50. https://doi.org/10.1038/ajg.2015.322.

13. Reavis KM, Morris CD, Gopal DV, Hunter JG, Jobe BA, Schirmer BD, et al. Laryngopharyngeal reflux symptoms better predict the presence of esophageal adenocarcinoma than typical gastroesophageal reflux symptoms. Annals of Surgery. 2004;239(6):849–58.

14. Shaheen NJ, Sharma P, Overholt BF, Wolfsen HC, Sampliner RE, Wang KK, et al. Radiofrequency ablation in Barrett's esophagus with dysplasia. N Engl J Med. 2009;360(22):2277–88. https://doi.org/10.1056/NEJMoa0808145.

15. Rex DK, Cummings OW, Shaw M, Cumings MD, Wong RKH, Vasudeva RS, et al. Screening for Barrett's esophagus in colonoscopy patients with and without heartburn. Gastroenterology. 2003;125(6):1670–7.

16. Ronkainen J, Aro P, Storskrubb T, Johansson SE, Lind T, Bolling-Sternevald E, et al. Prevalence of Barrett's esophagus in the general population: an endoscopic study. Gastroenterology. 2005;129(6):1825–31.

17. Atkinson M, Chak A. Unsedated small-caliber endoscopy--a new screening and surveillance tool for Barrett's esophagus? Nat Clin Pr Gastroenterol Hepatol. 2007;4(8):426–7.

18. Galmiche JP, Sacher-Huvelin S, Coron E, Cholet F, Ben SE, Sébille V, et al. Screening for esophagitis and Barrett's esophagus with wireless esophageal capsule endoscopy: a multicenter prospective trial in patients with reflux symptoms. Am J Gastroenterol. 2008;103(3):538–45.

19. Chak A, Alashkar BM, Isenberg GA, Chandar AK, Greer KB, Hepner A, et al. Comparative acceptability of transnasal esophagoscopy and esophageal capsule esophagoscopy: a randomized, controlled trial in veterans. Gastrointest Endosc. 2014;80(5):774–82.

20. Aedo MR, Zavala-González MÁ, Meixueiro-Daza A, Remes-Troche JM. Accuracy of transnasal endoscopy with a disposable esophagoscope compared to conventional endoscopy. World J Gastrointest Endosc. 2014;6(4):128–36. http://www.pubmedcentral.nih.gov/articlerender.fcgi?artid=3985153&tool=pmcentrez&rendertype=abstract.

21. Kadri PSR, Lao-Sirieix I, O'Donovan M, Debiram I, Das M, Blazeby JM, et al. Acceptability and accuracy of a non-endoscopic screening test for Barrett's oesophagus in primary care: cohort study. BMJ. 2010;341(7773):595.

22. Ross-Innes CS, Debiram-Beecham I, O'Donovan M, Walker E, Varghese S, Lao-Sirieix P, et al. Evaluation of a minimally invasive cell sampling device coupled with assessment of trefoil factor 3 expression for diagnosing Barrett's esophagus: a multi-center case-control study. PLoS Med. 2015;12(1):e1001780.
23. Streitz JM, Ellis FH, Tilden RL, Erickson RV. Endoscopic surveillance of Barrett's esophagus: a cost-effectiveness comparison with mammographic surveillance for breast cancer. Am J Gastroenterol. 1998;93(6):911–5.
24. Hvid-Jensen F, Pedersen L, Drewes AM, Sorensen HT, Funch-Jensen P. Incidence of adenocarcinoma among patients with Barrett's esophagus. N Engl J Med. 2011;365(15):1375–83. http://www.ncbi.nlm.nih.gov/pubmed/21995385%5Cnhttp://www.nejm.org/doi/pdf/10.1056/NEJMoa1103042
25. Komanduri S, Swanson G, Keefer L, Jakate S. Use of a new jumbo forceps improves tissue acquisition of Barrett's esophagus surveillance biopsies. Gastrointest Endosc. 2009;70(6):1072–8.e1.
26. Abela JE, Going JJ, Mackenzie JF, McKernan M, O'Mahoney S, Stuart RC. Systematic four-quadrant biopsy detects Barrett's dysplasia in more patients than nonsystematic biopsy. Am J Gastroenterol. 2008;103(4):850–5.
27. Wang KK, Sampliner RE. Updated guidelines 2008 for the diagnosis, surveillance and therapy of Barrett's esophagus. Am J Gastroenterol. 2008;103:788–97.
28. Sharma P. The development and validation of an endoscopic grading system for Barrett's esophagus: the Prague C & M criteria. Gastroenterology. 2006;131(5):1392–9.
29. Haidry RJ, Dunn JM, Butt MA, Burnell MG, Gupta A, Green S, et al. Radiofrequency ablation and endoscopic mucosal resection for dysplastic Barrett's esophagus and early esophageal adenocarcinoma: outcomes of the UK national halo RFA registry. Gastroenterology. 2013;145(1):87–95.
30. Phoa KN, van Vilsteren FGI, Weusten BLAM, Bisschops R, Schoon EJ, Ragunath K, et al. Radiofrequency ablation vs endoscopic surveillance for patients with Barrett esophagus and low-grade dysplasia. JAMA. 2014;311(12):1209. http://jama.jamanetwork.com/article.aspx?doi=10.1001/jama.2014.2511
31. Phoa KN, Pouw RE, Bisschops R, Pech O, Ragunath K, Weusten BLAM, et al. Multimodality endoscopic eradication for neoplastic Barrett oesophagus: results of an European multicentre study (EURO-II). Gut. 2016;65(4):555–62.
32. Haidry RJ, Lipman G, Banks MR, Butt MA, Sehgal V, Graham D, et al. Comparing outcome of radiofrequency ablation in Barrett's with high grade dysplasia and intramucosal carcinoma: a prospective multicenter UK registry. Endoscopy. 2015;47(11):980–7.
33. Weusten B, Bisschops R, Coron E, Dinis-Ribeiro M, Dumonceau J-M, Esteban J-M, et al. Endoscopic management of Barrett's esophagus: European Society of Gastrointestinal Endoscopy (ESGE) position statement. Endoscopy. 2017;49(2):191–8. http://www.thieme-connect.de/DOI/DOI?10.1055/s-0042-122140
34. Akiyama J, Roorda A, Triadafilopoulos G. Managing Barrett's esophagus with radiofrequency ablation. Gastroenterol Rep. 2013;1(2):95–104. https://academic.oup.com/gastro/article-lookup/doi/10.1093/gastro/got009
35. Lichtenstein DR. Role of endoscopy in the management of GERD. Gastrointest Endosc. 2007;66(2):219–24.
36. Triadafilopoulos G. Clinical experience with the Stretta® procedure. Gastrointest Endosc Clin N Am. 2003;13:147–55.
37. Bianco MA, et al. Endoscopic treatment of gastro-oesophageal reflux disease. Acta Otorhinolaryngol Ital. 2006;26(5):281–6.
38. Utley DS. The Stretta® procedure: device, technique, and pre-clinical study data. Gastrointest Endosc Clin N Am. 2003;13:135–45.
39. Arts J, Lerut T, Rutgeerts P, Sifrim D, Janssens J, Tack J. A one-year follow-up study of endoluminal gastroplication (Endocinch) in GERD patients refractory to proton pump inhibitor therapy. Dig Dis Sci. 2005;50(2):351–6.

40. Arts J, Sifrim D, Rutgeerts P, Lerut A, Janssens J, Tack J. Influence of radiofrequency energy delivery at the gastroesophageal junction (the Stretta procedure) on symptoms, acid exposure, and esophageal sensitivity to acid perfusion in gastroesophagal reflux disease. Dig Dis Sci. 2007;52(9):2170–7.
41. Singh PB, Das SK, Kumar A, Sharma GK, Pandey AK, Swain S, et al. Dorsal onlay lingual mucosal graft urethroplasty: comparison of two techniques. Int J Urol. 2008;15(11):1002–5.
42. Chuttani R, Sud R, Sachdev G, Puri R, Kozarek R, Haber G, et al. A novel endoscopic full-thickness plicator for the treatment of GERD: a pilot study. Gastrointest Endosc. 2003;58(5):770–6.
43. Pleskow D, Rothstein R, Kozarek R, Haber G, Gostout C, Lo S, et al. Endoscopic full-thickness plication for the treatment of GERD: five-year long-term multicenter results. Surg Endosc Other Interv Tech. 2008;22(2):326–32.
44. Von Renteln D, Schiefke I, Fuchs KH, Raczynski S, Philipper M, Breithaupt W, et al. Endoscopic full-thickness plication for the treatment of gastroesophageal reflux disease using multiple Plicator implants: 12-month multicenter study results. Surg Endosc Other Interv Tech. 2009;23(8):1866–75.
45. Leeds S, Reavis K. Endolumenal therapies for gastroesophageal reflux disease. Gastrointest Endosc Clin N Am. 2013;23:41–51.
46. Reavis KM, Perry KA. Transoral incisionless fundoplication for the treatment of gastro-esophageal reflux disease. Expert Rev Med Devices. 2014;11(4):341–50.
47. Louis H, Closset J, Deviere J. Enteryx. Best Pract Res Clin Gastroenterol. 2004;18(1):49–59.
48. Johnson DA. Enteryx® for gastroesophageal reflux disease. Expert Rev Med Devices. 2005;2(1):19–26.
49. Deviére J, Pastorelli A, Louis H, De Maertelaer V, Lehman G, Cicala M, et al. Endoscopic implantation of a biopolymer in the lower esophageal sphincter for gastroesophageal reflux: a pilot study. Gastrointest Endosc. 2002;55(3):335–41.
50. Corley DA, Katz P, Wo JM, Stefan A, Patti M, Rothstein R, et al. Improvement of gastro-esophageal reflux symptoms after radiofrequency energy: a randomized, sham-controlled trial. Gastroenterology. 2003;125(3):668–76.
51. Tam WCE, Schoeman MN, Zhang Q, Dent J, Rigda R, Utley D, et al. Delivery of radiofrequency energy to the lower oesophageal sphincter and gastric cardia inhibits transient lower oesophageal sphincter relaxations and gastro-oesophageal reflux in patients with reflux disease. Gut. 2003;52(4):479–85.
52. Dughera L, Rotondano G, De Cento M, Cassolino P, Cisarò F. Durability of stretta radiofrequency treatment for GERD: results of an 8-year follow-up. Gastroenterol Res Pract. 2014;2014
53. Wiersema MJ, Levy MJ, Harewood GC, Gostout CJ. Cost analysis of endoscopic antireflux procedures: Endoluminal plication vs. radiofrequency coagulation vs. treatment with a proton pump inhibitor [1] (multiple letters). Gastrointest Endosc. 2004;59:749–50.
54. Fry LC, Monkemuller K, Malfertheiner P. Systematic review: endoluminal therapy for gastro-oesophageal reflux disease: evidence from clinical trials. Eur J Gastroenterol Hepatol. 2007;19(12):1125–39.
55. Espino A, Cirocco M, DaCosta R, Marcon N. Advanced imaging technologies for the detection of dysplasia and early cancer in Barrett Esophagus. Clin Endosc. 2014;47(1):47–54.
56. Curvers WL, Peters FP, Elzer B, Schaap AJCM, Baak LC, Van Oijen A, et al. Quality of Barrett's surveillance in The Netherlands: a standardized review of endoscopy and pathology reports. Eur J Gastroenterol Hepatol. 2008;20(7):601–7.
57. Ramus JR, Caygill CPJ, Gatenby PAC, Watson A. Current United Kingdom practice in the diagnosis and management of columnar-lined oesophagus: results of the United Kingdom National Barrett Oesophagus Registry endoscopist questionnaire. Eur J Cancer Prev. 2008;17(5):422–5.
58. Das D, Ishaq S, Harrison R, Kosuri K, Harper E, DeCaestecker J, et al. Management of Barrett's esophagus in the UK: Overtreated and underbiopsied but improved by the introduction of a national randomized trial. Am J Gastroenterol. 2008;103(5):1079–89.

59. Garud SS, Willingham FF, Cai Q. Diagnosis and management of Barrett's esophagus for the endoscopist. Ther Adv Gastroenterol. 2010;3:227–38.
60. Alderson D. Observer variation in the diagnosis of superficial oesophageal adenocarcinoma: another spanner in the works? Gut. 2002;51:620–1.
61. Kara MA, Peters FP, Fockens P, ten Kate FJW, Bergman JJGHM. Endoscopic video-autofluorescence imaging followed by narrow band imaging for detecting early neoplasia in Barrett's esophagus. Gastrointest Endosc. 2006;64(2):176–85.
62. Gono K, Obi T, Yamaguchi M, Ohyama N, Machida H, Sano Y, et al. Appearance of enhanced tissue features in narrow-band endoscopic imaging. J Biomed Opt. 2004;9(3):568. http://biomedicaloptics.spiedigitallibrary.org/article.aspx?doi=10.1117/1.1695563
63. Mannath J, Subramanian V, Hawkey CJ, Ragunath K. Narrow band imaging for characterization of high grade dysplasia and specialized intestinal metaplasia in Barretts esophagus: a meta-analysis. Endoscopy. 2010;42(5):351–9.
64. Sharma P, Hawes RH, Bansal A, Gupta N, Curvers W, Rastogi A, et al. Standard endoscopy with random biopsies versus narrow band imaging targeted biopsies in Barrett's oesophagus: a prospective, international, randomised controlled trial. Gut. 2013;62(1):15–21.
65. Herrero LA, Curvers WL, Bansal A, Wani S, Kara M, Schenk E, et al. Zooming in on Barrett oesophagus using narrow-band imaging: an international observer agreement study. Eur J Gastroenterol Hepatol. 2009;21(9):1068–75.
66. Curvers WL, Bohmer CJ, Mallant-Hent RC, Naber AH, Ponsioen CIJ, Ragunath K, et al. Mucosal morphology in Barrett's esophagus: Interobserver agreement and role of narrow band imaging. Endoscopy. 2008;40(10):799–805.
67. Silva FB, Dinis-Ribeiro M, Vieth M, Rabenstein T, Goda K, Kiesslich R, et al. Endoscopic assessment and grading of Barrett's esophagus using magnification endoscopy and narrow-band imaging: accuracy and interobserver agreement of different classification systems (with videos). Gastrointest Endosc. 2011;73(1):7–14.
68. Leggett CL, Gorospe EC. Application of confocal laser endomicroscopy in the diagnosis and management of Barrett's esophagus. Ann Gastroenterol Q Publ Hell Soc Gastroenterol. 2014;27(3):193–9.
69. Kiesslich R, Gossner L, Goetz M, Dahlmann A, Vieth M, Stolte M, et al. In vivo histology of Barrett's esophagus and associated neoplasia by confocal laser endomicroscopy. Clin Gastroenterol Hepatol. 2006;4(8):979–87.
70. Canto MI, Anandasabapathy S, Brugge W, Falk GW, Dunbar KB, Zhang Z, et al. In vivo endomicroscopy improves detection of Barrett's esophagus-related neoplasia: a multicenter international randomized controlled trial (with video). Gastrointest Endosc. 2014;79(2):211–21.
71. Sharma P, Meining AR, Coron E, Lightdale CJ, Wolfsen HC, Bansal A, et al. Real-time increased detection of neoplastic tissue in Barrett's esophagus with probe-based confocal laser endomicroscopy: final results of an international multicenter, prospective, randomized, controlled trial. Gastrointest Endosc. 2011;74(3):465–72.
72. Bajbouj M, Vieth M, Rösch T, Miehlke S, Becker V, Anders M, et al. Probe-based confocal laser endomicroscopy compared with standard four-quadrant biopsy for evaluation of neoplasia in Barretts esophagus. Endoscopy. 2010;42(6):435–40.
73. Xiong YQ, Ma SJ, Hu HY, Ge J, Zhou LZ, Huo ST, Qiu MCQ. Comparison of narrow-band imaging and confocal laser endomicroscopy for the detection of neoplasia in Barrett's esophagus: a meta-analysis. Clin Res Hepatol Gastroenterol. 2017;S2210(17):30136–5.
74. Lee MH, Buterbaugh K, Richards-Kortum R, Anandasabapathy S. Advanced endoscopic imaging for Barrett's esophagus: current options and future directions. Curr Gastroenterol Rep. 2012;14(3):216–25.
75. Isenberg G, Sivak MV, Chak A, Wong RCK, Willis JE, Wolf B, et al. Accuracy of endoscopic optical coherence tomography in the detection of dysplasia in Barrett's esophagus: a prospective, double-blinded study. Gastrointest Endosc. 2005;62(6):825–31.
76. Qi X, Sivak MV, Isenberg G, Willis JE, Rollins AM. Computer-aided diagnosis of dysplasia in Barrett's esophagus using endoscopic optical coherence tomography. J Biomed Opt. 2006;11(4):44010. http://biomedicaloptics.spiedigitallibrary.org/article.aspx?doi=10.1117/1.2337314

77. Gill RS, Singh R. Endoscopic imaging in Barrett's esophagus: current practice and future applications. Ann Gastroenterol Q Publ Hell Soc Gastroenterol. 2012;25(2):89–95. http://www.ncbi.nlm.nih.gov/pubmed/24714225%5Cnhttp://www.pubmedcentral.nih.gov/articlerender.fcgi?artid=PMC3959381

78. Evans JA, Poneros JM, Bouma BE, Bressner J, Halpern EF, Shishkov M, et al. Optical coherence tomography to identify intramucosal carcinoma and high-grade dysplasia in Barrett's esophagus. Clin Gastroenterol Hepatol. 2006;4:38–43.

79. Clermont MP, et al. Impact of endoscopic mucosal resection in patients referred for endoscopic management of Barrett's esophagus. Gastrointest Interv. 2013;2(2):90–3.

80. Moss A, Bourke MJ, Hourigan LF, Gupta S, Williams SJ, Tran K, et al. Endoscopic resection for Barrett's high-grade dysplasia and early esophageal adenocarcinoma: an essential staging procedure with long-term therapeutic benefit. Am J Gastroenterol. 2010;105(6):1276–83.

81. Shimizu Y, Kato M, Yamamoto J, Ono Y, Katsurada T, Ono S, et al. Histologic results of EMR for esophageal lesions diagnosed as high-grade intraepithelial squamous neoplasia by endoscopic biopsy. Gastrointest Endosc. 2006;63:16–21.

82. Pech O, May A, Gossner L, Rabenstein T, Manner H, Huijsmans J, et al. Curative endoscopic therapy in patients with early esophageal squamous-cell carcinoma or high-grade intraepithelial neoplasia. Endoscopy. 2007;39(1):30–5. http://eutils.ncbi.nlm.nih.gov/entrez/eutils/elink.fcgi?dbfrom=pubmed&id=17252457&retmode=ref&cmd=prlinks%5Cnpapers3://publication/doi/10.1055/s-2006-945040

83. Savoy AD, Wallace MB. EUS in the management of the patient with dysplasia in Barrett's esophagus. J Clin Gastroenterol. 2005;39(4):263–7.

84. Attila T, Faigel DO. Role of endoscopic ultrasound in superficial esophageal cancer. Dis Esophagus. 2009;22(2):104–12. http://www.ncbi.nlm.nih.gov/pubmed/19021687

85. Thomas T, Gilbert D, Kaye PV, Penman I, Aithal GP, Ragunath K. High-resolution endoscopy and endoscopic ultrasound for evaluation of early neoplasia in Barrett's esophagus. Surg Endosc Other Interv Tech. 2010;24(5):1110–6.

86. Vazquez-Sequeiros E, Wiersema MJ, Clain JE, Norton ID, Levy MJ, Romero Y, et al. Impact of lymph node staging on therapy of esophageal carcinoma. Gastroenterology. 2003;125(6):1626–35.

87. Pech O, May A, Günter E, Gossner L, Ell C. The impact of endoscopic ultrasound and computed tomography on the TNM staging of early cancer in Barrett's esophagus. Am J Gastroenterol. 2006;101(10):2223–9.

88. Larghi A, Lightdale CJ, Memeo L, Bhagat G, Okpara N, Rotterdam H. EUS followed by EMR for staging of high-grade dysplasia and early cancer in Barrett's esophagus. Gastrointest Endosc. 2005;62(1):16–23.

89. Rampado S, Bocus P, Battaglia G, Ruol A, Portale G, Ancona E. Endoscopic ultrasound: accuracy in staging superficial carcinomas of the esophagus. Ann Thorac Surg. 2008;85(1):251–6.

90. Shimizu Y, Tsukagoshi H, Fujita M, Hosokawa M, Kato M, Asaka M. Long-term outcome after endoscopic mucosal resection in patients with esophageal squamous cell carcinoma invading the muscularis mucosae or deeper. Gastrointest Endosc. 2002;56(3):387–90.

91. He LJ, Shan HB, Luo GY, Li Y, Zhang R, Gao XY, et al. Endoscopic ultrasonography for staging of T1a and T1b esophageal squamous cell carcinoma. World J Gastroenterol. 2014;20(5):1340–7.

92. Wani S, Das A, Rastogi A, Drahos J, Ricker W, Parsons R, et al. Endoscopic ultrasonography in esophageal cancer leads to improved survival rates: results from a population-based study. Cancer. 2015;121(2):194–201.

93. Bailey BE, Freedenfeld RN, Kiser RS, Gatchel RJ. Lifetime physical and sexual abuse in chronic pain patients: psychosocial correlates and treatment outcomes. Disabil Rehabil. 2003;25(7):331–42.

94. Bennett C, Vakil N, Bergman J, Harrison R, Odze R, Vieth M, et al. Consensus statements for management of Barrett's dysplasia and early-stage esophageal adenocarcinoma, based on a delphi process. Gastroenterology. 2012;143(2):336–46.

95. Markar SR, Karthikesalingam A, Thrumurthy S, Low DE. Volume-outcome relationship in surgery for esophageal malignancy: systematic review and meta-analysis 2000-2011. J Gastrointest Surg. 2012;16:1055–63.
96. Ell C, May A, Gossner L, Pech O, Günter E, Mayer G, et al. Endoscopic mucosal resection of early cancer and high-grade dysplasia in Barrett's esophagus. Gastroenterology. 2000;118(4):670–7. http://www.ncbi.nlm.nih.gov/pubmed/10734018
97. Pech O, Bollschweiler E, Manner H, Leers J, Ell C, Hölscher AH. Comparison between endoscopic and surgical resection of mucosal esophageal adenocarcinoma in Barrett's esophagus at two high-volume centers. Ann Surg. 2011;254(1):67–72.
98. Prasad GA, Wu TT, Wigle DA, Buttar NS, Wongkeesong LM, Dunagan KT, et al. Endoscopic and surgical treatment of mucosal (T1a) esophageal adenocarcinoma in Barrett's esophagus. Gastroenterology. 2009;137(3):815–23.
99. Das A, et al. A comparison of endoscopic treatment and surgery in early esophageal cancer: an analysis of surveillance epidemiology and end results data. Am J Gastroenterol. 2008;103(6):1340–5.
100. Wani S, Drahos J, Cook MB, Rastogi A, Bansal A, Yen R, et al. Comparison of endoscopic therapies and surgical resection in patients with early esophageal cancer: a population-based study. Gastrointest Endosc. 2014;79(2):224–232.e1.
101. Pech O, Behrens A, May A, Nachbar L, Gossner L, Rabenstein T, et al. Long-term results and risk factor analysis for recurrence after curative endoscopic therapy in 349 patients with high-grade intraepithelial neoplasia and mucosal adenocarcinoma in Barrett's oesophagus. Gut. 2008;57(9):1200–6.
102. Larghi A, Lightdale CJ, Ross AS, Fedi P, Hart J, Rotterdam H, et al. Long-term follow-up of complete Barrett's eradication endoscopic mucosal resection (CBE-EMR) for the treatment of high grade dysplasia and intramucosal carcinoma. Endoscopy. 2007;39(12):1086–91.
103. Ell C, May A, Pech O, Gossner L, Guenter E, Behrens A, et al. Curative endoscopic resection of early esophageal adenocarcinomas (Barrett's cancer). Gastrointest Endosc. 2007;65(1):3–10.
104. May A, Gossner L, Pech O, Müller H, Vieth M, Stolte M, et al. Intraepithelial high-grade neoplasia and early adenocarcinoma in short-segment Barrett's esophagus (SSBE): curative treatment using local endoscopic treatment techniques. Endoscopy. 2002;34(8):604–10.
105. Pech O, May A, Manner H, Behrens A, Pohl J, Weferling M, et al. Long-term efficacy and safety of endoscopic resection for patients with mucosal adenocarcinoma of the esophagus. Gastroenterology. 2014;146(3):652–660.e1.
106. Manner H, Pech O, Heldmann Y, May A, Pohl J, Behrens A, et al. Efficacy, safety, and long-term results of endoscopic treatment for early stage adenocarcinoma of the esophagus with low-risk sm1 invasion. Clin Gastroenterol Hepatol. 2013;11(6):630–5.
107. Gamboa AM, Kim S, Woods KE, Force SD, Maithel SK, Staley C, et al. Treatment allocation in early stage esophageal adenocarcinoma: the national incidence rates and predictors of lymph node involvement. Gastrointest Endosc. 2014;79(5):AB133. http://www.embase.com/search/results?subaction=viewrecord&from=export&id=L71429238%5Cnhttp://dx.doi.org/10.1016/j.gie.2014.02.083%5Cnhttp://ca3cx5qj7w.search.serialssolutions.com?sid=EMBASE&issn=00165107&id=doi:10.1016%2Fj.gie.2014.02.083&atitle=Treatment+alloc
108. Esaki M, Matsumoto T, Hirakawa K, Nakamura S, Umeno J, Koga H, et al. Risk factors for local recurrence of superficial esophageal cancer after treatment by endoscopic mucosal resection. Endoscopy. 2007;39(1):41–5.
109. Pech O, Manner H, Ell C. Endoscopic resection. Gastrointest Endosc Clin N Am. 2011;21(1):81–94. http://www.ncbi.nlm.nih.gov/entrez/query.fcgi?cmd=Retrieve&db=PubMed&dopt=Citation&list_uids=21112499
110. Konda VJA, Gonzalez Haba Ruiz M, Koons A, Hart J, Xiao SY, Siddiqui UD, et al. Complete endoscopic mucosal resection is effective and durable treatment for barrett's-associated neoplasia. Clin Gastroenterol Hepatol. 2014;12(12):2002–10.

111. Ancona E, Rampado S, Cassaro M, Battaglia G, Ruol A, Castoro C, et al. Prediction of lymph node status in superficial esophageal carcinoma. Ann Surg Oncol. 2008;15(11):3278–88.
112. Westerterp M, Koppert LB, Buskens CJ, Tilanus HW, ten Kate FJW, JJHGM B, et al. Outcome of surgical treatment for early adenocarcinoma of the esophagus or gastro-esophageal junction. Virchows Arch. 2005;446(5):497–504. http://www.ncbi.nlm.nih.gov/pubmed/15838647
113. Eguchi T, Nakanishi Y, Shimoda T, Iwasaki M, Igaki H, Tachimori Y, et al. Histopathological criteria for additional treatment after endoscopic mucosal resection for esophageal cancer: analysis of 464 surgically resected cases. Mod Pathol. 2006;19(3):475–80.
114. Honda K, Akiho H. Endoscopic submucosal dissection for superficial esophageal squamous cell neoplasms. World J Gastrointest Pathophysiol. 2012;3(2):44–50.
115. Takahashi H, Arimura Y, Masao H, Okahara S, Tanuma T, Kodaira J, et al. Endoscopic submucosal dissection is superior to conventional endoscopic resection as a curative treatment for early squamous cell carcinoma of the esophagus (with video). Gastrointest Endosc. 2010;72(2):255–64.
116. Ishihara R, Iishi H, Takeuchi Y, Kato M, Yamamoto S, Yamamoto S, et al. Local recurrence of large squamous-cell carcinoma of the esophagus after endoscopic resection. Gastrointest Endosc. 2008;67(6):799–804.
117. Almond LM, Hodson J, Barr H. Meta-analysis of endoscopic therapy for low-grade dysplasia in Barrett's oesophagus. Br J Surg. 2014;101:1187–95.
118. Chadwick G, Groene O, Markar SR, Hoare J, Cromwell D, Hanna GB. Systematic review comparing radiofrequency ablation and complete endoscopic resection in treating dysplastic Barrett's esophagus: a critical assessment of histologic outcomes and adverse events. Gastrointest Endosc. 2014;79:718–731.e3.
119. Evans JA, Early DS, Fukami N, Ben-Menachem T, Chandrasekhara V, Chathadi KV, et al. The role of endoscopy in Barrett's esophagus and other premalignant conditions of the esophagus. Gastrointest Endosc. 2012;76(6):1087–94.
120. Orman ES, Li N, Shaheen NJ. Efficacy and durability of radiofrequency ablation for barrett's esophagus: systematic review and meta-analysis. Clin Gastroenterol Hepatol. 2013;11:1245–55.
121. Strauss AC, Agoston AT, Dulai PS, Srivastava A, Rothstein RI. Radiofrequency ablation for Barrett's-associated intramucosal carcinoma: a multi-center follow-up study. Surg Endosc Other Interv Tech. 2014;28(12):3366–72.
122. Titi M, Overhiser A, Ulusarac O, Falk GW, Chak A, Wang K, et al. Development of subsquamous high-grade dysplasia and adenocarcinoma after successful radiofrequency ablation of Barrett's esophagus. Gastroenterology. 2012;143(3):564–566.e1.
123. Kim HP, et al. Focal endoscopic mucosal resection before radiofrequency ablation is equally effective and safe compared with radiofrequency ablation alone for the eradication of Barrett's esophagus with advanced neoplasia. Gastrointest Endosc. 2012;76(4):733–9.
124. Bulsiewicz WJ, Kim HP, Dellon ES, Cotton CC, Pasricha S, Madanick RD, et al. Safety and efficacy of endoscopic mucosal therapy with radiofrequency ablation for patients with neoplastic barrett's esophagus. Clin Gastroenterol Hepatol. 2013;11(6):636–42.
125. Li N, Pasricha S, Bulsiewicz WJ, Pruitt RE, Komanduri S, Wolfsen HC, et al. Effects of preceding endoscopic mucosal resection on the efficacy and safety of radiofrequency ablation for treatment of Barrett's esophagus: results from the United States radiofrequency ablation registry. Dis Esophagus. 2016;29(6):537–43.

Principles and Approaches in Surgical Resection of Esophageal Cancer

9

Nassrene Elmadhun and Daniela Molena

History of Esophageal Resection

Resection of esophageal carcinoma was first successfully performed in 1913 in New York City by Franz Torek through a left chest approach. The patient survived with an esophagostomy and gastrostomy for 12 years [1]. While other surgeons described restoring enteric continuity subcutaneously using transverse colon or stomach, Japanese surgeon Oshawa in Kyoto performed the first successful esophagectomy with intrathoracic reconstitution of esophagogastric continuity in 1933. This technique was further popularized by Richard Sweet from Massachusetts General Hospital in 1945 with his descriptions of left-sided approach to transthoracic esophagectomy [2, 3]. In the same year, British surgeon Ivor Lewis was the first to describe an alternative right-sided approach for dissection and resection of the thoracic esophagus in 1946, which did not require a diaphragmatic incision, and would allow for dissection of the thoracic esophagus under direct visualization [4].

Ivor Lewis described his esophagectomy as a two-staged procedure. The first stage involved a midline laparotomy, mobilization of the gastric conduit, and closure. The right thoracotomy followed a week later with esophagectomy and esophagogastric anastomosis. The Ivor Lewis esophagectomy was refined in the decades that followed and has evolved into the one-stage procedure that still bears his name today. In the 1960s, British surgeon McKeown popularized a technique adding a third cervical phase to the Ivor Lewis esophagectomy moving the anastomosis from the chest into the neck [5]. Esophagectomy without thoracotomy was first described by the German surgeon Alwin von Ach and Austrian surgeon Wolfgang Denk in 1912 [6]. The so-called transhiatal esophagectomy which involves a gastric

N. Elmadhun · D. Molena (✉)
Thoracic Surgery Service, Department of Surgery, Memorial Sloan Kettering Cancer Center, New York, NY, USA
e-mail: Elmadhun@mskcc.org; Molenad@mskcc.org

© Springer Nature Switzerland AG 2020
N. F. Saba, B. F. El-Rayes (eds.), *Esophageal Cancer*,
https://doi.org/10.1007/978-3-030-29832-6_9

mobilization and transhiatal blunt esophageal mobilization followed by cervical anastomosis was revived and popularized by Japanese surgeon Hiroshi Akiyama from Tokyo and American surgeon Mark Orringer [7, 8]. Currently, esophagectomy is most commonly performed by an open technique with the transhiatal approach or Ivor Lewis approach being the most common techniques. The newest development in esophagectomy is minimally invasive esophagectomy wherein the abdominal mobilization of the gastric conduit and thoracic esophageal mobilization is all performed laparoscopically and thoracoscopically.

The Balance Between Technical Complications and Outcomes

Esophagectomies have historically been associated with a high incidence of morbidity and mortality, much of which can occur as a consequence of intraoperative technical complications, including anastomotic leaks, conduit failures, strictures, thoracic duct leaks, and recurrent nerve injuries. Some of these technical complications can be attributed to poor technique; others, however, are likely related to aspects of the surgical approaches discussed in this chapter. Although advances in pain management, respiratory physiotherapy, endoscopic and radiologic interventions, and intensive care management have all contributed to the overall improvements in morbidity and mortality seen in recent years, technical complications and their consequences persist. In addition to carrying immediate perioperative risks, technical complications can also have an insidious, long-lasting effect on survival, one that is masked by short-term improvements [9]. Consequently, when choosing an operative approach, consideration should be given to the incidence of the technical complications associated with the chosen approach, and the risk of these complications should be balanced against the oncologic and long-term symptomatic benefits of the approach.

In general, the aspects of esophagectomy that have been associated with a higher risk of complications include the use of thoracotomy, a more radical resection, a more extensive lymphadenectomy, and a cervical incision. Thoracotomies have been consistently associated with a higher risk of pneumonia, a finding seen in both retrospective studies [10] and a prospective randomized trial [11]. Likewise, more radical resections require longer operative times, which have been associated with increased incidence of respiratory complications [12]. More extensive lymphadenectomies also require longer operative times and are more likely to result in chyle leak. Last, rates of anastomotic leak and stricture are consistently higher the more proximal the anastomosis is: when the anastomosis is performed in the neck, the incidence of leaks is 8–15%, compared with 0–7% when the anastomosis is performed in the chest [13]. Furthermore, the more proximal the anastomosis, and when a cervical incision is used, the greater the likelihood of a recurrent nerve injury.

What is obvious regarding the associations between various aspects of esophagectomy and complications is that the aspects of an operation that are needed to achieve appropriate oncologic goals are often in direct conflict with the need to minimize technical complications. Thus, when selecting an operative approach, there needs to be careful consideration of both the risks of the operation and the oncologic benefits. Clearly, this would imply that, for some patients for whom an aggressive approach is unlikely to result in a significant oncologic benefit, the associated risks of aggressive surgery are not warranted. On the other hand, for patients who can gain a clear benefit from a more radical resection, an aggressive approach is likely worthwhile.

Operative Nomenclature

There are many possible surgical approaches for performing an esophagectomy, with the nomenclature variably describing the number of cavities opened (McKeown, Ivor Lewis, and transhiatal), the extent of lymphadenectomy (1-field, 2-field, modified 3-field, and 3-field), and the radicality of the resection (en bloc). With the introduction of minimally invasive techniques, a description of the type of access incision is now also used (open, minimally invasive, minimally invasive "assisted," and robotically assisted). Whereas the components of an en bloc resection are well described—and include resection of the pericardium, contralateral pleura, azygous vein, thoracic duct, and cuff of diaphragm (in junction tumors) [14]—the extent of lymphadenectomy is less well characterized. A "1-field lymphadenectomy," which refers to an intra-abdominal lymphadenectomy, does not define precisely which nodes need to be removed. Whereas many would agree that the equivalent of a gastric D1 lymphadenectomy is appropriate (N1 nodes—immediate perigastric nodes), others would argue for a more thorough approach, such as a D2 lymphadenectomy (N1 nodes + left gastric, celiac axis, common hepatic, splenic hilum, splenic artery, and hepatic artery nodes) [15]. The second field of a lymphadenectomy commonly refers to an infra-azygous nodal resection, including the subcarinal nodes and all periesophageal nodes from the subcarina down to the level of the hiatus. Last, the terminology used to describe the third field of a lymphadenectomy is inconsistent. A *standard* third field includes the intrathoracic component along the left and right recurrent laryngeal nerves, as well as a cervical component in which the remaining recurrent nerve nodal chain and the deep cervical nodes are removed [15]. An *extended* third field also includes the bilateral cervical and supraclavicular nodes.

Equally ambiguous in the terminology used to define lymphadenectomy is the designation of a "minimally invasive" approach. For instance, a "minimally invasive Ivor Lewis approach" could imply laparoscopic and thoracoscopic incisions, but for some, the use of either a laparotomy or a thoracotomy would still qualify as a minimally invasive "assisted" approach. Finally, although a surgical approach can limit the extent of the lymphadenectomy or the radicality of the procedure, the name of the approach does not necessarily imply the extent of the lymphadenectomy or the radicality of the operation. For instance, whereas a McKeown esophagectomy allows for a 1-, 2-, or 3-field lymphadenectomy with or without an en bloc component, an open transhiatal esophagectomy does not allow for a formal second- or third-field lymphadenectomy or an en bloc resection. Consequently, the most accurate way to describe an operative approach is by a combination of descriptors;

examples would include "a minimally invasive, McKeown esophagectomy with a 2-field lymphadenectomy with thoracoscopy and laparotomy" or "an open Ivor Lewis esophagectomy with en bloc resection and a 2-field lymphadenectomy."

Principles: Importance of Lymphadenectomy

There is accumulating evidence supporting an association between a more aggressive lymphadenectomy and survival in surgically treated patients with esophageal cancer [16, 17]. This association is strongest in patients with the highest risk of nodal disease [18]. That is, in patients who are least likely to have nodal metastases, fewer than ten nodes should be removed; in patients with a high risk of nodal disease, more than 30 nodes should be removed; and in patients with almost no risk (T1a) of nodal disease, as well as patients with many involved nodes (N3), removal of additional nodes has little bearing on survival. This better understanding of tumors with low and high risks of nodal metastases provides the necessary oncologic rationale for endoscopic resection of superficial tumors (T1a). Conversely, most patients currently undergoing surgery have a moderate-to-high risk of nodal metastases and performing an adequate lymphadenectomy in these patients mandates an aggressive approach. Level I support for this approach comes from the only prospective randomized trial that has addressed the effect of surgical approach on survival. This trial compared a "radical" transhiatal approach that is much more thorough than the typical transhiatal esophagectomy with an en bloc Ivor Lewis esophagectomy. The main difference between the two arms of this trial was the number of nodes removed (31 for en bloc, 16 for transhiatal). The results showed a trend toward improved survival for the en bloc Ivor Lewis approach, compared with the radical transhiatal approach [11]. Furthermore, an unplanned subgroup analysis found a statistically significant survival benefit in patients with 1–8 nodes involved, which is consistent with the concept that patients at risk of nodal disease benefit most from an aggressive lymphadenectomy [19].

When selecting a surgical approach, the choice should therefore take into account the need for an adequate lymphadenectomy. In some cases—for instance, when an endoscopic resection is not feasible—an approach that achieves a limited lymphadenectomy, such as a transhiatal approach, is adequate. On the other hand, in most patients, an adequate lymphadenectomy will consist of an aggressive intra-abdominal and intrathoracic lymphadenectomy (i.e., 2-field). The intra-abdominal component should include the celiac, splenic, and common hepatic lymph nodes, and the intrathoracic lymphadenectomy should include all the lymph nodes from the subcarinal space down to the hiatus. Because of these requirements, an intrathoracic approach is necessary to adequately remove all potentially involved lymph nodes, and an approach such as a transhiatal esophagectomy should be considered to be inadequate for these patients. It should be noted that an appropriate lymphadenectomy allows for either open or minimally invasive approaches, as long as an appropriate lymph node dissection is achieved.

Principles: Importance of Margins

The importance of margins has been vigorously debated despite little level I evidence supporting any one viewpoint. Most discussions regarding margins refer to radial margins, rather than proximal or distal margins. Regardless of which margins are being referenced, "nihilists" use retrospective studies to support the position that the presence of involved margins is an indication of aggressive tumor biology, for which more radical surgery would have little effect on outcome; supporters of radical resections (en bloc, 3-field lymphadenectomy), on the other hand, cite primarily single-center retrospective studies to show favorable survival outcomes in patients treated with more radical resection. Confounding many of these retrospective studies, however, is that they often fail to control for the depth of tumor invasion and that the issue of radial margins is relevant only for T3-T4 tumors. Furthermore, with the current widespread use of preoperative chemoradiation therapy, R0 resection rates from standard approaches are now comparable to those from en bloc esophagectomies without preoperative therapy, rendering the question of the importance of radial margins even more difficult to resolve. The proximal and distal margin distances needed to optimize survival are likewise not well defined. Retrospective studies that have evaluated these margins have recommended various distances. Of note, these studies tend to be small, and the results are likely confounded by other variables. Furthermore, as has been documented for gastric cancer, adequate margin distance seems to be relevant only in patients with a moderate tumor burden; it is less relevant in patients with either very advanced- or early-stage disease. Last, vigorous debate continues regarding the extent of proximal and distal margins needed for Siewert II and Siewert III tumors. The debate about these tumors primarily centers on whether a sufficient proximal margin is attainable for Siewert II tumors through a purely abdominal approach and whether a complete gastrectomy is necessary for Siewert III tumors. The only level I evidence addressing the operation type and margins, again, comes from the one randomized trial that compared two surgical approaches [11]. Although this trial did not answer the question of the importance of achieving R0 resection, it did show that similar rates of R0 resection can be achieved using either approach. The implication of this finding is that various aggressive, well-performed surgical approaches can achieve similar rates of R0 resection and that, since there are conflicting data on the importance of margin status, it would make sense to err on the side of an aggressive resection, in an attempt to achieve similar rates of R0 resection.

An issue particular to patients who have been treated with chemotherapy and radiation before surgery is the importance of establishing the extent of tumor extension before therapy. It is a generally accepted dictum that a resection should incorporate all sites of disease that are present before therapy. However, since most patients will have tumor regression after therapy, accurate assessment and mapping before chemoradiation therapy is critical. Furthermore, the operative plan should be based on the original assessment, rather than on a revised plan formulated from posttreatment imaging. This issue is most relevant in patients with disease extension into the gastric cardia and subcardia regions. In these patients, if a gastric conduit is to be used, the extent of a possible distal resection is limited because of technical considerations (conduit size, vascular supply). A separate technical issue, which arises more commonly in previously treated patients, is the intraoperative finding of an involved proximal or distal resection margin on frozen section. One reasonable approach in these patients, if achieving negative margins requires a significant extension of the procedure, is to defer the extended procedure until the final pathologic report is available; if the patient's prognosis is poor on the basis of the final pathologic report, then a more extensive and likely morbid procedure holds little potential benefit for the patient [20].

Surgical Management of the Pylorus and Conduit Size

The origin of the belief that a gastric emptying procedure is necessary during an esophagectomy stems from data on gastric surgeries for ulcer patients. In these patients, in whom vagotomies were performed to reduce acid production, a gastric emptying procedure was shown to be necessary [21], at the risk of gastric obstruction. What is often overlooked, however, is that these ulcer patients often also had an abnormal pylorus attributable to scarring from their ulcer disease; therefore, it is not clear that extrapolating this finding to esophagectomies is appropriate. Furthermore, although some studies have suggested that gastric emptying is important and that, when it is not performed, a postoperative gastric obstruction can result in a higher risk of aspiration pneumonia, anastomotic leak, and death [22], these findings are not definitive, and other studies have found no such associations [23]. Some of these studies also indicate that, by avoiding gastric emptying, one can perhaps achieve better long-term functional outcomes, with less dumping and bile reflux, two of the most debilitating long-term consequences of an esophagectomy with a gastric conduit. Confounding much of these data on gastric emptying is the possibility that the conduit diameter might also contribute to the emptying function of the gastric conduit, a variable that many of the studies fail to control for [24]. Whereas some surgeons prefer not to tubularize the gastric conduit, because of the concern that a narrow conduit will jeopardize the vascular supply and increase the risk of anastomotic leaks [25], others believe that a narrower conduit results in less stasis and bile reflux. One consistent finding among studies supporting gastric emptying procedures is that most patients treated without this procedure never develop a problem, and, furthermore, the vast majority of patients undergoing the procedure likely do not need it and are possibly subjected to long-term functional problems because of it. Therefore, two reasonable approaches to managing the pylorus arise: [1] non-surgically preempt problems by temporarily disabling the pylorus, either by use of a botulinum injection [26], or by use of pre-resection endoscopic balloon dilation of the pylorus [27]; [2] do nothing to the pylorus and use a postoperative nasogastric tube as a means of monitoring gastric emptying, with selective endoscopic management of the few patients who have gastric emptying problems [28]. With regard to the size of the gastric conduit, the data that show an association between diameter, perioperative complications, and long-term functional status are inconclusive; therefore, a reasonable surgical approach is to balance the varying recommendations and to create a reasonably narrow conduit (5–6 cm).

Surgical Techniques

Ivor Lewis Esophagectomy

Location of the tumor, surgeon preference, patient surgical history, choice of esophageal substitute, and previous radiation are all important considerations for the surgeon when selecting a surgical technique for esophagectomy. The most common indication for an Ivor Lewis esophagectomy is middle third or distal esophageal squamous or adenocarcinoma.

Ivor Lewis esophagectomy is performed in two phases: first, the abdominal phase followed by the thoracic phase. With the patient placed in supine position, an upper midline abdominal incision is made for abdominal exploration. A self-retaining retractor is placed and the left lobe of the liver is retracted cephalad to expose the hiatus. The gastrohepatic ligament is incised up to the right crus. The hiatus and distal esophagus are dissected anteriorly and posteriorly then the abdominal esophagus is encircled with a Penrose drain to assist in providing traction for dissection at the hiatus. The boundaries of the hiatal dissection include the aorta posteriorly, the pleura laterally, and the pericardium anteriorly.

The lesser sac is entered taking care to preserve the right gastroepiploic artery pedicle, which will ultimately provide the blood supply for the gastric conduit. Dissection along the greater curvature continues toward the spleen and the short gastric vessels are divided close to the spleen and taken to the left crus. The remainder of the phrenoesophageal ligament attachments are divided, and the abdominal esophagus and cardia are freed.

The stomach and duodenum are mobilized from retroperitoneal attachments and is deemed adequate when the pylorus can reach the right crus without tension. The left gastric artery is divided and all associated lymph nodes are swept from the common hepatic artery medially to the specimen side. Lymphadenectomy is continued to clear the lymphatic tissues along the splenic artery. Thus, all the nodal tissue from the common hepatic artery to the splenic artery is swept up toward the specimen to be removed en bloc.

Along the lesser curvature, the right gastric artery is divided. The stomach is then partially transected from the point where the right gastric artery is divided and carried up toward the fundus. The staple line is reinforced with interrupted lemberted sutures.

A feeding jejunostomy is inserted typically 40 cm distal to the ligament of Treitz. The feeding jejunostomy serves as definitive enteric access postoperatively and can be removed once the patient is tolerating an oral diet. The abdomen is closed and the patient is prepared for the thoracic phase.

The patient is re-positioned in the left lateral decubitus position with the right side up in preparation for a right thoracotomy. A posterolateral right thoracotomy is performed sparing the serratus muscle. The chest is entered in the fourth or fifth interspace. The lung is retracted anteriorly and the inferior pulmonary ligament is divided. The infracarinal lymph nodes are cleared from the right and left mainstem bronchi. The azygous vein is divided and the vagus nerve is identified at this level and divided to avoid traction injury to the recurrent laryngeal nerve. All periesophageal fatty and nodal tissue is swept toward the specimen side. The esophagus is dissected circumferentially from the vertebral body to the pericardium. Care should be taken to carefully clip or tie any lymphatics that are encountered to avoid possible chylothorax. Arterial branches originating directly from the aorta are also identified and divided. The proximal transection point is typically at the level of the transected azygous vein.

The anastomosis can be fashioned in a variety of ways at the discretion of the surgeon. Though we prefer the end-to-end stapled circular anastomosis, several anastomotic techniques have been described including hand-sewn (single layer vs. double layer), stapled (circular vs. side to side linear stapled anastomosis), and hybrid techniques [29–32]. Studies have not definitively proven one technique to be superior over another technique. In a meta-analysis evaluating 12 randomized control trials with over 1400 patients, there was no difference in the incidence of anastomotic leak or postoperative mortality [32] in circular stapled anastomosis compared to the hand-sewn technique. There was an increased incidence of anastomotic stricture and decreased operative time for the circular stapled anastomosis compared to the hand-sewn anastomosis.

After the anastomosis is completed, the remaining omentum is used to wrap around the conduit and tucked between the staple line and the airway to prevent possible fistula. Any redundant stomach is reduced back into the abdomen and the conduit is sutured to the diaphragmatic hiatus to prevent paraconduit hernia. The conduit is also secured to the mediastinal pleura to take some of the tension off the anastomosis. Chest tubes are placed anteriorly and posteriorly and the thoracotomy incision is closed.

Minimally Invasive Ivor Lewis Esophagectomy

Up until two decades ago, esophagectomy involved laparotomy and thoracotomy for Ivor Lewis esophagectomy or laparotomy and cervical incision for transhiatal esophagectomy or laparotomy, thoracotomy, and cervical incision for 3-hole McKeown esophagectomy. In attempts to reduce the morbidity and mortality of open esophagectomy, James Luketich adopted and refined the technique for minimally invasive esophagectomy [25, 33]. Though many hybrid approaches have been reported, minimally invasive esophagectomy typically includes laparoscopic transhiatal esophagectomy, laparoscopic-thoracoscopic 3-hole McKeown esophagectomy and laparoscopic-thoracoscopic Ivor Lewis esophagectomy. The majority of mid-esophageal to distal esophageal/gastroesophageal junction tumors can be resected with good exposure and adequate margins using the minimally invasive Ivor Lewis approach.

Similar to the open Ivor Lewis esophagectomy, the abdominal phase begins with the patient in supine position. Six abdominal ports are placed including one for the liver retractor, one for the laparoscopic camera, and two ports each for the surgeon and the first assistant. The abdomen is first insufflated with carbon dioxide and inspected for evidence of occult metastasis. Similar to open Ivor Lewis esophagectomy, the dissection begins at the hiatus. The gastrohepatic ligament is opened and the left gastric and celiac lymph node dissection is completed. The lower esophagus is circumferentially dissected at the level of the crus and into the mediastinum through the hiatus. The greater curve of the stomach is mobilized and the lesser sac is entered below the gastric antrum preserving the right gastroepiploic artery. The stomach is further mobilized from its retrogastric attachments. If needed, a Kocher maneuver is performed to mobilize the duodenum in order to allow for the pylorus to reach the right crus without tension. The left gastric pedicle is skeletonized and divided at the take-off from the celiac artery. All associated lymph node and fatty tissue is swept toward the specimen. The gastric conduit is created by first stapling the right gastric artery pedicle at the lesser curve and carrying the staple line up toward the fundus to create a tubular gastric conduit. A feeding jejunostomy is placed in the left lower quadrant using a modified Seldinger technique with a commercially available jejunostomy-tube kit.

The patient is then turned and positioned in the left lateral decubitus position. Five ports are placed in the chest: one port for the camera, one for the first assistant to provide suction, and two ports for the surgeon. The esophagus is mobilized in the chest similar to open esophagectomy with division of the inferior pulmonary ligament and division of the mediastinal pleura anterior and posterior to the esophagus. The azygous vein is divided and the esophagus is circumferentially dissected. The subcarinal lymph nodes are excised en bloc with the specimen. The vagus nerve is divided just above the azygous vein to avoid traction injury to the recurrent laryngeal nerve. Lymphatic tissue along the aortoesophageal branches and lymphatic tributaries are clipped to prevent chyle leak. The specimen with the attached gastric conduit is pulled into the chest taking care to preserve proper orientation of the conduit. At this time the anterior working port is enlarged to a 5-cm access incision. The specimen is transected proximal to the tumor and removed through the access incision. The stapled esophagogastric anastomosis is fashioned with an end-to-end stapler. Excess omentum is wrapped around the anastomosis especially between the conduit and airway to prevent fistula. The conduit is secured to the crus of the diaphragm to prevent conduit herniation through the esophageal hiatus. Chest tubes are placed and the incisions are closed.

Transhiatal Esophagectomy

Transhiatal esophagectomy can be considered as a safe, expeditious, and effective technique for resection of distal esophageal cancers with no evidence of subcarinal nodal disease on positron emission tomography or endoscopic ultrasound. The procedure is first performed through an upper midline laparotomy. After assessing for occult metastatic disease, the dissection proceeds similar to the abdominal phase of Ivor Lewis esophagectomy: the distal esophagus is circumferentially dissected free from the crus at the hiatus. The right gastroepiploic pedicle is preserved and the greater curvature is mobilized. The left gastric artery is identified and transected. Lymphadenectomy at the celiac axis is performed and swept toward the specimen. A Kocher maneuver is performed to ensure adequate mobilization of the gastric conduit. A feeding jejunostomy is placed.

The diaphragm is incised up to the pericardium to open the hiatus. The distal 10 cm of the esophagus is mobilized under direct vision while keeping the esophagus on tension. The surgeon's hand completes the remainder of the mediastinal mobilization with gentle blunt finger dissection to the level of the carina.

An oblique incision is made along the anterior border of the left sternocleidomastoid muscle extending down to the suprasternal notch. Dissection is carried down medially to the carotid sheath. The omohyoid muscle is divided and the middle thyroid vein and inferior thyroid artery are divided. The recurrent laryngeal nerve is identified and preserved. A plane is developed between the trachea and esophagus. The cervical esophagus is bluntly mobilized from adjacent tissues circumferentially with special attention not to injure the membranous portion of the trachea. The remainder of the mediastinal esophagus is dissected with blunt cervical dissection from the cervical incision. The esophagus is then transected at the level of the thoracic inlet in order to preserve as much of the cervical esophagus as possible.

The surgeon's hand is then inserted through the hiatus posterior to the esophagus to lyse any remaining adhesions in the mediastinum. The esophagus is delivered downward out of the hiatus. The stomach is separated from the esophagus with a linear stapler along the lesser curve and the specimen is removed from the field. A chest tube is passed through the cervical incision down through the mediastinum and out of the hiatus. The chest tube is then sutured to the gastric conduit and pulled up through the cervical incision taking care to ensure proper orientation of the gastric conduit. The cervical esophagogastric anastomosis is fashioned either using an end-to-end stapled anastomosis or hand-sewn in a single or double layer according to surgeon preference. The gastric conduit is secured to the hiatus to prevent herniation. A drain is placed in the neck near the anastomosis and bilateral anterior chest tubes are also placed. The abdominal and neck incisions are closed.

3-Hole McKeown Esophagectomy

The 3-hole esophagectomy is defined by thoracic esophageal mobilization, lymph node dissection, abdominal exploration, stomach mobilization, lymph node dissection, placement of feeding jejunostomy, and left cervical incision for cervical anastomosis. The advantage of the McKeown 3-hole approach is less morbidity if a leak occurs in the neck compared to leak in the chest. The McKeown esophagectomy is an appropriate surgical approach for Siewert type I and II tumors, as well as all patients with tumor above the gastroesophageal junction, up to the level of the clavicles. Advantages of the Ivor Lewis esophagectomy compared to the McKewon esophagectomy include lower stricture rate, lower leak, and lower aspiration rates [34].

With the patient positioned in left lateral decubitus position, a right posterolateral thoracotomy is made similar to Ivor Lewis esophagectomy in the fourth or fifth intercostal space. The thoracic esophagus is mobilized as described above, the azygous vein is divided, and the subcarinal and mediastinal lymph nodes are cleared. Two chest tubes are placed and the chest is closed. The patient is positioned in supine position and an upper midline incision is made. The gastric conduit is mobilized as described above and the celiac lymph nodes along the lesser curvature are swept toward the specimen. A feeding jejunostomy is placed.

Next, an oblique incision is made along the anterior border of the left sternocleidomastoid muscle. Similar to the transhiatal neck dissection, the omohyoid muscle is divided, the recurrent laryngeal nerve is identified and preserved, and the dissection is carried down to the cervical esophagus. The cervical esophagus is bluntly mobilized from the neck down into the mediastinum. The esophagus and attached gastric conduit is pulled up into the neck taking care to preserve the orientation of the conduit. The esophagus is transected and is passed off the field as specimen. The esophagogastric anastomosis is then fashioned either with a stapler or hand-sewn according to surgeon preference. A drain is placed in the neck near the cervical anastomosis, and the neck and abdominal incisions are closed.

Esophagectomy Complications

Conduit Ischemia

Conduit ischemia occurs as a result of compromise of the conduit blood supply, which typically presents with early clinical deterioration within the first 2–3 days of surgery. Initially, patients may develop tachycardia, arrhythmia, or an increased oxygen requirement. It is important to have a low threshold for performing esophagoscopy to evaluate for ischemia early since conduit ischemia can progress rapidly to sepsis and clinical lability. In the setting of gross ischemia and hemodynamic instability, reoperation is indicated with takedown of the conduit, cervical esophagostomy, wide drainage, and staged reconstruction at a later date [35].

Anastomotic Leaks

Anastomotic leak presents within the first week with signs of evolving clinical deterioration and sepsis with high chest tube output. Initial evaluation with esophagram with water-soluble contrast can reveal the location and size of the leak. Small leaks in a stable patient can be managed with percutaneous drainage, antibiotics, and bowel rest. Endoscopic placement of a covered stent can also be used to seal the leak while the anastomosis heals over the course of 4–6 weeks [36, 37]. In septic patients with large leaks, operative exploration including debridement, drainage, and possible diversion is indicated for source control.

Anastomotic Stricture

Anastomotic stricture can occur in the weeks to months following esophagectomy as a result of ischemia, leak, or use of a small diameter circular stapler [38, 39]. It is important to perform endoscopic evaluation to rule out recurrent disease, and dilation either with a tapered or balloon dilator. Commonly, patients will need more than one treatment in order to manage the anastomotic stricture. Alternatively, retrievable self-expanding esophageal stents can be placed temporarily for the management of anastomotic stricture [40].

Chylothorax

Chylothorax results from either direct injury to the thoracic duct or one of the lymphatic tributaries. Clinically, chylothorax presents as unusually high chest tube output that may be serous or milky in character. The diagnosis can be confirmed by checking the triglyceride level in the fluid after a fat challenge. Low-output chylothorax (defined as daily output less than 1 L in 24 h) can be managed conservatively with complete bowel rest and total parenteral nutrition. If the output persists, or if the chylothorax is high output (defined as daily output greater than 1 L in 24 h) then intervention may be required such as surgical thoracic duct ligation or lymphangiogram and thoracic duct embolization performed by interventional radiology [41].

Conclusions

The data supporting any one surgical approach for esophagectomy for cancer are mostly anecdotal. A prudent approach would be to balance aspects of the available data and to favor a more aggressive resection in patients who may benefit from it and a more limited resection in those who will not. The available data suggest that patients with T2-T3 tumors would most likely benefit from a resection that removes at least 30 local-regional lymph nodes in a manner that also obtains wide radial margins, whereas patients with T1 tumors or those with tumors with more than 7 involved lymph nodes should undergo a less aggressive nodal dissection (radial margins for such patients are either not relevant [T1] or do not contribute to survival [>7 nodes]). The consequence of being uniformly aggressive is that some patients will be unnecessarily exposed to added perioperative complications, with no added oncologic benefit. Likewise, a stomach conduit that is fashioned into a 5–6 cm tube should be wide enough to avoid concerns regarding ischemia, while being narrow enough to minimize the risk of stasis.

References

1. Dubecz A, Schwartz SI, Franz John A. Torek. Ann Thorac Surg. 2008;85(4):1497–9.
2. Churchill ED, Sweet RH. Transthoracic resection of tumors of the esophagus and stomach. Ann Surg. 1942;115(6):897–920.
3. Sweet RH. The treatment of carcinoma of the esophagus and cardiac end of the stomach by surgical extirpation; 203 cases of resection. Surgery. 1948;23(6):952–75.
4. Lewis I. The surgical treatment of carcinoma of the oesophagus; with special reference to a new operation for growths of the middle third. Br J Surg. 1946;34:18–31.
5. McKeown KC. Total three-stage oesophagectomy for cancer of the oesophagus. Br J Surg. 1976;63(4):259–62.
6. Dubecz A, Kun L, Stadlhuber RJ, Peters JH, Schwartz SI. The origins of an operation: a brief history of transhiatal esophagectomy. Ann Surg. 2009;249(3):535–40.
7. Akiyama H, Hiyama M, Miyazono H. Total esophageal reconstruction after extraction of the esophagus. Ann Surg. 1975;182(5):547–52.
8. Orringer MB, Sloan H. Esophagectomy without thoracotomy. J Thorac Cardiovasc Surg. 1978;76(5):643–54.
9. Rizk NP, Bach PB, Schrag D, Bains MS, Turnbull AD, Karpeh M, et al. The impact of complications on outcomes after resection for esophageal and gastroesophageal junction carcinoma. J Am Coll Surg. 2004;198(1):42–50.
10. Hulscher JB, Tijssen JG, Obertop H, van Lanschot JJ. Transthoracic versus transhiatal resection for carcinoma of the esophagus: a meta-analysis. Ann Thorac Surg. 2001;72(1):306–13.
11. Hulscher JB, van Sandick JW, de Boer AG, Wijnhoven BP, Tijssen JG, Fockens P, et al. Extended transthoracic resection compared with limited transhiatal resection for adenocarcinoma of the esophagus. N Engl J Med. 2002;347(21):1662–9.
12. Ayantunde AA, Ng MY, Pal S, Welch NT, Parsons SL. Analysis of blood transfusion predictors in patients undergoing elective oesophagectomy for cancer. BMC Surg. 2008;8:3.
13. Mitchell JD. Anastomotic leak after esophagectomy. Thorac Surg Clin. 2006;16(1):1–9.
14. Rizzetto C, DeMeester SR, Hagen JA, Peyre CG, Lipham JC, DeMeester TR. En bloc esophagectomy reduces local recurrence and improves survival compared with transhiatal resection after neoadjuvant therapy for esophageal adenocarcinoma. J Thorac Cardiovasc Surg. 2008;135(6):1228–36.
15. Altorki N, Kent M, Ferrara C, Port J. Three-field lymph node dissection for squamous cell and adenocarcinoma of the esophagus. Ann Surg. 2002;236(2):177–83.
16. Schwarz RE, Smith DD. Clinical impact of lymphadenectomy extent in resectable esophageal cancer. J Gastrointest Surg. 2007;11(11):1384–93. discussion 93-4
17. Peyre CG, Hagen JA, DeMeester SR, Altorki NK, Ancona E, Griffin SM, et al. The number of lymph nodes removed predicts survival in esophageal cancer: an international study on the impact of extent of surgical resection. Ann Surg. 2008;248(4):549–56.
18. Rizk NP, Ishwaran H, Rice TW, Chen LQ, Schipper PH, Kesler KA, et al. Optimum lymphadenectomy for esophageal cancer. Ann Surg. 2010;251(1):46–50.
19. Omloo JM, Lagarde SM, Hulscher JB, Reitsma JB, Fockens P, van Dekken H, et al. Extended transthoracic resection compared with limited transhiatal resection for adenocarcinoma of the mid/distal esophagus: five-year survival of a randomized clinical trial. Ann Surg. 2007;246(6):992–1000. discussion -1
20. Kim SH, Karpeh MS, Klimstra DS, Leung D, Brennan MF. Effect of microscopic resection line disease on gastric cancer survival. J Gastrointest Surg. 1999;3(1):24–33.
21. Burrows WM. Gastrointestinal function and related problems following esophagectomy. Semin Thorac Cardiovasc Surg. 2004;16(2):142–51.
22. Fok M, Cheng SW, Wong J. Pyloroplasty versus no drainage in gastric replacement of the esophagus. Am J Surg. 1991;162(5):447–52.
23. Nguyen NT, Dholakia C, Nguyen XM, Reavis K. Outcomes of minimally invasive esophagectomy without pyloroplasty: analysis of 109 cases. Am Surg. 2010;76(10):1135–8.

24. Lerut TE, van Lanschot JJ. Chronic symptoms after subtotal or partial oesophagectomy: diagnosis and treatment. Best Pract Res Clin Gastroenterol. 2004;18(5):901–15.
25. Luketich JD, Pennathur A, Awais O, Levy RM, Keeley S, Shende M, et al. Outcomes after minimally invasive esophagectomy: review of over 1000 patients. Ann Surg. 2012;256(1):95–103.
26. Cerfolio RJ, Bryant AS, Canon CL, Dhawan R, Eloubeidi MA. Is botulinum toxin injection of the pylorus during Ivor Lewis [corrected] esophagogastrectomy the optimal drainage strategy? J Thorac Cardiovasc Surg. 2009;137(3):565–72.
27. Swanson EW, Swanson SJ, Swanson RS. Endoscopic pyloric balloon dilatation obviates the need for pyloroplasty at esophagectomy. Surg Endosc. 2012;26(7):2023–8.
28. Lanuti M, DeDelva P, Morse CR, Wright CD, Wain JC, Gaissert HA, et al. Management of delayed gastric emptying after esophagectomy with endoscopic balloon dilatation of the pylorus. Ann Thorac Surg. 2011;91(4):1019–24.
29. Kim RH, Takabe K. Methods of esophagogastric anastomoses following esophagectomy for cancer: a systematic review. J Surg Oncol. 2010;101(6):527–33.
30. Law S, Fok M, Chu KM, Wong J. Comparison of hand-sewn and stapled esophagogastric anastomosis after esophageal resection for cancer: a prospective randomized controlled trial. Ann Surg. 1997;226(2):169–73.
31. Beitler AL, Urschel JD. Comparison of stapled and hand-sewn esophagogastric anastomoses. Am J Surg. 1998;175(4):337–40.
32. Honda M, Kuriyama A, Noma H, Nunobe S, Furukawa TA. Hand-sewn versus mechanical esophagogastric anastomosis after esophagectomy: a systematic review and meta-analysis. Ann Surg. 2013;257(2):238–48.
33. Luketich JD, Pennathur A, Franchetti Y, Catalano PJ, Swanson S, Sugarbaker DJ, et al. Minimally invasive esophagectomy: results of a prospective phase II multicenter trial-the eastern cooperative oncology group (E2202) study. Ann Surg. 2015;261(4):702–7.
34. D'Amico TA. Mckeown esophagogastrectomy. J Thorac Dis. 2014;6(Suppl 3):S322–4.
35. Wormuth JK, Heitmiller RF. Esophageal conduit necrosis. Thorac Surg Clin. 2006;16(1):11–22.
36. Dasari BV, Neely D, Kennedy A, Spence G, Rice P, Mackle E, et al. The role of esophageal stents in the management of esophageal anastomotic leaks and benign esophageal perforations. Ann Surg. 2014;259(5):852–60.
37. Salminen P, Gullichsen R, Laine S. Use of self-expandable metal stents for the treatment of esophageal perforations and anastomotic leaks. Surg Endosc. 2009;23(7):1526–30.
38. Cassivi SD. Leaks, strictures, and necrosis: a review of anastomotic complications following esophagectomy. Semin Thorac Cardiovasc Surg. 2004;16(2):124–32.
39. Park JY, Song HY, Kim JH, Park JH, Na HK, Kim YH, et al. Benign anastomotic strictures after esophagectomy: long-term effectiveness of balloon dilation and factors affecting recurrence in 155 patients. AJR Am J Roentgenol. 2012;198(5):1208–13.
40. Kim HC, Shin JH, Song HY, Park SI, Ko GY, Youn HK, et al. Fluoroscopically guided balloon dilation for benign anastomotic stricture after Ivor-Lewis esophagectomy: experience in 62 patients. J Vasc Interv Radiol. 2005;16(12):1699–704.
41. Mishra PK, Saluja SS, Ramaswamy D, Bains SS, Haque PD. Thoracic duct injury following esophagectomy in carcinoma of the esophagus: ligation by the abdominal approach. World J Surg. 2013;37(1):141–6.

Principles of Radiation Therapy

10

Neil Bryan Newman and A. Bapsi Chakravarthy

Introduction

The treatment design and delivery of radiation for esophageal cancer requires a comprehensive understanding of the natural history of disease, patterns of failure, anatomy, and principles of radiobiology. The use of pretreatment imaging, such as computerized axial tomography (CT) scans, endoscopic ultrasonography, and positron emission tomography (PET) scans, has improved target delineation. State-of-the-art equipment and advances in radiation planning software have improved treatment-related toxicities by allowing increasing dose to tumor while minimizing dose to surrounding normal structures.

Despite radical resection, a significant number of patients develop locoregional and/or distant recurrence leading to poor overall survival with surgery alone. This has led to the use of neoadjuvant therapies to complement resection. Over the past four decades, chemotherapy either alone or in combination with radiation therapy has been extensively studied. Although the role of radiation in the treatment of esophageal cancer has been clearly established, the integration of targeted agents as well as the ideal sequencing of chemotherapy, radiation, and surgery remain to be determined.

N. B. Newman
Vanderbilt Ingram Cancer Center Department of Radiation Oncology, Nashville, TN, USA
e-mail: neil.b.newman@vumc.org

A. B. Chakravarthy (✉)
Vanderbilt Ingram Cancer Center Department of Radiation Oncology, Nashville, USA
e-mail: bapsi.chak@vanderbilt.edu

© Springer Nature Switzerland AG 2020
N. F. Saba, B. F. El-Rayes (eds.), *Esophageal Cancer*,
https://doi.org/10.1007/978-3-030-29832-6_10

Radiation Alone

Historically, the results of radiation therapy alone in the treatment of localized esophageal cancer have been poor, with 2-year survival rates of approximately 10–20%, and 5-year survival rates approaching less than 5%.

A prospective trial, Radiation Therapy Oncology Group (RTOG) 85–01, found that concurrent chemoradiation (CRT) using 5000 cGy with 5-fluorouracil (5-FU) and cisplatin was superior to 6400 cGy of radiation alone in terms of local control, distant control, and survival [1]. Longer term follow-up confirmed these findings, with a 5-year survival rate of 27% in the combined modality group. The median survival duration was 9.3 months. On the other hand, no patients were alive at 5 years in the RT-alone group ($P < 0.0001$) [2]. Therefore, radiation alone is currently reserved for use primarily in the palliative setting.

Surgery Alone

Patients with early esophageal cancers (T1aN0 disease) that involve only the mucosa (lamina propria or into but not through the muscularis mucosae) have a less than 3% risk of nodal metastases and therefore may be considered for endoscopic mucosal resection alone. Patients with T1bN0M0 disease that invades the submucosa are currently treated with surgery alone. For those patients who are not surgical candidates, definitive CRT using 5040 cGy with concurrent carboplatin and paclitaxel can be considered.

Patients with higher stages of disease including T2–4, N0 or node-positive disease should be evaluated by a multidisciplinary team of surgeons, medical oncologists, and radiation oncologists to determine the best treatment plan for the individual patient, taking into consideration multiple factors including the location of the tumor, histology, comorbidities, and patient preferences. All patients should be evaluated for trimodality therapy.

Surgery With or Without Preoperative Radiation

Early attempts to improve local control and survival considered the addition of preoperative radiation alone to surgery. From 1977 to 1985, Wang and colleagues carried out a prospective randomized trial of 206 patients delivering 4000 cGy of radiation to the whole mediastinum and left gastroepiploic lymphatics followed by surgery versus surgery alone. The 5-year overall survival (OS) was 35% in the combined modality arm and 30% in the surgery alone arm. The primary pattern of failure in both arms was intra- or extra-thoracic lymph node metastasis (41% vs. 34%) [3]. The Gastrointestinal Tumor Study Group (GITSG) pooled five trials that reported one-year mortality data. No statistically significant difference in the risk of mortality with preoperative radiotherapy was found when compared to surgery alone (RR, 1.01; 95% CI, 0.88 to 1.16; $P = 0.87$) [4]. Therefore, preoperative radiation alone is currently not utilized.

Surgery With or Without Postoperative Radiation

Given the poor outcomes with surgery alone, multiple randomized trials have investigated resection followed by adjuvant radiation as compared to resection alone. In one such study, Teniere et al. randomized 221 patients to esophagectomy followed by 4500–5500 cGy vs. surgery alone. The median survival was 18 months in both arms and there was no significant difference in 5-year survival (21% vs. 19%) [5]. Although the rates of local recurrence with radiotherapy were slightly lower, this benefit was achieved at the expense of increased morbidity. Moreover, autopsy series have shown that systemic spread appears independent of achieving local control, thereby reinforcing the concept that esophageal cancer is often a local presentation of a systemic disease with occult metastasis at or around the time of diagnosis. Therefore, we no longer utilize postoperative radiation alone in the treatment of esophageal cancer.

Radiation With or Without Concurrent Chemotherapy

A landmark trial utilizing primary CRT was RTOG 85–01 [1]. One hundred and twenty-one individuals with T1-T3 N0-N1 M0, squamous cell carcinoma (SCC) (86%) or adenocarcinoma (14%) of the thoracic esophagus with no gastric involvement or distant metastases were randomized to receive either radiation alone to 6400 cGy or 5000 cGy with concurrent chemotherapy with 5-FU (1000 $mg/m^2/24hr$ for 4 days in weeks 1, 5, 8, 11) and cisplatin (75 mg/m^2 in weeks 1, 5, 8, 11). At 5-year follow-up, the OS for CRT was 26% (95% confidence interval [CI], 15%–37%) compared with 0% following RT alone. Median survival was 14.1 months in the CRT arm vs. 9.3 months in the RT alone arm on long-term follow-up [6]. Although persistent disease was the greatest cause of treatment failure in both groups, this was more common in the radiation alone arm. The results of RTOG 85-01 and several other randomized studies (Table 10.1) have demonstrated a survival advantage to combined modality therapy over radiation alone [7–9]. The improvement in survival in these trials was related in part to improvement in local control, but also to decreases in distant metastases. The distant metastases (with or without locoregional disease) accounted for the first site of treatment failure in 30% of the patients within the RT group versus 16% of patients in the combined modality group [6].

Table 10.1 Randomized studies comparing radiation alone with combined chemoradiation

Study	No. of patients	Radiation dose (Gy)	Chemotherapy	2-year survival (%)
Araujo et al.	28	50	None	22
[7]	31	50	5-FU, MMC, Bleo	38
Smith et al.	62	60	None	12
[8]	65	60	MMC, 5-FU	27
Roussel et al.	69	56.25	None	6 (3 YS)
[9]	75	56.25	MTX	12 (3 YS)
Herskovic	60	64	None	10
et al. [1]	61	50	5-FU, CDDP	38

As local failure rates even in the combined modality arm of RTOG 8501 were 50%, subsequent trials evaluated whether higher doses of radiation could improve on these results [10]. Two hundred and eighteen patients with either SCC (85%) or adenocarcinoma (15%) were randomized to receive combined modality therapy consisting of cisplatin and fluorouracil with concurrent radiation, either a high dose of 6480 cGy or standard doses of 5040 cGy, with the same chemotherapy. The trial was stopped after interim analysis due to 11 treatment-related deaths in the dose-escalation arm compared to 2 in the standard arm. Paradoxically, 7 of the 11 deaths in the high-dose arm had received 5040 cGy or less at the time of death. There was no significant difference in median survival (13 vs. 18.1 months), 2-year survival (31% vs. 40%), or locoregional failure (56% vs. 52%) between the high-dose and standard-dose arms, respectively. This trial established 5040 cGy as the standard dose for definitive CRT.

Another attempt at dose escalation included the use of a brachytherapy boost. In a phase II study, patients completed 5000 cGy of external beam radiation, which was followed 2 weeks later by high-dose-rate (HDR) or low-dose-rate (LDR) brachytherapy. Patients had concurrent cisplatin and continuous infusion 5-FU for four cycles. Due to life-threatening toxicities in 24% of patients, including 6 tracheo-esophageal fistulas, brachytherapy boost is no longer used in the United States [11].

Trimodality Therapy Compared to Surgery Alone

Given the improved survival and local control with the addition of chemotherapy to radiation, the question as to whether chemoradiation followed by surgery was superior to surgery alone needed further investigation. The major randomized controlled trials comparing CRT plus surgery to surgery alone are summarized in Table 10.2.

In the Walsh study, 113 patients were randomized to 4000 cGy in 15 fractions with concurrent 5-FU and cisplatin followed by surgery versus surgery alone. The median and 3-year survival rates were 16 months and 32% for the CRT group and 11 months and 6% for the surgery-only group ($P = 0.01$) [12]. This

Table 10.2 Selected trials of neoadjuvant chemoradiation versus surgery alone

Study	n	Dose	Chemotherapy	pCR (%)	Medn S (months)	3YOS (%)	P
Walsh et al. [12]	58	40 Gy/3 weeks	CDDP	25	16	32	0.01
	55	None	None		11	6	
Urba et al. [13]	50	45 Gy (1.5 bid)	CDDP/5-FU/VLB	28	17	30	0.15
	50	None	None		18	16	
Burmeister et al. [14]	128	35 Gy/3 weeks	CDDP/5-FU	12.5	22	42	0.57
	128	None	None		19	36	
Tepper et al. [15]	30	50.4 Gy/5.5 weeks	CDDP/5-FU	40	53.8	39	0.002
	26	None	None		21.5	15	
van Hagen et al. [16]	175	41.4 Gy/4.5 weeks	Carbo/Taxol	29	49	58	0.003
	188	None	None		24	44	

study was criticized for its short follow-up time (median 10 months), unconventional radiation dose, and fraction size as well as the poor survival outcomes in the surgery-alone arm compared to other randomized trials. The Urba study [13] was a small randomized study comparing 45 Gy of radiation BID with chemotherapy to surgery alone and found no difference in overall survival. The Burmeister Study [14] was a phase III study that found that the addition of chemotherapy to 35 Gy of radiation did not improve its primary outcome of progression free survival nor its secondary outcome of overall survival. Although this too was an unconventional radiation dose.

The CALGB 9781 trial randomized patients (both with and without nodal positivity) to neoadjuvant CRT using a standard radiation dose and fraction size (5040 cGy in 28 fractions) with concurrent cisplatin and 5-FU followed by surgery versus surgery alone. Although the trial was closed early due to poor accrual, the median and 5-year survival rates were 4.5 years and 39% for patients receiving CRT and 1.8 years and 16% for patients receiving surgery alone [15]. Multiple meta-analyses have examined the survival outcomes following CRT and surgery compared to surgery alone [16–20]. All but one analysis showed a significant reduction in mortality when CRT was added to surgery. Sjoquist et al. [20] reviewed 12 randomized controlled trials with a total of 1854 patients comparing CRT followed by surgery versus surgery alone. The HR for all-cause mortality for patients receiving neoadjuvant CRT was 0.78 (95% CI, 0.70–0.88; $P < 0.0001$) and this benefit was irrespective of histology. Urschel et al. evaluated 9 randomized trials with a total of 1116 patients and concluded that 3-year survival was improved with CRT (odds ratio [OR] = 0.66; 95% CI, 0.47–0.92; $P = 0.016$). Improvements in survival were most pronounced with concurrent CRT (OR = 0.45; 95% CI, 0.26–0.79; $P = 0.005$) compared with sequential therapy (OR = 0.82; 95% CI, 0.54–1.25; $P = 0.36$). In 2012, van Hagen et al. published the "ChemoRadiotherapy for Oesophageal cancer followed by Surgery Study" (CROSS) trial. Patients with resectable (T1N1 or T2–3/N0-N M0) esophageal or gastroesophageal junction (GEJ) tumors were randomized to neoadjuvant CRT with 4140 cGy in 23 fractions with concurrent carboplatin and paclitaxel followed by surgery versus surgery alone. A pathological complete response was achieved in 47 of 161 patients (29%) who underwent resection following CRT. Median OS was 49.4 months in the trimodality arm versus 24.0 months in the surgery-alone group. At a median follow-up of 45.4 months, the 3- and 5-year OS rates, respectively, were 58% vs. 44% and 47% vs. 24% for trimodality therapy vs. surgery-alone arms ($p = 0.003$) [21]. Interestingly, subset analysis showed that patients with SCC benefited the most from this regimen. The benefit of trimodality therapy was associated with a HR of 0.74 for adenocarcinoma histology while it was 0.42 for patients receiving trimodality therapy for SCC.Follow-up data on the CROSS study revealed that overall and locoregional recurrence rates were 58% and 34% in the surgery arm, respectively, while they were 35% and 14% in the trimodality arm [22]. Despite concerns regarding the lower doses of radiation used in the trimodality arm, the incidence of in-field recurrence was less than 5%. The predominant pattern of failure remained distant failures at 31% as compared to 14% local-regional failures. Although concerns have also been raised about the lower doses of chemotherapy, the CRT arm resulted in significant decrease in both peritoneal carcinomatosis from 14% to 4% ($P < 0.001$) as well as hematogenous spread (35% vs. 29%; $P = 0.025$). On the other hand, the lower doses of both radiation and chemotherapy have resulted in a much improved side effect profile as compared to RTOG 8501.While neoadjuvant CRT improves outcomes, it is less clear which subsets of patients benefit the most. To determine whether patients with adenocarcinoma histology had similar outcomes when stratified by nodal status a retrospective analysis using the NCDB database was performed [23]. This study reviewed outcomes on 1301 patients and compared those who received trimodality therapy vs. surgery alone. Three-year OS was better for trimodality therapy over surgery alone (49% vs. 38%). However, when stratified by nodal status, the survival advantage of receiving trimodality therapy was greater for node-positive patients. HR in node-positive patients ($n = 618$) was 0.52, $p < 0.001$. Interestingly, with node-negative patients ($n = 691$), the adjusted HR of receiving trimodality therapy was 0.84 and was not significant. While this data is potentially clinically relevant, it would be difficult to implement due to mismatch between clinical and surgical staging.

Definitive Chemoradiation Compared to Neoadjuvant Chemoradiation

Stahl et al. compared CRT with or without surgery. Patients with locally advanced SCC were randomized to induction chemotherapy (5-FU, leucovorin, etoposide, cisplatin) followed by CRT (4000 cGy with concurrent cisplatin/etoposide) followed by surgery versus the same induction chemotherapy followed by CRT (6500 cGy with cisplatin and etoposide) [24]. There was no significant difference between treatment arms in terms of OS at 2 years (40% vs. 35%). Although there was no survival benefit in favor of surgery, those patients had better 2-year progression-free survival (PFS; 64% vs. 41%, $p = 0.03$). Of note though, treatment-related mortality was higher in the surgery arm (13% vs. 4%, p = 0.03). Cox regression analysis revealed clinical tumor response to induction chemotherapy to be the single independent prognostic factor for OS (hazard ratio [HR], 0.30; 95% CI, 0.19–0.47; $P < 0.0001$). In a French trial by Bedenne et al., 444 patients with SCC underwent concurrent CRT with two cycles of cisplatin and 5-FU. Patients who demonstrated a partial or complete response to treatment were then randomized to receive either surgery or additional CRT. Only 259 (58%) of the patients treated with this regimen went on to randomization. The median survival time was 17.7 months in the surgery group versus 19.3 months in the definitive CRT group. Similar to the Stahl study, local control was improved in the surgery arm, 66.4% vs 57%. However, the trial suffered from poor accrual and suboptimal design. The randomization of these patients did not take place at the time of diagnosis, rather after they were treated with CRT. Therefore, those who were unresponsive to CRT went on to surgery, but were not followed on the trial; this may have limited the quality of the analysis as these patients would have likely benefited most from surgery as part of the treatment regimen [25].

Surgery With or Without Neoadjuvant Chemotherapy Alone

To determine whether neoadjuvant chemotherapy alone could replace neoadjuvant CRT, the MRC conducted a trial randomizing patients to cisplatin 80 mg/m^2 plus fluorouracil 1000 mg/m^2 daily by continuous infusion for 4 days followed by surgery or surgery alone. Preoperative radiation was left to the discretion of the treating physician. Only 9% of patients received radiation and this was similar in both arms. There was a significant improvement in 2-year survival with the addition of chemotherapy (43% to 34%, $p = 0.004$) [26].

In contrast to the MRC study, the Intergroup trial 0113, RTOG 8911, which also randomized patients to either preoperative 5-FU and cisplatin followed by surgery or surgery alone, found no difference in 2-year survival (38–40%) and a high rate of local failure in both arms (27–29%) [27]. The rate of local failure was much higher than in the neoadjuvant CRT arm of the CROSS trial (5%) [21].

In the phase III PreOperative therapy in Esophagogastric adenocarcinoma Trial (POET), patients with adenocarcinomas of the GE junction were randomized to either induction chemotherapy (cisplatin, leucovorin, 5-FU) followed by surgery or the same induction chemotherapy followed by CRT (concurrent cisplatin/etoposide with 3000 cGy in 15 fractions) followed by surgery. Although the study closed early due to poor accrual, the preoperative CRT arm had an improved 3-year survival over chemotherapy alone of 47.4% to 27.7% ($p = 0.07$) [28].

Adjuvant vs. Neoadjuvant Therapy

The Pasquali meta-analysis pooled together 33 randomized trials with 6072 patients who were able to receive either surgery-alone, neoadjuvant chemotherapy/radiation therapy/CRT, or adjuvant chemotherapy/radiation therapy/CRT. Surgery along with adjuvant regimens showed no significant survival advantage, while neoadjuvant CRT was superior to surgery (HR 0.77, $p < 0.001$). Neoadjuvant chemotherapy demonstrated a HR of 0.89 ($p = 0.051$). This supports neoadjuvant CRT with surgery as the superior regimen when esophagectomy is feasible [29].

Cancer of the Cervical Esophagus

Squamous cell carcinomas of the cervical esophagus that extend from the hypopharynx to the sternal notch are a unique challenge due to the associated surgical morbidity. These tumors represent 5–6% of esophageal cancers. Surgery may require removal of a portion of the pharynx, larynx, and radical neck dissection causing severe functional deficits and impairment of quality of life. Therefore, cervical esophageal tumors are treated with primary CRT similarly to locally advanced cancers of the hypopharynx and larynx, with surgery reserved for salvage.

Multiple series have demonstrated similar survival outcomes between surgery and CRT in this population [30, 31]. In a phase II trial by Bidoli et al., 101 patients were treated with cisplatin and 5-FU with concurrent radiation to 3000 cGy. Patients with potentially resectable tumors were then assessed for curative surgery; the remaining patients received two more cycles of chemotherapy and additional radiation to a total dose of 5000 cGy. Of the 40 patients who were candidates for surgery, 32 patients underwent resection with a reported surgical mortality of 22%. Of the 61 nonsurgical patients, 37 patients (61%) achieved complete clinical remission, and 14 patients (23%) achieved partial remission. The median survival for the entire group was 15 months. At 10 years, freedom from disease progression was similar in the two groups (24%), whereas the median survival (22 months vs. 12 months) and the OS rates (17% vs. 9%) were superior in the nonsurgical compared with the surgical patients, a factor likely explained by the high surgical mortality rate [30].

Cancers of the Gastroesophageal Junction

The incidence of adenocarcinoma of the GEJ continues to increase over the last few decades. Cancers of the GEJ have been included in gastric and esophageal trials, and therefore the optimal treatment approach for these patients remains unclear. Four major trials that have included patients with GEJ tumors are the US Intergroup 0116 trial, the MAGIC trial, the German POET trial, and the CROSS trial. The US Intergroup 0116 trial provides the most compelling data for the use of adjuvant CRT. Following resection, patients ($n = 556$) were randomly assigned to either observation alone or adjuvant chemoradiotherapy. Three-year disease-free (48% vs. 31%) and overall (50% vs. 41%) survival rates were significantly better with combined modality therapy. This benefit was confirmed with longer follow-up with 5-year OS being 43% vs. 28%, HR for survival 1.32 (95% CI 1.10–1.60) [32].

Another study of patients with gastric cancer (74%) included patients with both distal esophageal tumors (11%) as well as GEJ tumors (15%). The Medical Research Council Adjuvant Gastric Infusional Chemotherapy (MAGIC) trial randomized 503 patients to surgery-alone or surgery-plus perioperative chemotherapy consisting of 3 cycles of epirubicin, cisplatin, and infusional 5-FU (ECF). The OS was significantly better in the chemotherapy group (HR for death 0.75, 95% CI 0.60–0.93) as was PFS (HR for progression 0.66). The 25% reduction in the risk of death favoring chemotherapy translated into an improvement in 5-year survival from 23 to 36% [33].

The German multicenter POET trial was the first randomized study exclusively for patients with adenocarcinomas of the GEJ. Patients with locally advanced (EUS-staged T3–4, N0, M0) adenocarcinoma of the lower esophagus, GEJ or gastric cardia were randomized to neoadjuvant chemotherapy (12 weeks) followed by surgery, or induction chemotherapy followed by 3 weeks of concurrent chemoradiotherapy followed by surgery. Although the study was closed prematurely due to poor accrual, there was a trend toward improved 3-year survival with chemoradiotherapy (47% vs. 28%; $p = 0.07$). The rate of complete (R0) resection was similar in both arms (72% vs. 70%) but the pathologic complete response rate was higher with chemoradiotherapy (16% vs. 2%), as was the rate of negative lymph nodes (64% vs. 38%). Moreover, the local failure rate in the chemotherapy-alone group was high (41%), a finding that has been reported by others when radiation was not a component of trimodality therapy [28].

   Therefore, cancers of the GEJ can be treated with either perioperative chemotherapy as outlined in the MAGIC trial or postoperative CRT as outlined in the Intergroup 0116 study. The CROSS trial also favored the trimodality approach with improvement in survival compared to surgery alone. Therefore, the trimodality approach using neoadjuvant chemotherapy with weekly carboplatin and paclitaxel with radiation is the favored approach. In patients where the tumor comes to within 2 cm of the GEJ, suggesting a primary esophageal origin, neoadjuvant CRT using weekly carboplatin/paclitaxel is preferred. On the other hand, for patients whose tumors are located primarily in the stomach and can tolerate aggressive chemotherapy, the perioperative approach (per MAGIC) is the favored approach. If patients are not good candidates for the aggressive chemotherapy regimen outlined by MAGIC, surgery followed by CRT (per Intergroup 0116) is recommended. Finally, patients who are not surgical candidates are considered for primary CRT.

Palliative Radiotherapy Alone in the Metastatic Setting

More than 50% of patients present with unresectable or metastatic disease at the time of presentation [34]. Historically, radiotherapy has played an important role in the management of unresectable or metastatic disease, both for palliation of dysphagia, pain, and bleeding.

   Recently, a phase III study performed by the Trans-Tasman Radiation Oncology Group (TROG) 03.01 and National Cancer Institute of Canada (NCIC) CTG ES.2 trial found that CRT led to increased toxicity without additional symptom control or improved survival compared to radiation alone. This study enrolled 220 patients, the majority with metastatic disease, and randomized them to palliative radiation alone (3000–3500 cGy) or concurrent CRT (with cisplatin and 5-FU) in order to evaluate symptomatic dysphagia control, quality of life, and survival. There was no statistically significant difference in median dysphagia-free survival or median OS between the two groups. On the other hand, the grade 3–4 acute toxicity was significantly worse for patients receiving CRT (36% vs. 16%, $p = 0.0017$) [34]. Therefore, we favor radiation alone in the metastatic setting.

   We favor the use of either radiation alone or CRT for relief of dysphagia over the placement of stents. Stents often result in pain with swallowing as well as severe reflux symptoms. Over 70% of patients can achieve relief of dysphagia and remain dysphagia-free until death. There can be transient worsening prior to improvement of symptoms and patients should be warned to anticipate this.

Chemoradiation Therapy in the Metastatic Setting

Although the majority of patients with metastatic esophageal cancer are best treated by radiation alone, there is a wide spectrum of presentations of this disease. In patients with good performance status and oligometastatic disease, a more aggressive approach utilizing CRT may be considered.

There is some retrospective data suggesting that definitive CRT therapy to the primary site may confer a survival advantage in this group of patients.

In an analysis of stage IV patients (n = 12,683) using the NCDB, patients were grouped into three cohorts: (1) chemotherapy plus conventional palliative dose radiotherapy (<5040 cGy); (2) chemotherapy plus definitive dose radiotherapy (≥5040 cGy); or (3) chemotherapy alone. Compared with chemotherapy alone, patients who received chemotherapy plus definitive dose radiotherapy(>5040 cGy) had improved survival with a median OS of 8.3 vs. 11.3 months [HR = 0.72, 95% confidence interval: 0.70–0.74, p ≤ 0.001). As in all retrospective analyses, there is a risk of selection bias as patients with better performance status as well as fewer sites of metastatic disease are more likely to receive a definitive course of CRT [35].

A prospective phase II trial of 60 patients comparing definitive CRT to chemotherapy alone in stage IV disease has also suggested a statistically significant advantage for definitive CRT in terms of tumor response rate (83.3% vs. 46.7%, p = 0.001) as well as PFS (9.3 vs. 4.7 months, p = 0.021) and OS (18.3 vs 10.2 months at 18 months of follow-up [36]. For the subgroup of patients with low volume oligometastatic disease, we recommend 5040 cGy to the gross tumor volume alone without inclusion of regional nodes and concurrent weekly carboplatin/paclitaxel.

Esophageal Cancer in Older Patients

Patients over 65 are becoming an increasingly prevalent group of esophageal cancer patients and require additional consideration prior to undergoing esophagectomy. Lester et al. designed a large retrospective study comparing outcomes of trimodality therapy for patients older than 65 (n = 202) with those younger than 65 (n = 369) to see whether the therapeutic gains conferred by trimodality therapy were offset by morbidity of esophagectomy in elderly populations [37]. Interestingly, in terms of OS, DFS, and FFEC (freedom from esophageal cancer) there was no significant difference noted in terms of hazard ratios on multivariable cox regression analyses. Median OS was 4.2 years for the older patient cohort vs. 5.3 years for the younger cohort. However, of note, older patients had a significant increase on multivariable analysis of morbidity for both cardiac and pulmonary issues (HR~2.0). Both morbidities were linearly associated with age. This data suggests that in carefully selected elderly patients, especially those without comorbid conditions, trimodality therapy should be considered.

Xu et al. compared patients over the age of 80 who underwent CRT with two younger patient cohorts to see how well they were able to tolerate therapy. While older patients had more comorbidities and the median survival was approximately 15 months compared to over 20 months in younger patient cohorts, there were no statistically significant differences in OS and recurrence-free survival between the two groups. The main difference was an 11% rate of radiation pneumonitis among the older patients vs. less than 4% in the younger group [38]. This underscores that the elderly may do well with definitive CRT alone if they are unwilling or unable to undergo an esophagectomy.

Radiation Techniques

Imaging

Today, 3D planning by computed tomography helps better outline both the target and normal tissues to help minimize side effects such as acute esophagitis and pneumonitis without compromising clinical outcomes. Further improvements in local disease characterization can be achieved by PET/CT imaging. A retrospective definition of tumor volumes in 21 cases of esophageal cancer by both CT and PET/CT showed the former inadequately covered disease in 36% of patients and treatment plan modifications based on the latter reduced dosage to the lungs and heart [39].

Treatment planning of esophageal cancer is further complicated by its location in the thorax, where chest and diaphragm movements can alter location with each respiratory cycle, up to 6 mm in any direction [40]. Four-dimensional CT planning is one approach to overcome this problem. This requires imaging being acquired throughout a breathing cycle. These images can then be interpolated to generate an expanded treatment volume called the internal target volume (ITV). Patients should be simulated after not eating or drinking for 4 h prior to simulation (as well as daily treatments) to avoid variations in stomach filling. Oral and intravenous contrast during CT simulation allows for better visualization of both tumor and nodal chains as well as the stomach and small bowel.

Contouring

Contouring begins by identifying the tumor volume using a combination of endoscopic ultrasound, CT, and PET imaging. This defines the "gross tumor volume" (GTV), which includes both the gross tumor as well as involved lymph nodes. Margins are typically expanded to include microscopic disease in what is termed the "clinical tumor volume" (CTV). In esophageal cancer, margins of 4 cm in the superior and inferior directions along with a 1.0 cm to 1.5 cm in the radial directions are used to account for subclinical submucosal spread. Superior and inferior expansions follow the contour of the esophagus and stomach. Dose to uninvolved stomach should be kept to a minimum as it may be used for future reconstruction. Using four-dimensional CT scans, an "internal target volume" (ITV) can be mapped to set boundaries of where the tumor could be at any point of respiration during treatment. The CTV also includes high-risk nodal stations. Elective nodal coverage of the peri-esophageal nodes should be included in all patients. When the tumor is proximal, the supraclavicular nodes are included, para-esophageal nodes are treated for tumors of the middle third, while for distal tumors celiac nodes are included. Tumors that extend into the stomach may require inclusion of nodes of the lesser curvature as well as spleen [41]. The inclusion or exclusion of uninvolved nodal basins is often made on pragmatic grounds of field size that result in acceptable normal tissue tolerance.

A further expansion is placed on the CTV or the ITV when considering daily variations in patient positioning, yielding a "planning target volume" (PTV) that is used to design treatment fields. The expansion placed on the PTV takes into account daily setup errors and can range from 0.5 to 1.0 cm. The current standard of care in the United States is to deliver either 5000 cGy in 25 fractions or 5040 cGy in 28 fractions with concurrent chemotherapy. Currently in Asia, total doses are generally higher in the range of 6000 cGy.

Dose Constraints

For tumors in the upper esophagus, the relevant nearby structures that must be accounted for include the spinal cord and larynx. Likewise, treatment of tumors in the lower esophagus requires attention to dose to the lung, kidneys, liver, and heart. The volume of lung receiving more than 20 Gy (V20) is kept to less than 35%. The volume of lung receiving more than 5Gy (V5) should be less than 60%. As pulmonary complications increase with increasing mean lung dose, it should be kept to less than 2000 cGy [42].

In a multivariate analysis of patients with locally advanced lung cancer treated with either standard dose radiation to 6000 cGy or high-dose radiation of 7400 cGy with concurrent carboplatin/paclitaxel, heart V40 was a significant independent predictor of survival [43]. In a pooled analysis of six dose escalation trials in Stage III non-small cell lung cancer (NSCLC), 2-year cardiac events increased with increasing mean heart dose [44]. Therefore, the volume of heart receiving more than 50 Gy (V50) is kept to less than 30% and the volume receiving more than 30 Gy (V30) is less than 100%. Mean heart dose should be less than 2000 cGy. These constraints avoid acute toxicities such as radiation pneumonitis in the lungs as well as long-term cardiac deaths and are used to limit normal tissue toxicity when treating esophageal cancers with radiation.

Respiratory gating is capable of reducing the ITV margin by turning the radiation treatment beam on during specified times of the respiratory cycle [45]. This leads to radiating less normal tissue and lowering heart V30 as well as lung V20.

Intensity-Modulated Radiation Therapy vs. 3D Conformal Radiation Therapy

Three-dimensional conformal radiation therapy (3D-CRT) is currently the mainstay of treatment, delivering precisely shaped radiation beams from varying angles to the diseased tissue while reducing exposure to nearby healthy tissue. Intensity-modulated radiation therapy (IMRT) increases both the number of concurrent beams used and modulates their intensity so as to conform to the treatment volume. This further improves dose conformality and minimizes dose to healthy tissues. In a retrospective analysis of patients at MD Anderson who underwent 3D-CRT or IMRT treatment, patients undergoing 3D-CRT had a greater risk of death overall (72.6% vs. 52.9%) with an increased incidence of cardiac death and locoregional recurrence [46]. Unlike patients who are treated with IMRT for lung cancer where few proceed to surgery, patients with esophageal cancer are often being treated in the neoadjuvant setting. The risk of radiation pneumonitis has been suggested retrospectively to increase with the volume of lung receiving doses of radiation of more than 500 cGy [47]. The use of volumetric modulated arc therapy (VMAT) allows for adequate treatment as the gantry rotates with conformal or modulated fields and has the potential to reduce heart dose V30 (31% vs. 55%, $p = 0.02$) as compared to 3D conformal therapy [48]. Although VMAT decreases high doses to critical structures such as the heart and lung, low doses are often given to larger volumes of both lungs (see Fig. 10.1). Despite encouraging single-institution retrospective studies, there are no large trials that have confirmed the superiority of IMRT to 3D CRT in esophageal cancer [46, 49]. As the CROSS regimen resulted in excellent pathologic response of 29% and a local-regional recurrence rate of only 14% in patients, it is reasonable to consider sparing patients the toxicity by limiting the total dose to 4140 cGy for patients who clearly have resectable tumor [21].

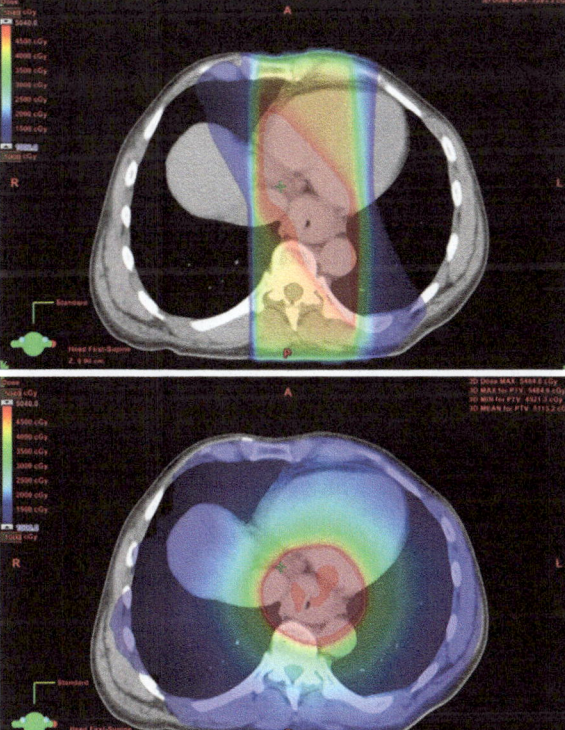

Fig. 10.1 A comparison of Isodose lines for 3D-CRT (top) to IMRT (bottom)

Brachytherapy

In patients who are in need of palliation where external beam radiation cannot be used, high-dose rate brachytherapy can be utilized using 600 cGy in 3 fractions or 800 cGy in 2 fractions to palliate dysphagia. Brachytherapy should not be used with external beam radiation or concurrent chemotherapy. In this procedure, a catheter is directed through the nose or mouth into the esophagus and to the tumor site under fluoroscopic guidance. The catheter is secured in place and the patient undergoes CT simulation for treatment planning. Once planning is complete, the radioactive source is advanced through the tube and treatment is initiated using high–dose-rate brachytherapy.

A randomized trial involving 209 patients with inoperable esophageal cancer examined the outcomes of brachytherapy (1200 cGy) versus stent placement for esophageal obstruction. While the stented group showed rapid improvement, the brachytherapy effect was more durable, extending relief to 115 days vs. 82 days. The brachytherapy group also demonstrated better quality of life scores and fewer complications, especially that of hemorrhage (5% vs. 13%) [50].

A prospective study by Sur et al. examined the placement of high-dose brachy-therapy seed prescribed to 1 cm from the source axis using three different dose levels in 121 patients. Higher doses of 1800 cGy in three fractions led to greater OS at 12 months compared to lower dose regimens such as 1200 cGy in one fraction (35% vs. 9.8%). Furthermore, higher dose rate led to better dysphagia free survival. On multivariate analysis, it appeared that tumor length was most significant in predicting disease-free survival [51].

Additionally, a meta-analysis of six prospective studies for palliation of dysphagia with brachytherapy [52] examined 623 patients with doses ranging from 1200 to 2100 cGy and found that DFS was 86.9% at 3 months, 67.2% at 6 months, and 29.4% at 12 months. Main side effects included esophageal stenosis (12.3%) and fistula formation in about 8.1% of patients.

Targeted Therapies

Epidermal growth factor receptor (EGFR) is known to be overexpressed in up to 50% of esophageal cancer cases. Unfortunately, EGFR-targeted agents have failed to improve outcomes in multiple clinical trials including REAL-3 (panitumumab) [53], SCOPE1 [54], and RTOG 0436 [55] (cetuximab).

RTOG 0436 [55] randomized 344 patients with inoperable esophageal cancer to cisplatin, paclitaxel, and radiation (5040 cGy) with or without cetuximab. The addition of cetuximab failed to improve OS at 2- or 3-year endpoints or clinical response as measured by repeat endoscopy 6–8 weeks following treatment completion. Therefore, strategies utilizing EGFR-targeted agents added to standard concurrent regimens in unselected patients are no longer being investigated.

The ongoing RTOG 1010 phase III trial is examining the addition of trastuzumab (Herceptin) to trimodality therapy of HER2 overexpressing esophageal adenocarci-noma. Patients with HER2-amplified tumors are randomized to paclitaxel, carbopla-tin, and radiation with or without trastuzumab. Patients randomized to the trastuzumab arm continue maintenance therapy every 3 weeks for 13 treatments [56].

Immune checkpoint inhibitors in the PD1/PDL1 inhibitor class have been shown to improve DFS, PFS, and OS as a monotherapy in advanced solid tumors including esophageal and gastric cancers. Currently, there are several ongoing trials examining the benefits of adding immunotherapy in cancers of the esophagus. The Checkmate-577 (NCT02743494) study is an ongoing phase III trial, which is randomizing patients with localized cancers of the esophagus and GEJ following neoadjuvant CRT and surgery to nivolumab or placebo. The primary endpoints being evaluated are OS and DFS [57]. Another phase III trial (NCT02730546) is examining the addition of pembrolizumab in combination with chemotherapy and radiation in the neoadjuvant setting. Primary endpoints are OS and DFS [58].

Proton Therapy

Using particle beams comprised of protons instead of photons has potential advantages to conventional therapy but still requires further study before it is established as a standard of care. Proton beam therapy (PBT) allows a sharp dose fall off following depositing most of its energy at the desired of depth, known as the Bragg peak. This may allow further reductions in dose to normal tissue while allowing for dose escalation to the tumor. The dose at the target is not compromised while normal tissues are spared allowing for a greater therapeutic ratio.

A prospective study by Lin et al. evaluated 62 patients who were treated with PBT to median dose of 50.4 Gy with concurrent chemotherapy. The median follow-up time for survivors was 20.1 months and 28% of patients had a complete pathologic response, which is similar to that seen with traditional treatment modalities. Outcomes in terms of acute radiation side effects were encouraging with most side effects, usually over 80%, being grade 1–2 esophagitis, fatigue, and dermatitis. No differences in OS or distant metastasis among patients receiving neoadjuvant proton therapy vs. definitive proton therapy were observed [59]. This small series serves as a basis for further prospective comparisons to conventional therapies.

Another retrospective dosimetric analysis compared doses to the heart in 727 patients who received either IMRT or proton therapy. Volumes of the heart receiving doses between 20 and 40 Gy were significantly lower with proton therapy. Doses to the left circumflex artery, left main coronary, left atrium, and right atrium and mean heart dose were significantly less with proton therapy. Whether this cardiac sparing effect results in long-term survival benefit for esophageal cancer patients remains to be determined [60]. There are currently several ongoing phase II and III trials of concurrent carboplatin/paclitaxel with proton therapy followed by surgery such as (NCT01684904) [61].

Imaging Biomarkers of Response

In addition to improving chemotherapy agents by the use of targeted agents and newer radiation techniques, another strategy is tailoring treatment to an individual patient's response to induction chemotherapy prior to preop chemoradiation. An ongoing multicenter phase II study (CALGB 80803) is randomizing patients to modified FOLFOX6 (100 mg/m^2 oxaliplatin and 100 mg/m^2 leucovorin (LV) as a 2-h intravenous infusion on day 1, followed by 5-FU at 2000 mg/m^2 as a 46-h continuous infusion) for three cycles versus two cycles of carboplatin and paclitaxel as induction therapy. Pre- and posttreatment PET scans are obtained. Patients who have greater than 35% decrease in SUV_{max} continue on the same chemotherapy regimen during preop chemoradiation, otherwise they cross over to the other chemotherapy arm. Interim results of this study have demonstrated that for patients who were nonresponders based on PET and crossed over to alternative chemotherapy during CRT that the pCR was 15.6% and the resulting efficacy endpoint was met [62].

Radiomics

Radiomics is a method of quantifying tumor phenotypes by extracting a large amount of imaging characteristics using advanced computer algorithms. The use of advanced algorithms attempts to characterize the tumor as well as its microenvironment by assessing features such as heterogeneity, which can reveal features known to correlate with resistance and angiogenesis. In a retrospective study of patients treated with definitive CRT, features were assessed before and after therapy in a set of 36 patients and correlated with OS. Patients who had more irregularly shaped tumors that were more heterogeneous (indicating relative hypoxia and perhaps resistance) had a marked survival disadvantage of a difference of nearly 20 months [63]. Whether posttreatment imaging can at some point be used to facilitate salvage therapy remains to be further investigated.

In one study, 4D-CT scans were used to help identify tumor-related features, which correlated with OS [64]. Nearly 1045 features were identified in esophageal cancer and modeled using specialized software along with 3-dimensional reconstructions of image sets. These software programs are able to characterize key tumor imaging features such as tumor shape/size, geometric boundaries, gray zone borders, and spatial voxel intensity and identify which features are most relevant. Large data-set imaging features may soon be able to prognosticate which tumors are more responsive to therapy.

Biomarker-Driven Therapy

In an effort to individualize therapy, molecular biomarkers that can predict response are being evaluated. Cytotoxic T cells (lymphocytes) are known to mediate host immunity against neoplastic cells [65]. A meta-analysis of several studies in esophageal cancer has shown that in a combined group of 1540 patients treated with trimodality therapy, higher neutrophil to lymphocyte ratios predict a poorer survival outcome. This is thought to stem from poor immune response against the tumor [66]. Recently, a retrospective study evaluating 512 patients with esophageal cancer found that patients who develop grade 4 lymphopenia during definitive CRT for esophageal cancer have a median OS of 2.8 years vs. 5.0 years for those with grade 0–2 lymphopenia (HR 1.58) [67]. Furthermore, patients who received PBT (which reduces total body dose due to its physical properties of depositing energy more locally) were less likely to have grade 4 lymphopenia. Additional prospective studies need to be performed to determine the relative effect on declining immune system progenitor cells and whether sparing of bone marrow and/or circulating lymphocytes via lower mean body dose is a method of mitigating this side effect.

Another biomarker that has been investigated is excision repair cross-complementing protein (ERCC1). ERCC1 is used to repair platinum-damaged DNA through the nucleotide excision repair pathway. The SouthWest Oncology Group SWOG 0353 trial was a prospective phase II study that evaluated the effect of mRNA levels of ERCC1 as well as thymidylate synthase in trimodality therapy of esophageal cancer. Levels of ERCC1 were inversely related to 2-year OS (16% to 62%) while thymidylate synthase was not associated with survival [68].

Two promising biomarkers are transcription factors BMI1 and Gli-1. BMI1 is a transcription repressor oncoprotein known to be involved with cancer stem cell self-renewal and proliferation [69]. Yoshikawa et al. analyzed 78 patients, of whom 24 were positive for BMI1 expression. All patients were treated with standard-of-care trimodality therapy and interestingly mean OS and DFS were 21.8 vs. 76.6 months ($p = 0.002$) and 16.8 vs. 76.2 months ($p = 0.005$), respectively, for patients with positive expression of BMI1 compared to those without [70]. These dramatic differences could potentially be explained by the self-renewal capacity induced by the transcription factor. Similarly, Gli-1 is a transcription factor in the hedgehog pathway that has been shown to be elevated in esophageal cancer. Gli-1 has been shown to be involved in maintaining cancer stem cell populations and promoting hedgehog pathway transcription through mTOR [71].

One study performed at MD Anderson Cancer center followed 167 patients for pathological complete response following trimodality therapy. They correlated the levels of Gli-1 in tissue samples with pathological complete response and found that increased levels of Gli-1 inversely correlated with obtaining a pathological complete response (OR 0.84, $p = 0.001$) at a mean follow-up time of 81.5 months [72]. These biomarkers are starting to show promise toward understanding why some cancers are more resistant to traditional therapy.

Conclusions

The ideal treatment approach for patients with locally advanced esophageal cancer is controversial and requires a multidisciplinary approach involving surgeons, medical oncologists, and radiation oncologists. For the operable patient, a trimodality approach using preoperative chemoradiation followed by surgical resection is favored. For inoperable patients, primary chemoradiation is recommended. All patients should undergo CT-based treatment planning. Intensity-modulated radiation therapy (IMRT) may be utilized when dose to critical organs such as heart and lung cannot be achieved using 3-D techniques. Although there are many areas of active investigation including combining chemoradiation with targeted agents, immunotherapy, radiomics, biomarker-driven treatment approaches, and the use of protons in the treatment of esophageal cancer, their role has yet to be established in the care of esophageal cancer patients.

References

1. Herskovic A, Martz K, al-Sarraf M, Leichman L, Brindle J, Vaitkevicius V, et al. Combined chemotherapy and radiotherapy compared with radiotherapy alone in patients with cancer of the esophagus. N Engl J Med. 1992;326(24):1593–8.
2. al-Sarraf M, Martz K, Herskovic A, Leichman L, Brindle JS, Vaitkevicius VK, et al. Progress report of combined chemoradiotherapy versus radiotherapy alone in patients with esophageal cancer: an intergroup study. J Clin Oncol. 1997;15(1):277–84.
3. Wang M, Gu XZ, Yin WB, Huang GJ, Wang LJ, Zhang DW. Randomized clinical trial on the combination of preoperative irradiation and surgery in the treatment of esophageal carcinoma: report on 206 patients. Int J Radiat Oncol Biol Phys. 1989;16(2):325–7.
4. Malthaner RA, Wong RK, Rumble RB, Zuraw L, Gastrointestinal Cancer Disease Site Group of Cancer Care Ontario's Program in Evidence-based C. Neoadjuvant or adjuvant therapy for resectable esophageal cancer: a clinical practice guideline. BMC Cancer. 2004;4:67.
5. Teniere P, Hay JM, Fingerhut A, Fagniez PL. Postoperative radiation therapy does not increase survival after curative resection for squamous cell carcinoma of the middle and lower esophagus as shown by a multicenter controlled trial. French University Association for Surgical Research. Surg Gynecol Obstet. 1991;173(2):123–30.
6. Cooper JS, Guo MD, Herskovic A, Macdonald JS, Martenson JA Jr, Al-Sarraf M, et al. Chemoradiotherapy of locally advanced esophageal cancer: long-term follow-up of a prospective randomized trial (RTOG 85-01). Radiation Therapy Oncology Group. JAMA. 1999;281(17):1623–7.
7. Araujo CM, Souhami L, Gil RA, Carvalho R, Garcia JA, Froimtchuk MJ, et al. A randomized trial comparing radiation therapy versus concomitant radiation therapy and chemotherapy in carcinoma of the thoracic esophagus. Cancer. 1991;67(9):2258–61.
8. Smith TJ, Ryan LM, Douglass HO Jr, Haller DG, Dayal Y, Kirkwood J, et al. Combined chemoradiotherapy vs. radiotherapy alone for early stage squamous cell carcinoma of the esophagus: a study of the Eastern Cooperative Oncology Group. Int J Radiat Oncol Biol Phys. 1998;42(2):269–76.
9. Roussel A, Bleiberg H, Dalesio O, Jacob JH, Haegele P, Jung GM, et al. Palliative therapy of inoperable oesophageal carcinoma with radiotherapy and methotrexate: final results of a controlled clinical trial. Int J Radiat Oncol Biol Phys. 1989;16(1):67–72.
10. Minsky BD, Pajak TF, Ginsberg RJ, Pisansky TM, Martenson J, Komaki R, et al. INT 0123 (Radiation Therapy Oncology Group 94-05) phase III trial of combined-modality therapy for esophageal cancer: high-dose versus standard-dose radiation therapy. J Clin Oncol. 2002;20(5):1167–74.
11. Gaspar LE, Qian C, Kocha WI, Coia LR, Herskovic A, Graham M. A phase I/II study of external beam radiation, brachytherapy and concurrent chemotherapy in localized cancer of the esophagus (RTOG 92-07): preliminary toxicity report. Int J Radiat Oncol Biol Phys. 1997;37(3):593–9.
12. Walsh TN, Noonan N, Hollywood D, Kelly A, Keeling N, Hennessy TP. A comparison of multimodal therapy and surgery for esophageal adenocarcinoma. N Engl J Med. 1996;335(7):462–7.
13. Urba SG, Orringer MB, Turrisi A, Iannettoni M, Forastiere A, Strawderman M. Randomized trial of preoperative chemoradiation versus surgery alone in patients with locoregional esophageal carcinoma. J Clin Oncol. 2001;19(2):305–13.
14. Burmeister BH, Smithers BM, Gebski V, Fitzgerald L, Simes RJ, Devitt P, et al. Surgery alone versus chemoradiotherapy followed by surgery for resectable cancer of the oesophagus: a randomised controlled phase III trial. Lancet Oncol. 2005;6(9):659–68.
15. Tepper J, Krasna MJ, Niedzwiecki D, Hollis D, Reed CE, Goldberg R, et al. Phase III trial of trimodality therapy with cisplatin, fluorouracil, radiotherapy, and surgery compared with surgery alone for esophageal cancer: CALGB 9781. J Clin Oncol. 2008;26(7):1086–92.
16. Kranzfelder M, Schuster T, Geinitz H, Friess H, Buchler P. Meta-analysis of neoadjuvant treatment modalities and definitive non-surgical therapy for oesophageal squamous cell cancer. Br J Surg. 2011;98(6):768–83.

17. Jin HL, Zhu H, Ling TS, Zhang HJ, Shi RH. Neoadjuvant chemoradiotherapy for resectable esophageal carcinoma: a meta-analysis. World J Gastroenterol. 2009;15(47):5983–91.
18. Urschel JD, Vasan H. A meta-analysis of randomized controlled trials that compared neoadjuvant chemoradiation and surgery to surgery alone for resectable esophageal cancer. Am J Surg. 2003;185(6):538–43.
19. Gebski V, Burmeister B, Smithers BM, Foo K, Zalcberg J, Simes J, et al. Survival benefits from neoadjuvant chemoradiotherapy or chemotherapy in oesophageal carcinoma: a meta-analysis. Lancet Oncol. 2007;8(3):226–34.
20. Sjoquist KM, Burmeister BH, Smithers BM, Zalcberg JR, Simes RJ, Barbour A, et al. Survival after neoadjuvant chemotherapy or chemoradiotherapy for resectable oesophageal carcinoma: an updated meta-analysis. Lancet Oncol. 2011;12(7):681–92.
21. van Hagen P, Hulshof MC, van Lanschot JJ, Steyerberg EW, van Berge Henegouwen MI, Wijnhoven BP, et al. Preoperative chemoradiotherapy for esophageal or junctional cancer. N Engl J Med. 2012;366(22):2074–84.
22. Oppedijk V, van der Gaast A, van Lanschot JJ, van Hagen P, van Os R, van Rij CM, et al. Patterns of recurrence after surgery alone versus preoperative chemoradiotherapy and surgery in the CROSS trials. J Clin Oncol. 2014;32(5):385–91.
23. Gabriel E, Attwood K, Du W, Tuttle R, Alnaji RM, Nurkin S, et al. Association between clinically staged node-negative esophageal adenocarcinoma and overall survival benefit from neoadjuvant chemoradiation. JAMA Surg. 2016;151(3):234–45.
24. Stahl M, Stuschke M, Lehmann N, Meyer H-J, Walz MK, Seeber S, et al. Chemoradiation with and without surgery in patients with locally advanced squamous cell carcinoma of the esophagus. J Clin Oncol. 2005;23(10):2310–7.
25. Bedenne L, Michel P, Bouche O, Milan C, Mariette C, Conroy T, et al. Chemoradiation followed by surgery compared with chemoradiation alone in squamous cancer of the esophagus: FFCD 9102. J Clin Oncol. 2007;25(10):1160–8.
26. Medical Research Council Oesophageal Cancer Working G. Surgical resection with or without preoperative chemotherapy in oesophageal cancer: a randomised controlled trial. Lancet. 2002;359(9319):1727–33.
27. Kelsen DP, Ginsberg R, Pajak TF, Sheahan DG, Gunderson L, Mortimer J, et al. Chemotherapy followed by surgery compared with surgery alone for localized esophageal cancer. N Engl J Med. 1998;339(27):1979–84.
28. Stahl M, Walz MK, Stuschke M, Lehmann N, Meyer HJ, Riera-Knorrenschild J, et al. Phase III comparison of preoperative chemotherapy compared with chemoradiotherapy in patients with locally advanced adenocarcinoma of the esophagogastric junction. J Clin Oncol. 2009;27(6):851–6.
29. Pasquali S, Yim G, Vohra RS, Mocellin S, Nyanhongo D, Marriott P, et al. Survival after neoadjuvant and adjuvant treatments compared to surgery alone for resectable esophageal carcinoma: a network metaanalysis. Ann Surg. 2017;265(3):481–91.
30. Bidoli P, Bajetta E, Stani SC, De CD, Santoro A, Valente M, et al. Ten-year survival with chemotherapy and radiotherapy in patients with squamous cell carcinoma of the esophagus. Cancer. 2002;94(2):352–61.
31. Stuschke M, Stahl M, Wilke H, Walz MK, Oldenburg AR, Stuben G, et al. Induction chemotherapy followed by concurrent chemotherapy and high-dose radiotherapy for locally advanced squamous cell carcinoma of the cervical oesophagus. Oncology. 1999;57(2):99–105.
32. Macdonald JS, Smalley SR, Benedetti J, Hundahl SA, Estes NC, Stemmermann GN, et al. Chemoradiotherapy after surgery compared with surgery alone for adenocarcinoma of the stomach or gastroesophageal junction. N Engl J Med. 2001;345(10):725–30.
33. Cunningham D, Allum WH, Stenning SP, Thompson JN, Van de Velde CJ, Nicolson M, et al. Perioperative chemotherapy versus surgery alone for resectable gastroesophageal cancer. N Engl J Med. 2006;355(1):11–20.
34. Penniment MG, De Ieso PB, Harvey JA, Stephens S, Au HJ, O'Callaghan CJ, et al. Palliative chemoradiotherapy versus radiotherapy alone for dysphagia in advanced oesophageal cancer:

a multicentre randomised controlled trial (TROG 03.01). Lancet Gastroenterol Hepatol. 2018;3(2):114–24.

35. Guttmann DM, Mitra N, Bekelman J, Metz JM, Plastaras J, Feng W, et al. Improved overall survival with aggressive primary tumor radiotherapy for patients with metastatic esophageal cancer. J Thorac Oncol. 2017;12(7):1131–42.

36. Li T, Jiahua L, et al. Prospective randomized phase 2 study of concurrent chemoradiation therapy (CCRT) versus chemotherapy alone in stage IV esophageal squamous cell carcinoma (ESCC). Int J Radiat Oncol Biol Phys. 2016;96:S1.

37. Lester SC, Lin SH, Chuong M, Bhooshan N, Liao Z, Arnett AL, et al. A multi-institutional analysis of trimodality therapy for esophageal cancer in elderly patients. Int J Radiat Oncol Biol Phys. 2017;98(4):820–8.

38. Xu C, Xi M, Moreno A, Shiraishi Y, Hobbs BP, Huang M, et al. Definitive chemoradiation therapy for esophageal cancer in the elderly: clinical outcomes for patients exceeding 80 years old. Int J Radiat Oncol Biol Phys. 2017;98(4):811–9.

39. Mackley HB, Adelstein JS, Reddy CA, Adelstein DJ, Rice TW, Saxton JP, et al. Choice of radiotherapy planning modality influences toxicity in the treatment of locally advanced esophageal cancer. J Gastrointest Cancer. 2008;39(1–4):130–7.

40. Wang J, Lin SH, Dong L, Balter P, Mohan R, Komaki R, et al. Quantifying the interfractional displacement of the gastroesophageal junction during radiation therapy for esophageal cancer. Int J Radiat Oncol Biol Phys. 2012;83(2):e273–80.

41. Lee NY, Lu JJ. Target volume delineation and field setup : a practical guide for conformal and intensity-modulated radiation therapy, vol. vii. Heidelberg: Springer; 2013. p. 321.

42. Wang J, Wei C, Tucker SL, Myles B, Palmer M, Hofstetter WL, et al. Predictors of postoperative complications after trimodality therapy for esophageal cancer. Int J Radiat Oncol Biol Phys. 2013;86(5):885–91.

43. Bradley JD, Paulus R, Komaki R, Masters G, Blumenschein G, Schild S, et al. Standard-dose versus high-dose conformal radiotherapy with concurrent and consolidation carboplatin plus paclitaxel with or without cetuximab for patients with stage IIIA or IIIB non-small-cell lung cancer (RTOG 0617): a randomised, two-by-two factorial phase 3 study. Lancet Oncol. 2015;16(2):187–99.

44. Wang K, Eblan MJ, Deal AM, Lipner M, Zagar TM, Wang Y, et al. Cardiac toxicity after radiotherapy for stage III non-small-cell lung cancer: pooled analysis of dose-escalation trials delivering 70 to 90 Gy. J Clin Oncol. 2017;35(13):1387–94.

45. Yoganathan SA, Maria Das KJ, Agarwal A, Kumar S. Magnitude, impact, and management of respiration-induced target motion in radiotherapy treatment: a comprehensive review. J Med Phys. 2017;42(3):101–15.

46. Lin SH, Wang L, Myles B, Thall PF, Hofstetter WL, Swisher SG, et al. Propensity score-based comparison of long-term outcomes with 3-dimensional conformal radiotherapy vs intensity-modulated radiotherapy for esophageal cancer. Int J Radiat Oncol Biol Phys. 2012;84(5):1078–85.

47. Wang SL, Liao Z, Vaporciyan AA, Tucker SL, Liu H, Wei X, et al. Investigation of clinical and dosimetric factors associated with postoperative pulmonary complications in esophageal cancer patients treated with concurrent chemoradiotherapy followed by surgery. Int J Radiat Oncol Biol Phys. 2006;64(3):692–9.

48. Hawkins MA, Bedford JL, Warrington AP, Tait DM. Volumetric modulated arc therapy planning for distal oesophageal malignancies. Br J Radiol. 2012;85(1009):44–52.

49. Zhang M, Wu AJ. Radiation techniques for esophageal cancer. Chin Clin Oncol. 2017;6(5):45. https://doi.org/10.21037/cco.2017.06.33.

50. Homs MY, Steyerberg EW, Eijkenboom WM, Tilanus HW, Stalpers LJ, Bartelsman JF, et al. Single-dose brachytherapy versus metal stent placement for the palliation of dysphagia from oesophageal cancer: multicentre randomised trial. Lancet. 2004;364(9444):1497–504.

51. Sur RK, Donde B, Levin VC, Mannell A. Fractionated high dose rate intraluminal brachytherapy in palliation of advanced esophageal cancer. Int J Radiat Oncol Biol Phys. 1998;40(2):447–53.

52. Fuccio L, Mandolesi D, Farioli A, Hassan C, Frazzoni L, Guido A, et al. Brachytherapy for the palliation of dysphagia owing to esophageal cancer: a systematic review and meta-analysis of prospective studies. Radiother Oncol. 2017;122(3):332–9.
53. Waddell T, Chau I, Cunningham D, Gonzalez D, Okines AF, Okines C, et al. Epirubicin, oxaliplatin, and capecitabine with or without panitumumab for patients with previously untreated advanced oesophagogastric cancer (REAL3): a randomised, open-label phase 3 trial. Lancet Oncol. 2013;14(6):481–9.
54. Tomblyn MB, Goldman BH, Thomas CR Jr, Benedetti JK, Lenz HJ, Mehta V, et al. Cetuximab plus cisplatin, irinotecan, and thoracic radiotherapy as definitive treatment for locally advanced, unresectable esophageal cancer: a phase-II study of the SWOG (S0414). J Thorac Oncol. 2012;7(5):906–12.
55. Suntharalingam M, Winter K, Ilson D, Dicker AP, Kachnic L, Konski A, et al. Effect of the addition of cetuximab to paclitaxel, cisplatin, and radiation therapy for patients with esophageal Cancer: the NRG oncology RTOG 0436 phase 3 randomized clinical trial. JAMA Oncol. 2017;3(11):1520–8.
56. RTOG 1010: a Phase III Trial evaluating the addition of Trastuzumab to Trimodality treatment of Her2-overexpressing esophageal adenocarcinoma. https://clinicaltrials.gov/ct2/show/NCT01196390?term=RTOG+1010&rank=1.
57. Ronan Joseph Kelly ACL, Jonker DJ, Melichar B, Andre T, Chau I, Clarke SJ, Cleary JM, Doki Y, Franke FA, Kitagawa Y, Mariette C, Montenegro PC, Roca EL, Ciprotti M, Moehler M. An investigational immuno-therapy study of nivolumab or placebo in patients with resected esophageal or gastroesophageal junction cancer (CheckMate 577). J Clin Oncol. 2017;35(4):suppl TPS212-TPS.
58. Pembrolizumab, combination chemotherapy, and radiation therapy before surgery in treating adult patients with locally advanced gastroesophageal junction or gastric cardia cancer that can be removed by surgery. NCT02730546: ClinicalTrials.gov: National Library of Medicine(US); 2016. p. 4. https://clinicaltrials.gov/ct2/show/NCT02730546.
59. Lin SH, Komaki R, Liao Z, Wei C, Myles B, Guo X, et al. Proton beam therapy and concurrent chemotherapy for esophageal cancer. Int J Radiat Oncol Biol Phys. 2012;83(3):e345–51.
60. Shiraishi Y, Xu C, Yang J, Komaki R, Lin SH. Dosimetric comparison to the heart and cardiac substructure in a large cohort of esophageal cancer patients treated with proton beam therapy or intensity-modulated radiation therapy. Radiother Oncol. 2017;25(1):48–54.
61. A Phase II Trial of Proton Chemotherapy (PCT) for resectable esophageal or esophagogastric junction cancer. NCT01684904: ClinicalTrials.gov: National Library of Medicine (US). https://clinicaltrials.gov/ct2/show/NCT01684904.
62. Karyn A, Goodman DN, Hall N, Bekaii-Saab TS, Ye X, Meyers MO, Mitchell-Richards K, Boffa DJ, Frankel WL, Venook AP, Hochster HS, Crane CH, O'Reilly EM, Ilson DH. Initial results of CALGB 80803 (Alliance): a randomized phase II trial of PET scan-directed combined modality therapy for esophageal cancer. J Clin Oncol. 2017;35(4):suppl 1.
63. Yip C, Landau D, Kozarski R, Ganeshan B, Thomas R, Michaelidou A, et al. Primary esophageal cancer: heterogeneity as potential prognostic biomarker in patients treated with definitive chemotherapy and radiation therapy. Radiology. 2014;270(1):141–8.
64. Larue R, Van De Voorde L, van Timmeren JE, Leijenaar RTH, Berbee M, Sosef MN, et al. 4DCT imaging to assess radiomics feature stability: an investigation for thoracic cancers. Radiother Oncol. 2017;125(1):147–53.
65. Hung K, Hayashi R, Lafond-Walker A, Lowenstein C, Pardoll D, Levitsky H. The central role of CD4(+) T cells in the antitumor immune response. J Exp Med. 1998;188(12):2357–68.
66. Yodying H, Matsuda A, Miyashita M, Matsumoto S, Sakurazawa N, Yamada M, et al. Prognostic significance of neutrophil-to-lymphocyte ratio and platelet-to-lymphocyte ratio in oncologic outcomes of esophageal cancer: a systematic review and meta-analysis. Ann Surg Oncol. 2016;23(2):646–54.
67. Davuluri R, Jiang W, Fang P, Xu C, Komaki R, Gomez DR, et al. Lymphocyte nadir and esophageal cancer survival outcomes after chemoradiation therapy. Int J Radiat Oncol Biol Phys. 2017;99(1):128–35.

68. Leichman LP, Goldman BH, Bohanes PO, Lenz HJ, Thomas CR, Billingsley KG, et al. S0356: a phase II clinical and prospective molecular trial with oxaliplatin, fluorouracil, and external-beam radiation therapy before surgery for patients with esophageal adenocarcinoma. J Clin Oncol. 2011;29(34):4555–60.
69. Liu S, Dontu G, Mantle ID, Patel S, Ahn NS, Jackson KW, et al. Hedgehog signaling and Bmi-1 regulate self-renewal of normal and malignant human mammary stem cells. Cancer Res. 2006;66(12):6063–71.
70. Yoshikawa R, Tsujimura T, Tao L, Kamikonya N, Fujiwara Y. The oncoprotein and stem cell renewal factor BMI1 associates with poor clinical outcome in oesophageal cancer patients undergoing preoperative chemoradiotherapy. BMC Cancer. 2012;12(1)
71. Po A, Ferretti E, Miele E, De Smaele E, Paganelli A, Canettieri G, et al. Hedgehog controls neural stem cells through p53-independent regulation of Nanog. EMBO J. 2010;29(15):2646–58.
72. Wadhwa R, Wang X, Baladandayuthapani V, Liu B, Shiozaki H, Shimodaira Y, et al. Nuclear expression of Gli-1 is predictive of pathologic complete response to chemoradiation in trimodality treated oesophageal cancer patients. Br J Cancer. 2017;117(5):648–55.

The Multidisciplinary Management of Early-Stage Cervical Esophageal Cancer

Jarred P. Tanksley, Jordan A. Torok, Joseph K. Salama, and Manisha Palta

Introduction

Cervical esophageal cancer (CEC) was historically treated with primary surgery, typically a pharyngo-laryngo-esophagectomy (PLE), a morbid procedure with substantial impact on a patient's long-term quality of life. More recently, a paradigm shift has occurred such that now the preferred initial approach is treatment with definitive, concurrent chemotherapy and radiation (CRT), with a goal of preserving a functional larynx while not compromising survival. As the cervical esophagus lies at the junction of the hypopharynx and proximal esophagus, there has been ongoing debate as to whether CEC should be treated with CRT schedules used in locally advanced head and neck squamous cell cancers (HNSCC) as opposed to the CRT schedules used in more distal esophageal cancers. This chapter will briefly review the anatomy, risk factors, clinical presentation, and diagnostic work-up of CEC, and will close with a more detailed discussion of the data that have informed the current, however variable, approach to the treatment of CEC.

Anatomy

The cervical esophagus originates at the upper esophageal sphincter, just caudal to the hypopharynx, and posterior to the cricoid cartilage (Fig. 11.1). The upper sphincter comprises muscle fibers from the inferior pharyngeal constrictors, the cricopharyngeus muscle, and the cervical esophagus. It is lined by a layer of stratified squamous epithelium, and in turn virtually all (95%) of the cancers that originate in the cervical esophagus are squamous cell carcinomas (SCCs) [1]. The cervical

J. P. Tanksley · J. A. Torok · J. K. Salama (✉) · M. Palta
Department of Radiation Oncology, Duke University, Durham, NC, USA
e-mail: Joseph.salama@duke.edu; manisha.palta@dm.duke.edu

© Springer Nature Switzerland AG 2020
N. F. Saba, B. F. El-Rayes (eds.), *Esophageal Cancer*,
https://doi.org/10.1007/978-3-030-29832-6_11

AJCC regions of the esophagus

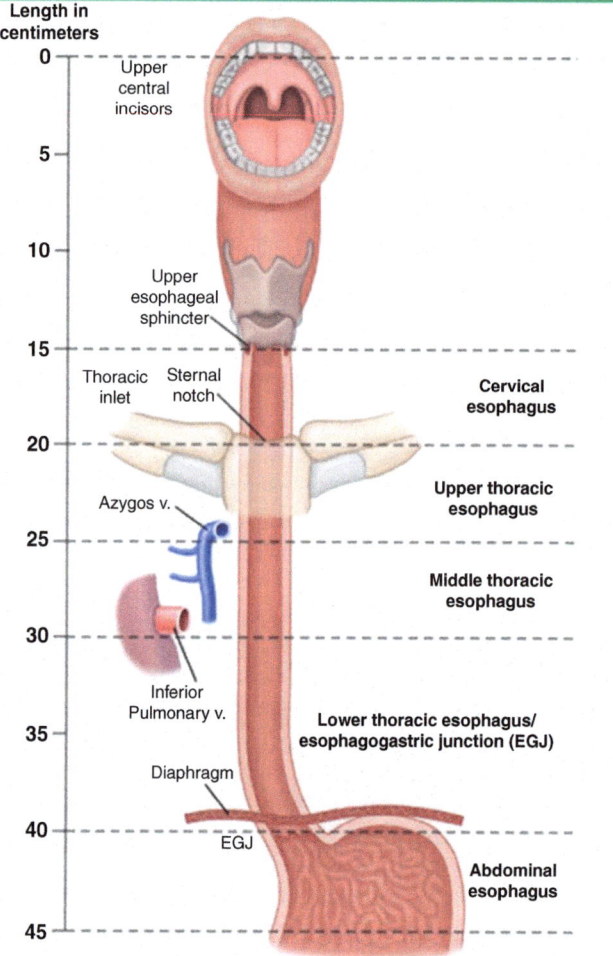

The American Joint Committee on Caner (AJCC) divides the esophagus into four areas. The cervical esophagus extends from the lower border of the cricoid cartilage to the thoracic inlet. The upper thoracic esophagus extends from the thoracic inlet to the tracheal bifurcation. The mid-thoracic esophagus extends from the tracheal bifurcation to a level approximately 32 cm from the incisors. The lower thoracic and abdominal esophagus extends from the mid-thoracic esophagus to the EG junction, approximately 40 cm from the incisors.
Data from: Esophagus. In: AJCC Cancer Staging Manual, 6th edition, 2002.

Fig. 11.1 Divisions of the esophagus. The esophagus is commonly divided into four regions including: the cervical, upper, middle, and lower thoracic/abdominal esophagus

esophagus is around 5 cm in length, and extends 15–20 cm from the incisors on endoscopy. The transition between the cervical and thoracic esophagus is generally considered to be the point at which the esophagus enters the thoracic inlet. Osseous landmarks approximating the cervical esophagus include the C6/C7 vertebral body, demarcating the origin, and the sternal notch or T3 vertebral body, indicating its termination.

The lymphatic drainage of the cervical esophagus includes the lower cervical chain and supraclavicular nodes, the extensive submucosal lymphatics of the proximal esophagus, and the paratracheal and paraesophageal lymph nodes in the upper mediastinum. Surgical series have found metastases to the cervical lymph nodes in 25% of cases, and to mediastinal lymph nodes in 60% of cases [2]. Compared to hypopharynx primaries, isolated CECs have a lower tendency to involve the cervical lymphatics, and are more likely to metastasize to lymph nodes in the mediastinum. The primary pattern of pathologic lymph node involvement is to the supraclavicular fossa and cervical levels II–IV. Involvement of cervical levels I, V, and VI is rare. Unlike other esophageal sites, involvement of the upper abdominal lymph nodes (i.e., celiac/para-aortic) does not commonly occur [3].

Epidemiology

Only 5% of esophageal tumors arise in the cervical segment, making it the least common site for esophageal cancer [1]. The incidence in men is twice as common as in women. Risk factors for CEC are similar to those of HNSCC, including a history of alcohol and/or tobacco use and betel nut chewing. These common risk factors lead to a second malignancy rate of 30%, primarily in other portions of the upper aero-digestive tract [4]. Certain cultural practices, such as the frequent ingestion of hot beverages, may also add to the risk through repetitive thermal injury [5].

In the last decade, the human papilloma virus (HPV), which is rapidly becoming the leading cause of some HNSCCs, has been proposed as a causal factor in CEC. It has been associated with a three- to sixfold increase in the risk of SCC of the esophagus; however, it has also been found in a small minority of cases in the United States in some retrospective series [6, 7]. While it is known in HNSCC that HPV-associated malignancies have a more robust treatment response and more favorable prognosis, the influence of HPV on response to therapy and survival in CEC remains unknown [8]. Overall, the prognosis of CEC has historically been poor, with a population-based registry study demonstrating a median overall survival (OS) of 14 months [9].

There have been no studies focused on the molecular changes underlying the development and progression of CEC specifically. The Cancer Genome Atlas (TCGA) Research Network has published a comprehensive analysis of the molecular features of esophageal carcinoma [10]. In this study, 90 esophageal SCCs and more than 100 esophageal or gastroesophageal junction adenocarcinomas were subjected to next-generation sequencing, gene expression and epigenetic profiling, and in some cases proteomic analysis. The findings suggested that esophageal SCC and esophageal adenocarcinoma are two distinct molecular diseases. Interestingly, esophageal SCC shares more molecular features with HNSCCs, of which the majority were oral cavity and oropharynx cancers, than with esophageal adenocarcinoma, which had a genetic landscape more similar to gastric cancers.

Also, important with respect to potential therapeutic options for CEC, TCGA analysis found that HER2 overexpression, a targetable molecular aberration, was relatively common in esophageal adenocarcinomas (32%), but was virtually absent (3%) in esophageal SCCs. Trastuzumab, an anti-HER2 antibody, has been shown to be beneficial in the treatment of gastro-esophageal and gastric tumors overexpressing the receptor [11]. Another targetable aberration, EGFR overexpression, was found in approximately 20% of esophageal SCCs. Cetuximab, an anti-EGFR antibody, has shown no benefit for patients with esophageal cancers, which is in contrast to HNSCCs, where its addition to RT improved OS when compared to RT alone [12, 13].

Presentation

Cervical esophageal cancer patients most often present with dysphagia, which can be due to obstruction of the esophageal lumen or dysfunction of the muscles of deglutition as a consequence of tumor infiltration. The incidences of the most common symptoms at presentation are as follows: dysphagia (96%), weight loss (61%), neck pain (32%), neck mass (28%), and vocal cord paralysis (24%) [1]. Most CECs extend superiorly into the hypopharynx or inferiorly into the thoracic esophagus, and are locally advanced at presentation, commonly involving nearby anatomic structures, including the thyroid gland, thyroid and cricoid cartilages, and recurrent laryngeal nerve [14].

Diagnosis, Workup, and Staging

The work-up for CEC, in the setting of the aforementioned symptoms, typically starts with an upper endoscopy with biopsy to establish the diagnosis. Endoscopic ultrasound should be utilized to more accurately assess the T-stage and regional nodal involvement. Accuracy in defining the T-stage of esophageal SCC with endoscopic ultrasound (EUS) is approximately 80% [15]. The accuracy and specificity of EUS in detecting more proximal lymph node groups, such as the cervical, upper paraesophageal, and supraclavicular nodes is over 90%, while sensitivity is more variable, ranging from 30 to 60% [16]. A contrast-enhanced CT of the neck, chest, and abdomen should be performed in order to assess the extent of locoregional disease. If PET/CT is available, it should be utilized for initial staging, as it has been reported to upstage 20% of patients when compared to CT alone, thus potentially altering treatment management [17].

Bronchoscopy is recommended to rule out tracheoesophageal fistula, as up to 35% of cervical esophageal patients have been noted to have tracheal invasion [1]. Esophageal dilation, if feasible, may be done at the time of initial evaluation in order to improve dysphagia and prevent the need for feeding tube placement during CRT. Alternative methods for alimentation, such as a jejunostomy tube, should be considered prior to the initiation of treatment, especially for those with obstructive lesions, and for those who are planned to be managed surgically. Jejunostomy tube placement during treatment can prolong the treatment duration or alter the chemotherapy schedule, either of which could lead to suboptimal outcomes. Percutaneous endoscopic gastrostomy tubes should be avoided, as they may interfere with the subsequent surgical anastomosis. Given the rarity and complexity of CEC, the National Comprehensive Cancer Network (NCCN) has recommended that a multidisciplinary team should evaluate all of these patients prior to the initiation of treatment in order to coordinate procedures and therapy, and tailor their sequence to the needs of each individual patient.

Management

Surgery

Historically, surgical management was the sole treatment modality for CEC. The extent of surgical resection for CECs typically requires removal of portions of the pharynx, the larynx, and the proximal to entire esophagus in a procedure known as a pharyngo-laryngo-esophagectomy (PLE). A small proportion of patients with CEC are eligible for larynx-sparing surgeries. A PLE requires a permanent tracheostomy, a mediastinal dissection, and commonly a bilateral radical neck dissection. Gastrointestinal continuity is accomplished with a gastric pull-up anastomosis or an interposition free jejunal graft [18].

Most published surgical series of PLE are heterogeneous, and in addition to CEC also include cancers of the larynx and hypopharynx. Further limiting our ability to interpret the success of surgery alone in addressing the locoregional disease is the fact that few of these historical series have reported these critical data. Importantly, historical series of surgery alone typically report high rates of operative mortality and relatively low rates of long-term survival (Table 11.1). In one of the largest series of surgery alone, including both hypopharynx and CEC primaries, the overall 5-year actuarial survival was 16% when excluding the in-hospital mortality of

Table 11.1 Select historical series of surgery alone for CEC

Series	Patients (n)	Operative mortality	Survival
Gunnlaugsson et al. [20]	17	24%	12% (5 years)
Peracchia et al. [21]	74	19%	15% (3 years)
Pearson et al. [22]	25	NR	16% (5 years)

5.5% [19]. In patients who underwent a complete resection, those with cervical esophageal primaries had a worse 5-year survival when compared to those with hypopharynx primaries (17 vs. 26%).

Overall reports of hospital mortality rates for PLE have ranged from 5 to 30%, but have decreased in recent years with more modern surgical capabilities and better postoperative care [23, 24]. Morbidity associated with PLE includes anastomotic leaks, wound infection, pneumonia, and cardiovascular complications in the perioperative period, in addition to the near universal psychological sequelae of a laryngectomy. Local control with surgery alone is approximately 50%, and the predominant pattern of failure is locoregional (80%) [14, 25]. The sum of these data suggests that surgery alone is often an inadequate treatment with significant short- and long-term morbidity.

Surgery with Adjuvant Therapy

Given the poor survival outcomes in patients with CEC who were treated with surgery alone, a number of retrospective series have evaluated the efficacy of postoperative therapy. One of the larger contemporary surgical series of PLE with adjuvant therapy included 209 patients, 78 of whom had CEC [26]. In this series, the majority of patients received combined modality treatment (20% received neoadjuvant chemotherapy and/or radiation, 73% received postoperative radiotherapy). The in-hospital mortality rate was 5%, with significant complications occurring in 38% of patients. The 5-year survival rate for patients with CEC remained low, at 14%. On multivariate analysis, predictors for poorer outcomes included a primary in the cervical esophagus, a T3- or T4-stage tumor, and lack of postoperative radiation therapy. Neither overall nor treatment-specific rates of local control were reported.

Furthermore, in an experience of 41 patients treated with PLE for SCC involving the pharyngoesophageal junction, 51% of patients received postoperative radiotherapy, generally 3–4 weeks after surgery to a mean dose of 47.5 Gy. The patient group was further subdivided into two groups based upon the likely site of origin of the primary tumor, be it hypopharynx ($n = 26$) or cervical esophagus ($n = 15$). In this study, the 5-year OS in this series was 32%, but was only 13% in the patients with primary cervical esophagus tumors [27]. On multivariate analysis, as in the previous trial, a primary location in the cervical esophagus and lack of adjuvant radiotherapy were found to be poor prognostic factors.

Lastly, an institution in Hong Kong with significant experience with PLE published a comprehensive report of the immediate surgical outcomes of 62 patients who underwent primary resection for CEC [23]. In this report, an R0 resection was achieved in 60% of the cases, and 60% of patients received adjuvant radiation therapy. In-hospital mortality was 7% and the 2-year OS was 38%. Neither rates of local control nor the prognostic impact of adjuvant therapy were reported.

Concurrent Chemotherapy and Radiation Therapy in Esophageal Cancer

As discussed above, PLE is an inherently morbid procedure that leaves permanent functional alterations, and in turn, has a substantial impact on the patient's long-term quality of life in addition to relatively high potential for postoperative mortality. Consequently, there is a need for alternative approaches allowing for functional organ preservation without compromising survival. Definitive CRT has evolved as an alternative, and often preferred initial modality, given the possibility of functional larynx preservation. CRT is now recommended as the first-line treatment modality for SCC of the cervical esophagus by the NCCN, with surgery reserved for salvage of recurrent or progressive disease.

Randomized trials evaluating concurrent CRT in the treatment of esophageal cancer, in both the definitive and neoadjuvant setting, have influenced the treatment approach for CEC. These trials primarily, if not exclusively, included middle and lower esophageal and gastroesophageal junction cancers, with variable rates of SCCs versus adenocarcinomas.

In the landmark Radiation Therapy Oncology Group (RTOG) 85-01 trial, 129 patients with esophageal cancer were randomized to 64 Gy alone or 50 Gy concurrent with combination cisplatin and 5-fluorouracil (5-FU) followed by adjuvant chemotherapy. The majority of patients in this trial had cancers that originated in the upper to middle thoracic esophagus, while only one case was noted to originate in the cervical esophagus. Nearly 90% of these patients had SCC. The combination of chemotherapy and radiation therapy resulted in a significant OS improvement, with 26% of patients in the combined modality arm alive after 5 years as compared to 0% in the arm assigned to receive radiation alone [28]. The addition of chemotherapy also decreased the incidence of both local and distant recurrence, albeit with more toxicity. The results of this trial established CRT as superior to RT alone in the nonsurgical, definitive treatment of esophageal cancer, in particular SCCs.

Neoadjuvant CRT followed by surgery has also been shown to be superior to surgery alone in two randomized trials. The CALGB 9781 and CROSS trials both randomized patients with locally advanced esophageal cancers to receive neoadjuvant CRT prior to surgery or to proceed directly to esophagectomy [29, 30]. Each used different chemo regimens, though both were platinum-based, and the CALGB study used a higher dose of RT (50.4 vs. 41.4 Gy). These trials, which predominantly included adenocarcinomas (approximately 75%), noted a doubling of median survival in patients receiving CRT, from approximately 2 to 4 years. In the context of CEC, it is important to consider the pathologic analysis of the surgical specimens following esophagectomy in the patients treated with neoadjuvant CRT in these two trials. The CALGB study noted a 40% pathologic complete response (pCR), without differentiating between the SCCs and adenocarcinomas. The CROSS trial noted an overall 29% pCR rate, with a pCR of 49% in SCC versus a pCR of 23% in adenocarcinomas.

As CRT alone has better outcomes than RT alone, and as neoadjuvant CRT followed by surgery has better outcomes than surgery alone, the question remains as to whether CRT alone has comparable outcomes to triple modality therapy. There have been two randomized trials that have attempted to answer this question. Firstly, a study from France compared neoadjuvant CRT to definitive CRT in thoracic esophageal cancers, predominantly SCCs, though it did exclude cancers originating within 18 cm of the dental ridge. In this trial, patients were randomized following an initial course of CRT and clinical reassessment. Those noted to have responded to treatment were then randomized to surgery versus definitive CRT. Those who received definitive CRT received either a split-course regimen or a total dose of 66 Gy in daily 2 Gy fractions with concurrent 5-FU and cisplatin. Two-year survival was not statistically different, with 34% alive in the arm receiving neoadjuvant CRT, and 40% in the arm receiving CRT alone [31]. Locoregional recurrence was reduced with trimodality therapy (34 vs. 43%), but three-month mortality was higher in the same group (9 vs. 1%). A German study also compared neoadjuvant CRT to definitive CRT in 172 patients with cancers of squamous histology involving the upper/ mid esophagus, though in this trial, inclusion was not dependent upon disease response to initial therapy [32]. Again, no significant difference in OS was noted; however, local progression was reduced with trimodality therapy. Notably, each of these trials used radiation techniques that are not considered standard for esophageal cancer, including split-courses, twice daily fractionation, and/or brachytherapy. Nevertheless, the use of surgery after neoadjuvant CRT did not improve survival in these patients when compared to CRT alone.

Concurrent Chemotherapy and Radiation Therapy in Hypopharynx Cancer

Just as trials focused on treatment regimens for cancers of the lower esophagus have influenced the approach for CEC, randomized trials evaluating CRT in the treatment of hypopharynx cancer, and other HNSCCs, have also influenced the practice. In patients with hypopharynx cancers being treated with a larynx preserving strategy, French investigators randomized patients to induction chemotherapy followed by RT, or to a concurrent CRT approach with cisplatin and a planned dose of 70 Gy to gross disease. The number of patients included in the trial was relatively low, limiting power to detect survival differences; however, the concurrent CRT arm had significantly higher rates of functional larynx preservation (92 vs. 68% at 2 years) [33].

A large meta-analysis of chemotherapy in head and neck cancer (MACH-NC) has reported the benefit of the addition of chemotherapy to radiotherapy across several tumor sub-sites. In patients with hypopharynx cancer, the hazard ratio of death associated with the addition of chemotherapy was 0.88 (95% CI: 0.80–0.96), with an absolute 5-year OS benefit of 4% [34]. This survival benefit was primarily attributed to the use of concurrent chemotherapy with platinum-agent monotherapy or combination chemotherapy regimens.

The European Organisation for Research and Treatment of Cancer (EORTC) conducted a randomized trial in patients with predominantly hypopharynx primaries, comparing a surgical approach (total laryngectomy, partial pharyngectomy, and neck dissection followed by postoperative RT) to induction chemotherapy followed by definitive RT to 70 Gy. At 10 years of follow-up, there was no statistically significant difference in OS, and more than half of survivors in the non-operative arm retained a functional larynx [35].

Studies Focused on Cervical Esophageal Cancer

Randomized trials addressing disease sites above and below the cervical esophagus would support an organ-preserving strategy, which could be an effective initial approach in CEC. Findings in line with this idea come from relatively large retrospective institutional series, focused more specifically on CEC, which have compared CRT to PLE with or without adjuvant therapy. Investigators from Hong Kong reported their institutional experience of patients with CEC treated with CRT or PLE. From 1995 to 2008, a total of 107 patients were treated with PLE, CRT, or palliative treatment. The patients receiving up-front CRT were treated to a total dose of 60–68 Gy with concurrent cisplatin and 5-FU. Of these patients, 30% had a clinical complete response, while 50% had a partial response significant enough to result in down-staging. Of the entire cohort receiving up-front CRT, 24% ultimately required salvage PLE. The median survival of patients in the PLE and CRT arms were not significantly different (20 vs. 25 months, respectively) [23].

A prospective trial from Italy examined the effects of a combined modality approach for patients with SCC of the esophagus, approximately one-third of which were located in the cervical esophagus. Patients were treated with combination cisplatin ($100 \text{ mg/m}^2\text{/day}$) on day 1 and fluorouracil ($1000 \text{ mg/m}^2\text{/day}$) on days 1–4 for two cycles with concurrent RT to a total dose of 30 Gy. Patients were subsequently assessed for surgery, and those not deemed to be operative candidates were treated with additional chemotherapy and 20 Gy RT (50 Gy total). In this trial, a nonoperative approach was favored for CEC, with PLE reserved as salvage treatment for recurrent or persistent disease. Of the nonsurgical patients, 61% achieved complete clinical remission [36]. The median survival in the surgical and nonsurgical groups were 12 and 22 months, respectively, with significant procedure-related mortality likely contributing to worse survival in the surgical group. Larynx preservation was achieved in 30% of the patients with CEC in this trial.

These series suggest definitive CRT has equivalent to improved outcomes when compared to a primary surgical approach. Following CRT, patients with persistent or recurrent disease should be assessed for salvage surgery, although outcomes are generally poor in this population. For example, at one high volume surgical center, the outcomes of 12 patients treated with salvage surgery between 1990 and 2005 were analyzed, with 42% of patients having one or more postoperative complications. While only one patient died of postoperative complications, the cause of death was recurrent cancer in 83%, with a median survival of 21 months [37]. PLE is technically more demanding in an irradiated neck, and postoperative complications are more likely, in turn limiting the success of this strategy.

Seeking improved outcomes by limiting the extent of surgery, an alternative approach was described by German investigators where patients underwent preoperative CRT followed by a limited resection and free jejunal graft interposition. Prior to 2000, patients were treated to 30 Gy in 2-Gy daily fractions with continuous infusional 5-FU. Since then, patients have been treated to 45 Gy in 1.8-Gy daily fractions with concurrent 5-FU with or without cisplatin. In this series, a pCR was seen in 29% of patients, with 76% having an R0 resection [38]. Despite high complication rates, in-hospital mortality was low, and a median survival of 30 months was reported. Similar to other neoadjuvant results, patients with a complete tumor response had a more favorable prognosis.

Several retrospective series have reported the outcomes of patients treated with definitive CRT for CEC (Table 11.2). Burmeister et al. reported on 34 patients treated with CRT, the majority of which had stage I–II disease. Local complete response rates were 91%, with a 5-year OS of 55% [39]. Yamada et al. reported their institutional experience with 27 patients treated with CRT, including more locally advanced tumors than the Burmeister study. Median survival was 14 months, with a 5-year OS of 38% [40]. German investigators have described a sequential approach where patients with locally advanced CEC are treated with induction chemotherapy, followed by concurrent CRT. OS was appreciably lower in these trials, although the tumors appeared to be more advanced [41, 42].

More recently, a comprehensive, retrospective analysis from Peking Union Medical College in China evaluated the outcomes of primary CRT with or without surgery and primary surgery with or without adjuvant treatment [43]. In this analysis, 224 patients were included, 161 of whom received primary RT (the majority received >60 Gy), and 63 of whom received primary surgery (27 had no adjuvant treatment). The operative mortality rate was low, at 1.5%, and the 2-year OS was 50.7%. No differences were noted between the two groups for local, regional, and distant failure-free survival. A subset of patients matched for age, grade, and stage showed a trend toward an improvement in regional recurrence-free survival in the primary RT group. This finding is in line with several other recently reported retrospective studies in which the 3-year OS for CEC is now commonly greater than 50%, with a Japanese study noting a 10-year OS of 35.6% [44–46].

Table 11.2 Selected series of concurrent chemotherapy and radiation therapy alone for the definitive treatment of cervical esophagus cancer

Study	N	Chemotherapy regimen	RT dose	CR	OS
Burmeister et al. [39]	34	CDDP/5FU or 5FU alone	61.2 Gy	91%	55% (5 years)
Yamada et al. [40]	27	CDDP/5FU	66 Gy		38% (5 years)
Stuschke et al. [42]	17	CDDP/Etop	60–66 Gy		24% (3 years)
Cao et al. [43]	161	CDDP/5FU	>60 Gy		51% (2 years)
Zenda et al. [47]	30	CDDP/5FU	60 Gy	73%	67% (3 years)

The outcomes of a multicenter Phase II trial further support the idea that an attempt at organ preservation with CRT should be the initial approach in the treatment of CEC. In this trial, 30 patients, predominantly with locally advanced disease, were treated with CRT consisting of a CDDP/5FU-based chemotherapy regimen given concurrently with 60 Gy 3DCRT in 30 fractions, and followed by two additional cycles of chemotherapy [47]. In this trial, the 3-year OS and laryngectomy-free survival were 67% and 53%, respectively, but lower in patients with T4 disease. Nonhematologic grade 3 toxicities were less than 15% during CRT.

Radiation Dose for Cervical Esophagus Cancer

Given the overall poor outcomes of CEC patients, attempts at further optimizing the CRT platform have been undertaken. RT dose escalation in esophageal cancer was investigated in INT-0123, which randomized patients with clinical stage T1-T4, N0-N1 esophageal carcinoma to 50.4 or 64.8 Gy, both with concurrent cisplatin and 5-FU chemotherapy. The majority of these patients had SCC (~85%). The study closed early after an interim analysis revealed little chance for the high dose arm to show a survival advantage. For the 218 eligible patients, there was no significant difference in median or 2-year survival or local/regional recurrence [48]. A higher number of treatment-related deaths were seen in the high-dose arm; however, the majority of these deaths occurred prior to reaching 50.4 Gy.

While INT-0123 included all locations of esophageal cancer, retrospective evidence suggests high-dose conformal CRT is feasible in CEC. Investigators from Princess Margaret Hospital reported their experience comparing their prior institutional protocol of 54 Gy in 20 fractions with 5-FU on days 1–4 and cisplatin or mitomycin C on day one to their updated institutional protocol of 70 Gy in 35 fractions delivered concurrent with high-dose cisplatin every 3 weeks using a conformal RT technique. After a median follow-up of 3 years, no significant differences in survival or locoregional recurrence were seen [49]. Severe dysphagia requiring insertion of an enteral feeding tube, stent, or esophageal dilation was seen in 45% of patients with no significant difference between dose arms. In contrast, a retrospective series from China suggests improved OS with radiation doses of 66 Gy [50].

A recent National Cancer Data Base analysis of CEC, which categorized patients as receiving standard (50–50.4 Gy), medium (>50.4 to <66 Gy), or high (>66 Gy) doses of RT, found no difference in OS among the groups [51]. This is in contrast to some of the aforementioned retrospective studies that have suggested that outcomes are dose-dependent [44, 46]. Therefore, there is no clear evidence for dose-escalated radiotherapy. Furthermore, there is no clear evidence for a preferred concurrent chemotherapy platform. Most series have utilized a combination of 5-FU and cisplatin. Outcomes utilizing weekly carboplatin and paclitaxel, as in the CROSS trial, have not been reported for CEC.

Radiotherapy Technique

The optimal radiation technique for CEC is typically either 3D-conformal RT (3DCRT) or intensity-modulated radiotherapy (IMRT). IMRT is a technique allowing for variation of the intensity and shape of each beam, typically accomplished by the use of computer-controlled dynamic multileaf collimators. This allows for improved conformality and dose homogeneity, and decreased dose to normal structures such as the spinal cord, brain stem, and parotid glands (Fig. 11.2) [52].

Recent retrospective studies have supported the dosimetric advantages of using IMRT or volumetric-modulated arc therapy (VMAT) over 3DCRT, and have suggested a survival advantage. A Chinese study noted similar survival outcomes overall with lower lung V20, and lower maximum doses to the spinal cord and brachial plexus when IMRT or VMAT was used [53]. At Princess Margaret, patients with CEC who were treated from 1997 to 2013 with 2D RT, 3DCRT, and IMRT, all with concurrent chemotherapy, were analyzed for differences in OS, locoregional, and distant control [54]. There were no differences in locoregional control among the groups, but notably there was a nonsignificant trend for improved 5-year OS in the IMRT group as compared to the 3DCRT group (43% vs. 22%).

Our institutional practice is to treat a single volume including the primary tumor/esophagus with a 3 cm superior expansion to include the hypopharynx and larynx and a 3 cm inferior expansion to account for submucosal spread of disease. The radial volume encompasses the soft tissues of the mediastinum inferiorly and the cervical levels III–V lymph nodes superiorly. These volumes are expanded to create the planning target volume to account for daily setup uncertainty. This single volume is treated to a total dose of 50.4 Gy with concurrent carboplatin and paclitaxel. The supraclavicular nodes are covered, with further elective neck coverage based on the extent of lymphatic involvement. Radiation treatment volumes and dose distribution for a typical CEC patient are shown in Fig. 11.2.

Acute adverse effects from RT include mucositis and esophagitis resulting in odynophagia. While typically relieved by topical and oral analgesics, patients occasionally require placement of a feeding tube for adequate alimentation. One of the more common late effects is esophageal stricture. Of those who do develop a stricture, they are often mild requiring no specific treatment. Moderate cases can be treated with repeated dilation. Severe strictures are rare, but may require palliative PLE in certain cases for relief of dysphagia. Another common late effect is hypothyroidism requiring life-long thyroid supplementation. Chemotherapeutic side effects relate to the particular agents delivered, but predominantly include myelosuppression.

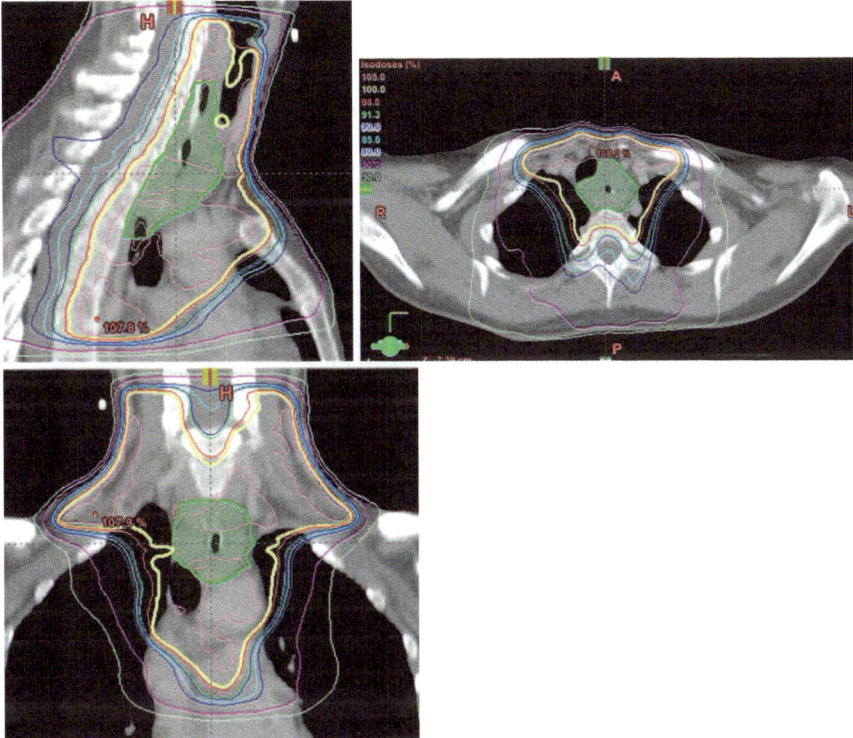

Fig. 11.2 Sagittal, axial, and coronal images of a treatment plan for CEC. Gross tumor volume is demarcated by the solid green volume, and the yellow line represents the 100% isodose line

Conclusions

The lack of high-level evidence for the management of CEC has led to a variety of treatment protocols. Findings extrapolated from trials including HNSCC patients versus those focusing on more distal esophageal cancers have led to varying opinions on the optimal selection of concurrent chemotherapeutic agents and radiation dose. Retrospective studies of CEC are hampered by selection bias and significant heterogeneity of the patient population, in addition to relatively limited outcome data. Despite these difficulties, the predominant management strategy has become definitive CRT in an effort to preserve a functional larynx, with PLE reserved for salvage in the setting of recurrent disease. Unfortunately, the optimal concurrent chemotherapy regimen and radiation dose is unknown, and more carefully analyzed studies addressing the question of which CRT regimen to implement are needed if we hope to improve survival outcomes in this challenging disease.

References

1. Collin CF, Spiro RH. Carcinoma of the cervical esophagus: changing therapeutic trends. Am J Surg. 1984;148(4):460–6.
2. Martins AS. Neck and mediastinal node dissection in pharyngolaryngoesophageal tumors. Head Neck. 2001;23(9):772–9.
3. Fujita H, Kakegawa T, Yamana H, Sueyoshi S, Hikita S, Mine T, et al. Total esophagectomy versus proximal esophagectomy for esophageal cancer at the cervicothoracic junction. World J Surg. 1999;23(5):486–91.
4. Mendenhall WM, Sombeck MD, Parsons JT, Kasper ME, Stringer SP, Vogel SB. Management of cervical esophageal carcinoma. Semin Radiat Oncol. 1994;4(3):179–91.
5. Islami F, Boffetta P, Ren JS, Pedoeim L, Khatib D, Kamangar F. High-temperature beverages and foods and esophageal cancer risk--a systematic review. Int J Cancer. 2009;125(3):491–524.
6. Liyanage SS, Rahman B, Ridda I, Newall AT, Tabrizi SN, Garland SM, et al. The aetiological role of human papillomavirus in oesophageal squamous cell carcinoma: a meta-analysis. PLoS One. 2013;8(7):e69238.
7. Ludmir EB, Palta M, Zhang X, Wu Y, Willett CG, Czito BG. Incidence and prognostic impact of high-risk HPV tumor infection in cervical esophageal carcinoma. J Gastrointest Oncol. 2014;5(6):401–7.
8. Ang KK, Harris J, Wheeler R, Weber R, Rosenthal DI, Nguyen-Tan PF, et al. Human papillomavirus and survival of patients with oropharyngeal cancer. N Engl J Med. 2010;363(1):24–35.
9. Grass GD, Cooper SL, Armeson K, Garrett-Mayer E, Sharma A. Cervical esophageal cancer: a population-based study. Head Neck. 2015;37(6):808–14.
10. Cancer Genome Atlas Research N, Analysis Working Group: Asan U, Agency BCC, Brigham, Women's H, Broad I, et al. Integrated genomic characterization of oesophageal carcinoma. Nature. 2017;541(7636):169–75.
11. Bang YJ, Van Cutsem E, Feyereislova A, Chung HC, Shen L, Sawaki A, et al. Trastuzumab in combination with chemotherapy versus chemotherapy alone for treatment of HER2-positive advanced gastric or gastro-oesophageal junction cancer (ToGA): a phase 3, open-label, randomised controlled trial. Lancet. 2010;376(9742):687–97.
12. Bonner JA, Harari PM, Giralt J, Azarnia N, Shin DM, Cohen RB, et al. Radiotherapy plus cetuximab for squamous-cell carcinoma of the head and neck. N Engl J Med. 2006;354(6):567–78.
13. Suntharalingam M, Winter K, Ilson D, Dicker AP, Kachnic L, Konski A, et al. Effect of the addition of cetuximab to paclitaxel, cisplatin, and radiation therapy for patients with esophageal cancer: the NRG oncology RTOG 0436 phase 3 randomized clinical trial. JAMA Oncol. 2017;3(11):1520–8.
14. Daiko H, Hayashi R, Saikawa M, Sakuraba M, Yamazaki M, Miyazaki M, et al. Surgical management of carcinoma of the cervical esophagus. J Surg Oncol. 2007;96(2):166–72.
15. Thosani N, Singh H, Kapadia A, Ochi N, Lee JH, Ajani J, et al. Diagnostic accuracy of EUS in differentiating mucosal versus submucosal invasion of superficial esophageal cancers: a systematic review and meta-analysis. Gastrointest Endosc. 2012;75(2):242–53.
16. Chandawarkar RY, Kakegawa T, Fujita H, Yamana H, Toh Y, Fujitoh H. Endosonography for preoperative staging of specific nodal groups associated with esophageal cancer. World J Surg. 1996;20(6):700–2.
17. Heeren PA, Jager PL, Bongaerts F, van Dullemen H, Sluiter W, Plukker JT. Detection of distant metastases in esophageal cancer with (18)F-FDG PET. J Nucl Med. 2004;45(6):980–7.
18. Zhao D, Gao X, Guan L, Su W, Gao J, Liu C, et al. Free jejunal graft for reconstruction of defects in the hypopharynx and cervical esophagus following the cancer resections. J Gastrointest Surg. 2009;13(7):1368–72.
19. Peracchia A, Bardini R, Ruol A, Segalin A, Castoro C, Asolati M, et al. Surgical management of carcinoma of the hypopharynx and cervical esophagus. Hepato-Gastroenterology. 1990;37(4):371–5.

20. Gunnlaugsson GH, Wychulis AR, Roland C, Ellis FH Jr. Analysis of the records of 1,657 patients with carcinoma of the esophagus and cardia of the stomach. Surg Gynecol Obstet. 1970;130(6):997–1005.
21. Peracchia A, Ancona E, Buin F. The surgical treatment of cancer of the cervical esophagus: complications and preliminary results. Int Surg. 1982;67(2):135–7.
22. Pearson JG. Radiotherapy for esophageal carcinoma. World J Surg. 1981;5(4):489–97.
23. Tong DK, Law S, Kwong DL, Wei WI, Ng RW, Wong KH. Current management of cervical esophageal cancer. World J Surg. 2011;35(3):600–7.
24. Wei WI, Lam LK, Yuen PW, Wong J. Current status of pharyngolaryngo-esophagectomy and pharyngogastric anastomosis. Head Neck. 1998;20(3):240–4.
25. Marmuse JP, Koka VN, Guedon C, Benhamou G. Surgical treatment of carcinoma of the proximal esophagus. Am J Surg. 1995;169(4):386–90.
26. Triboulet JP, Mariette C, Chevalier D, Amrouni H. Surgical management of carcinoma of the hypopharynx and cervical esophagus: analysis of 209 cases. Arch Surg. 2001;136(10):1164–70.
27. Wang HW, Chu PY, Kuo KT, Yang CH, Chang SY, Hsu WH, et al. A reappraisal of surgical management for squamous cell carcinoma in the pharyngoesophageal junction. J Surg Oncol. 2006;93(6):468–76.
28. Cooper JS, Guo MD, Herskovic A, Macdonald JS, Martenson JA Jr, Al-Sarraf M, et al. Chemoradiotherapy of locally advanced esophageal cancer: long-term follow-up of a prospective randomized trial (RTOG 85-01). Radiation therapy oncology group. JAMA. 1999;281(17):1623–7.
29. Tepper J, Krasna MJ, Niedzwiecki D, Hollis D, Reed CE, Goldberg R, et al. Phase III trial of trimodality therapy with cisplatin, fluorouracil, radiotherapy, and surgery compared with surgery alone for esophageal cancer: CALGB 9781. J Clin Oncol. 2008;26(7):1086–92.
30. van Hagen P, Hulshof MC, van Lanschot JJ, Steyerberg EW, van Berge Henegouwen MI, Wijnhoven BP, et al. Preoperative chemoradiotherapy for esophageal or junctional cancer. N Engl J Med. 2012;366(22):2074–84.
31. Bedenne L, Michel P, Bouche O, Milan C, Mariette C, Conroy T, et al. Chemoradiation followed by surgery compared with chemoradiation alone in squamous cancer of the esophagus: FFCD 9102. J Clin Oncol. 2007;25(10):1160–8.
32. Stahl M, Stuschke M, Lehmann N, Meyer HJ, Walz MK, Seeber S, et al. Chemoradiation with and without surgery in patients with locally advanced squamous cell carcinoma of the esophagus. J Clin Oncol. 2005;23(10):2310–7.
33. Prades JM, Lallemant B, Garrel R, Reyt E, Righini C, Schmitt T, et al. Randomized phase III trial comparing induction chemotherapy followed by radiotherapy to concomitant chemoradiotherapy for laryngeal preservation in T3M0 pyriform sinus carcinoma. Acta Otolaryngol. 2010;130(1):150–5.
34. Blanchard P, Baujat B, Holostenco V, Bourredjem A, Baey C, Bourhis J, et al. Meta-analysis of chemotherapy in head and neck cancer (MACH-NC): a comprehensive analysis by tumour site. Radiother Oncol. 2011;100(1):33–40.
35. Lefebvre JL, Andry G, Chevalier D, Luboinski B, Collette L, Traissac L, et al. Laryngeal preservation with induction chemotherapy for hypopharyngeal squamous cell carcinoma: 10-year results of EORTC trial 24891. Ann Oncol. 2012;23(10):2708–14.
36. Bidoli P, Bajetta E, Stani SC, De CD, Santoro A, Valente M, et al. Ten-year survival with chemotherapy and radiotherapy in patients with squamous cell carcinoma of the esophagus. Cancer. 2002;94(2):352–61.
37. Schieman C, Wigle DA, Deschamps C, Nichols FC 3rd, Cassivi SD, Shen KR, et al. Salvage resections for recurrent or persistent cancer of the proximal esophagus after chemoradiotherapy. Ann Thorac Surg. 2013;95(2):459–63.
38. Ott K, Lordick F, Molls M, Bartels H, Biemer E, Siewert JR. Limited resection and free jejunal graft interposition for squamous cell carcinoma of the cervical oesophagus. Br J Surg. 2009;96(3):258–66.

39. Burmeister BH, Dickie G, Smithers BM, Hodge R, Morton K. Thirty-four patients with carcinoma of the cervical esophagus treated with chemoradiation therapy. Arch Otolaryngol Head Neck Surg. 2000;126(2):205–8.
40. Yamada K, Murakami M, Okamoto Y, Okuno Y, Nakajima T, Kusumi F, et al. Treatment results of radiotherapy for carcinoma of the cervical esophagus. Acta Oncol. 2006;45(8):1120–5.
41. Gkika E, Gauler T, Eberhardt W, Stahl M, Stuschke M, Pottgen C. Long-term results of definitive radiochemotherapy in locally advanced cancers of the cervical esophagus. Dis Esophagus. 2014;27(7):678–84.
42. Stuschke M, Stahl M, Wilke H, Walz MK, Oldenburg AR, Stuben G, et al. Induction chemotherapy followed by concurrent chemotherapy and high-dose radiotherapy for locally advanced squamous cell carcinoma of the cervical oesophagus. Oncology. 1999;57(2):99–105.
43. Cao CN, Luo JW, Gao L, Xu GZ, Yi JL, Huang XD, et al. Primary radiotherapy compared with primary surgery in cervical esophageal cancer. JAMA Otolaryngol Head Neck Surg. 2014;140(10):918–26.
44. Zhao L, Zhou Y, Mu Y, Chai G, Xiao F, Tan L, et al. Patterns of failure and clinical outcomes of definitive radiotherapy for cervical esophageal cancer. Oncotarget. 2017;8(13):21852–60.
45. Kumabe A, Zenda S, Motegi A, Onozawa M, Nakamura N, Kojima T, et al. Long-term clinical results of concurrent chemoradiotherapy for patients with cervical esophageal squamous cell carcinoma. Anticancer Res. 2017;37(9):5039–44.
46. Herrmann E, Mertineit N, De Bari B, Hoeng L, Caparotti F, Leiser D, et al. Outcome of proximal esophageal cancer after definitive combined chemo-radiation: a Swiss multicenter retrospective study. Radiat Oncol. 2017;12(1):97.
47. Zenda S, Kojima T, Kato K, Izumi S, Ozawa T, Kiyota N, et al. Multicenter phase 2 study of cisplatin and 5-fluorouracil with concurrent radiation therapy as an organ preservation approach in patients with squamous cell carcinoma of the cervical esophagus. Int J Radiat Oncol Biol Phys. 2016;96(5):976–84.
48. Minsky BD, Pajak TF, Ginsberg RJ, Pisansky TM, Martenson J, Komaki R, et al. INT 0123 (Radiation Therapy Oncology Group 94-05) phase III trial of combined-modality therapy for esophageal cancer: high-dose versus standard-dose radiation therapy. J Clin Oncol. 2002;20(5):1167–74.
49. Huang SH, Lockwood G, Brierley J, Cummings B, Kim J, Wong R, et al. Effect of concurrent high-dose cisplatin chemotherapy and conformal radiotherapy on cervical esophageal cancer survival. Int J Radiat Oncol Biol Phys. 2008;71(3):735–40.
50. Cao C, Luo J, Gao L, Xu G, Yi J, Huang X, et al. Definitive radiotherapy for cervical esophageal cancer. Head Neck. 2015;37(2):151–5.
51. De B, Rhome R, Doucette J, Buckstein M. Dose escalation of definitive radiation is not associated with improved survival for cervical esophageal cancer: a National Cancer Data Base (NCDB) analysis. Dis Esophagus. 2017;30(4):1–10.
52. Fenkell L, Kaminsky I, Breen S, Huang S, Van Prooijen M, Ringash J. Dosimetric comparison of IMRT vs. 3D conformal radiotherapy in the treatment of cancer of the cervical esophagus. Radiother Oncol. 2008;89(3):287–91.
53. Yang H, Feng C, Cai BN, Yang J, Liu HX, Ma L. Comparison of three-dimensional conformal radiation therapy, intensity-modulated radiation therapy, and volumetric-modulated arc therapy in the treatment of cervical esophageal carcinoma. Dis Esophagus. 2017;30(2):1–8.
54. McDowell LJ, Huang SH, Xu W, Che J, Wong RKS, Brierley J, et al. Effect of intensity modulated radiation therapy with concurrent chemotherapy on survival for patients with cervical esophageal carcinoma. Int J Radiat Oncol Biol Phys. 2017;98(1):186–95.

The Multidisciplinary Management of Early-Stage Thoracic Esophageal Cancer

12

Brandon Mahal and Theodore S. Hong

Diagnosis

The appropriate work-up and staging of thoracic esophageal carcinoma is essential for appropriate treatment recommendations. Initial work-up includes history and physical exam, upper GI endoscopy with biopsy, CT chest/abdomen with oral and IV contrast, PET-CT, endoscopic ultrasound, and bronchoscopy for masses located at or above the carina.

Anatomy

The esophagus is anatomically defined into four regions based on measured distance from the incisors. The cervical esophagus is located from the cricoid cartilage to the thoracic inlet (~15 to 18 cm from the incisors). The upper thoracic esophagus is located from the thoracic inlet to tracheal bifurcation (~18 to 24 cm from incisors). The mid thoracic esophagus is located from the tracheal bifurcation to the midway of the gastroesophageal junction (~24 to 32 cm from incisors). The lower thoracic or abdominal esophagus encompasses the gastroesophageal junction (~32 to 40 cm from incisors). The esophagus lacks a serosal layer and has an extensive lymphatic drainage. Cancers that arise in the upper third of the esophagus drain predominately to the supraclavicular, cervical, and superior mediastinal nodes, while cancers in the lower esophagus can drain to the lower mediastinum and celiac

B. Mahal
Harvard Radiation Oncology Program, Harvard Medical School, Boston, MA, USA

T. S. Hong (✉)
Department of Radiation Oncology, Massachusetts General Hospital, Boston, MA, USA
e-mail: Tshong1@mgh.harvard.edu

© Springer Nature Switzerland AG 2020
N. F. Saba, B. F. El-Rayes (eds.), *Esophageal Cancer*,
https://doi.org/10.1007/978-3-030-29832-6_12

gastric or hepatic nodes. Influenced by location, middle thoracic cancers can drain superiorly or inferiorly. Nodal stations at risk must be taken into account during surgical node dissection and radiation planning. The majority of upper to mid thoracic esophageal cancers are SCC, while lower thoracic and gastroesophageal are predominantly adenocarcinoma (see Chap. 1).

Surgical Management

Appropriate candidates for surgical resection of thoracic esophageal carcinoma include patients with early clinically staged disease (T1N0–T2N0) and patients planned for trimodality therapy following chemoradiation therapy (Chap. 9). Surgical resection options include open and laparoscopic or minimally invasive approaches. Surgeon preference, tumor location, planned lymph node dissection, and planned anastomosis dictate surgical approach and type (transhiatal, transthoracic (Ivor Lewis), and tri-incisional).

Transhiatal esophagectomy is accomplished with a midline laparotomy and left neck incision with blunt dissection of the thoracic esophagus and a cervical anastomosis generated [1]. Due to difficulty with complete visualization with blunt dissection, a complete lymphadenectomy is typically not accomplished. Modern experiences show post-operative mortality of ~1% and anastomotic leak rates of ~10% [2–5].

Transthoracic (Ivor Lewis) esophagectomy is performed with laparotomy and right thoracotomy that allows direction visualization of the thoracic esophagus and enables a full thoracic lymphadenectomy. This approach may be limited to cancers of the lower thoracic esophagus due to the proximal/superior resection that generates an intrathoracic esophagogastric anastomosis. Post-operative mortality is less than 4% with similar outcomes compared to a transhiatal approach [6, 7]. Post-operative complications include severe reflux (3–20%), risk of intrathoracic anastomotic leakage that can result in severe morbidity, and close proximal margins [8–10].

Tri-incisional esophagectomy is a less commonly used approach and is accomplished with a right posterolateral thoracotomy/thoracoscopy, laparotomy, and left neck incision. This approach permits direct visualization during mediastinal and upper abdominal lymphadenectomy with the generation of a cervical esophagogastric anastomosis. Post-operative mortality is less than 4% with anastomotic leak rates of ~5% [11].

Evolution of Multimodality Therapy

Management of localized esophageal cancers with surgery or radiotherapy alone has historically poor survival outcomes, with 5-year survival rates ranging from 0 to 20% [12–15]. Locoregional failure rates from modern reported trials range from 32 to 45% of patients that undergo resection [2, 15–17]. Modern surgical advances and post-operative care have mildly improved survival rates for patients that undergo resection alone (5-year overall survival rates 20–25%). A vast majority of patients with esophageal cancer are unresectable (~60–70%) at presentation, and only ~20% of patients are ultimately able to proceed to surgery [18]. Based on these observations, the rationale for preoperative radiation therapy (RT) in an attempt to increase resectability and survival has been investigated. Data from multiple prospective trials of patients treated with preoperative RT have failed to show improvements in survival outcomes or resection rates [19, 20]. A meta-analysis of 5 randomized trials including 1147 patients showed a non-statistically significant trend toward survival benefit for patients treated with preoperative RT (HR 0.89, $p = 0.06$) [21]. Post-operative RT has been evaluated in two randomized trials that failed to demonstrate a survival benefit [22, 23]. Despite improvements in staging, surgical techniques, post-operative care, and radiation delivery, the risks of locoregional recurrences and metastatic disease have formed the rationale for combined modality therapy with the addition of chemotherapy.

Preoperative Chemotherapy

Preoperative chemotherapy has been tested in multiple randomized controlled trials for patients with resectable esophageal cancer. Intergroup 0133 (Radiation Therapy Oncology Group 8911) randomized 443 patients with resectable esophageal cancer (adenocarcinoma or SCC) to surgery alone or three cycles of preoperative cisplatin and 5-fluorouracil followed by surgery and two additional cycles of chemotherapy [15]. There was no observed benefit associated with the preoperative chemotherapy arm for median survival (15 months vs. 16 months), 4-year overall survival (26% vs. 23%), or R0 resection rate (59% vs. 63%) [24]. Regardless of treatment arm, patients with a complete resection (R0 vs. R1) had improved 5-year survival (32% vs. 5%).

The Medical Research Council Oesophageal Cancer Working Party reported on 802 patients with resectable esophageal cancer (adenocarcinoma or SCC) treated with surgery alone or two cycles of preoperative cisplatin and 5-fluorouracil and surgery [25]. Patients in the preoperative chemotherapy arm had statistically significant improved 2-year (43% vs. 34%) and 5-year overall survival rates (23% vs. 17%) and R0 resection rates (60% vs. 54%). The differences in outcomes between the INT-0113 and MRC trials may be explained in part by the slightly higher rate of patients with adenocarcinoma enrolled in the MRC study (MRC 66% adenocarcinoma, 31% SCC; INT-0133 54% adenocarcinoma, 46% SCC).

Two randomized trials have evaluated the role of preoperative chemotherapy (cisplatin and 5-fluorouracil) in patients with esophageal SCC and failed to observe a survival benefit [16, 26].

A meta-analysis of 8 randomized trials encompassing 1724 patients with resectable esophageal cancer demonstrated a 2-year overall survival benefit of 7% (HR 0.9, $p = 0.05$) with benefit limited to patients with adenocarcinoma [27]. A recent updated meta-analysis of 9 randomized trials (1981 patients) demonstrated a survival benefit for neoadjuvant chemotherapy compared to surgery alone (HR 0.87,

$p = 0.005$), with observed benefit for adenocarcinoma (HR 0.83, $p = 0.01$) but not statistically significant for SCC (HR 0.92, $p = 0.18$) [28].

Preoperative Chemoradiation Therapy

Preoperative chemoradiation has been evaluated with multiple randomized trials (Table 12.1). The EORTC randomized 282 patients with T1-3N0 and T1-2N1 SCC to surgery alone or preoperative chemoradiation therapy and surgery. Chemoradiation consisted of two cycles of cisplatin, and radiation was delivered using a split course of 37 Gy in 10 fractions. There was no difference in overall survival, and median survival was 18.6 months for both treatment arms [30]. Preoperative chemoradiation was associated with an improved disease-free survival, higher rate of curative resection, and more post-operative deaths.

The FFCD 9901 trial randomized 195 patients with early-stage esophageal cancer to surgery versus neoadjuvant chemoradiation therapy (45 Gy in 25 fractions with 2 cycles of cisplatin and fluorouracil). Seventy percent of patients enrolled had SCC. With a median follow-up of ~93 months, there were no observed differences between surgery and combined modality arms for overall survival (53% vs. 48%) or complete resection rates (92% vs. 94%). Local regional control was improved in patients in the combined modality arm (29% vs. 15%). After interim analysis, the trial was stopped due to futility of either treatment arm reaching superiority. Post-operative mortality was significantly increased for patients in the combined modality arm (11% vs. 3.4%, $p = 0.049$) [34].

Table 12.1 Trials of neoadjuvant chemoradiation vs. surgery in esophageal carcinoma

Reference	Year	Path	Arm	N	OS	MS	pCR	RT	Chemo
[29]	1988–1991	SCC 100%	S	45	3y 14%	11 m	9.8%	20 Gy	CDDP, 5FU
			CRT	41	3y 19%	10.5 m			
[2]	1989–1994	SCC 25% AC 75%	S	50	3y 16%	17.6 m	28%	45 Gy (BID)	CDDP, 5FU, vinblastine
			CRT	50	3y 30% NS	16.9 m NS			
[30]	1989–1995	SCC 100%	S	139	3y 34%	18.6 m	21%	37 Gy	CDDP
			CRT	143	3y 37% NS	18.6 m NS			
[31]	1994–2000	SCC 35% AC 63%	S	128	3y 36%	22.2 m	13%	35 Gy	CDDP, 5FU
			CRT	128	3y 31% NS	19.3 m NS			
[32]	1997–2000	SCC 25% AC 75%	S	30	5y 16%	7.8 m	33%	50.4 Gy	CDDP/5FU
			CRT	26	5y 39% SS	19.4 m SS			
[33]	2004–2008	SCC/AC	S	188	5y 34%	49 m	29%	41.4 Gy	Carboplatin, paclitaxel
			CRT	178	5y 47% SS	24 m SS			

CALGB 9781 randomized patients with stage I–III SCC or adenocarcinoma of the thoracic esophagus and GEJ to surgery alone or neoadjuvant chemoradiation (50.4 Gy in 28 fractions) with concurrent cisplatin and 5-fluorouracil followed by surgery. The trial enrolled 56 of a target 500 patients and closed early due to non-accrual. A pathologic complete response was observed in 40% of patients on the combined modality arm. Intent to treat analysis with a median follow-up of 6 years showed an improvement in median overall survival (4.5 years vs. 1.8 years) and 5-year overall survival (39% vs. 16%) for patients on the combined modality treatment arm [32].

The landmark CROSS study randomized 366 patients with resectable (T1N1, T2-3N0–1) esophageal or GEJ cancer to surgery alone or weekly carboplatin and paclitaxel with concurrent radiation therapy (41.4 Gy in 23 fractions) followed by surgery, with stratification by performance status, nodal stage, histology, and treatment center [33]. Baseline patient characteristics included 75% esophagus versus 22% GEJ tumors and 75% adenocarcinoma versus 23% SCC tumor histology. Patients on the combined modality arm had improved median survival (49.4 months vs. 24 months) and complete resection rate (92% vs. 69%, $p < 0.001$), with a pathologic complete response rate of 29% in the neoadjuvant chemoradiation arm and significantly lower local recurrence rates and hematogenous spread for patients in the combined modality arm (34% vs. 14%, $p < 0.001$, and 35% vs. 29%, $p = 0.025$, respectively). Overall survival was significantly improved for the combined modality arm (HR 0.657, $p = 0.003$), with an absolute 5-year survival benefit of 13% observed for patients in the combined modality arm (47% vs. 34%). Notably, postoperative mortality was 4% in both arms. Long-term follow-up results confirmed the overall survival benefits associated with neoadjuvant chemoradiation when added to surgery (HR 0.68, $p = 0.003$), with clinically relevant improvements in both SCC (median OS 81.6 months with trimodality therapy, HR 0.48, $p = 0.008$) and adenocarcinoma subtypes (median OS 43.2 months with trimodality, HR 0.73, 0.038) [35]. This landmark trial established preoperative chemoradiation as the standard of care for early-stage localized adenocarcinoma of the thoracic esophagus and suggests that the observed survival benefit is due to improved local control associated with combined modality therapy [17]. Notably, a meta-analysis that included 1854 patients from 12 randomized trials of neoadjuvant chemotherapy versus surgery alone (including the CROSS trial) similarly showed a survival benefit for patients treated with neoadjuvant chemoradiotherapy over surgery alone (0.78, $p = 0.0001$), with observed benefit for both esophageal SCC (HR 0.80, $p = 0.004$) and adenocarcinoma (HR 0.75, $p = 0.02$) [28].

Chemoradiation Versus Trimodality Therapy

Trimodality therapy (neoadjuvant chemoradiation followed by surgery) versus definitive chemoradiation therapy has been evaluated in two randomized European trials. A French study, FF9102, randomized 259 patients with resectable (T3–4, N0–1) esophageal cancer (SCC and adenocarcinoma, with nearly 90% SCC) to trimodality therapy versus definitive chemoradiation. All patients received neoadjuvant cisplatin and 5-fluorouracil and radiation therapy (46 Gy in 23 fractions or a split course 15 Gy in 5 fractions). Patients with a partial or complete clinical response were then randomized to surgery or additional chemoradiation therapy (cisplatin and 5-fluorouracil and 20 Gy in 10 fractions or split course 15 Gy in 5 fractions). No difference was observed in median survival for trimodality versus definitive chemoradiation (17.7 months vs. 19.3 months) or 2-year overall survival (34% vs. 40%). An improvement in local control at 2 years was observed for trimodality vs. definitive chemoradiation (65% vs. 57%), and treatment-related mortality was increased in patients treated with trimodality therapy (9% vs. 1%, $p = 0.002$) [36].

Stahl et al. reported on 172 patients with T3–4, N0–1 (EUS staged) SCC of the upper and mid esophagus [37]. Patients were treated with induction chemotherapy (three cycles of 5-fluorouracil, leucovorin, etoposide, and cisplatin) followed by chemoradiation (40 Gy with concurrent cisplatin and etoposide) and then randomized to surgery or definitive chemoradiation to >65 Gy. There was no difference in median overall survival (16 months vs. 15 months) or 3-year overall survival (28% vs. 20%) for the surgery or chemoradiation arm. Improved freedom from local progression (64% vs. 41%) and treatment-related mortality (13% vs. 4%) were statistically significant between the surgery and chemoradiation arms.

Additional randomized trials have observed no difference in survival outcomes for patients with resectable esophageal cancer treated with surgery versus definitive chemoradiation [38, 39]. Collectively these data suggest that the addition of surgery to chemoradiation does not provide a survival benefit, at least for SCC histologies. Based on these observations, some argue that definitive chemoradiation is a standard of care and that surgery may serve as a salvage therapy, in particular for SCC histologies. The same conclusions are not widely applied to adenocarcinoma histologies given that this histology was not adequately represented in these studies.

The phase II RTOG 0246 study enrolled 43 patients treated with induction chemotherapy (2 cycles of 5-fluorouracil, cisplatin, and paclitaxel) followed by chemoradiation (50.4 Gy with concurrent 5-fluorouracil, cisplatin) and salvage esophagectomy for persistent or recurrent disease. With a median follow-up of 6.7 years, the estimated 5-year survival rate was 37%. Salvage resection was attempted in 51% of patients due to residual or recurrent disease or patient choice [40].

The role of surgery for salvage therapy following persistent disease or failure after definitive chemoradiation therapy in patients with early-stage SCC may be a reasonable management option in appropriately selected early-stage patients [41, 42].

Cumulatively, these data suggest that trimodality therapy is an appropriate treatment option for patients with resectable thoracic esophageal malignancies. The underlying biological differences between SCC and adenocarcinoma likely contribute in part to observed differences in treatment outcomes from reported trials, where SCC histology may be more responsive to chemoradiation and therefore benefit to a lesser degree from trimodality therapy. Baseline patient characteristics and risk factors associated with SCC (tobacco and alcohol use) or adenocarcinoma (obesity, GERD, Barrett's disease) may also contribute to observed survival outcomes and post-operative mortality risk.

Radiation Dose Escalation and Chemotherapy Regimens

With chemoradiation established as a standard of care approach to therapy, Intergroup 0123 investigated the role of radiation dose escalation by randomizing patients with clinical stage T1–T4, N0–N1 SCC or adenocarcinoma to concurrent chemoradiation therapy (fluorouracil and cisplatin) to a total dose of 64.8 Gy vs. 50.4 Gy. Median survival (13 vs. 18 months), 2-year survival (31% vs. 40%), and locoregional failure rates (56% vs. 52%) were similar when comparing high-dose and low-dose treatment arms, respectively. There were 11 treatment-related deaths in the high-dose arm, and 7 of the deaths occurred at doses less than 50.4 Gy [43]. As such, the standard of care radiation dose has remained 50.4 Gy due to concern for treatment-related toxicity.

To study optimal chemotherapy regimens, the multicenter phase II–III PRODIGE5/ACCORD17 trial compared definitive chemoradiotherapy with 50 Gy in 25 fractions in combination with FOLFOX (fluorouracil, leucovorin, oxaliplatin) versus fluorouracil and cisplatin in patients with localized esophageal cancer. With a median follow-up of 25.3 months, there were no significant differences in median progression-free survival (9.7 months in FOLFOX arm vs. 9.4 months in fluorouracil/cisplatin arm, $p = 0.64$) or median overall survival (20.2 months in FOLFOX arm vs. 17.5 months in fluorouracil/cisplatin arm, $p = 0.70$). Treatment arms were similar in regard to completion of all chemotherapy (71% in FOLFOX arm vs. 76% in fluorouracil/cisplatin arm). While no significant differences were noted in toxicity profiles, there were more toxicity-related deaths in the fluorouracil/cisplatin arm versus the FOLFOX arm (6 vs. 1, $p = 0.66$) [44]. As such, FOLFOX and fluorouracil/cisplatin remain reasonable standard of care radiotherapy options.

Potential Toxicity and Treatment Planning

Historically, radiation treatment fields for esophageal cancer have included large cranio-caudal borders in order to cover at-risk nodal volumes (ranging from supra-clavicular to celiac stations) and standard superior-inferior tumor expansion (routinely 5 cm) using 3D planning techniques. A standard treatment design included anterior-posterior/posterior-anterior (AP-PA) limited by spinal cord constraints followed with a boost using an off-cord multi-field arrangement. In addition to the spinal cord, organs at risk include the lungs, heart, liver, and kidneys. Dose-volume histogram constraints for lung metrics have been studied in relation to risk of radiation pneumonitis with models based on testing the normal tissue complication probability models [45]. Notably, technical advances in radiation delivery techniques including intensity-modulated radiation therapy (IMRT) have enabled improved conformal dose distributions with the ability to limit dose to adjacent normal tissues; Fig. 12.1 depicts a representative IMRT generated plan for a patient with SCC of the thoracic esophagus. While no randomized evidence is available for comparison of 3D versus IMRT, improved dose homogeneity and dose-volume histogram (DVH) parameters can be accomplished with IMRT planning [46]. Lung and cardiac dosage has been shown to be significantly reduced with IMRT compared to 3D

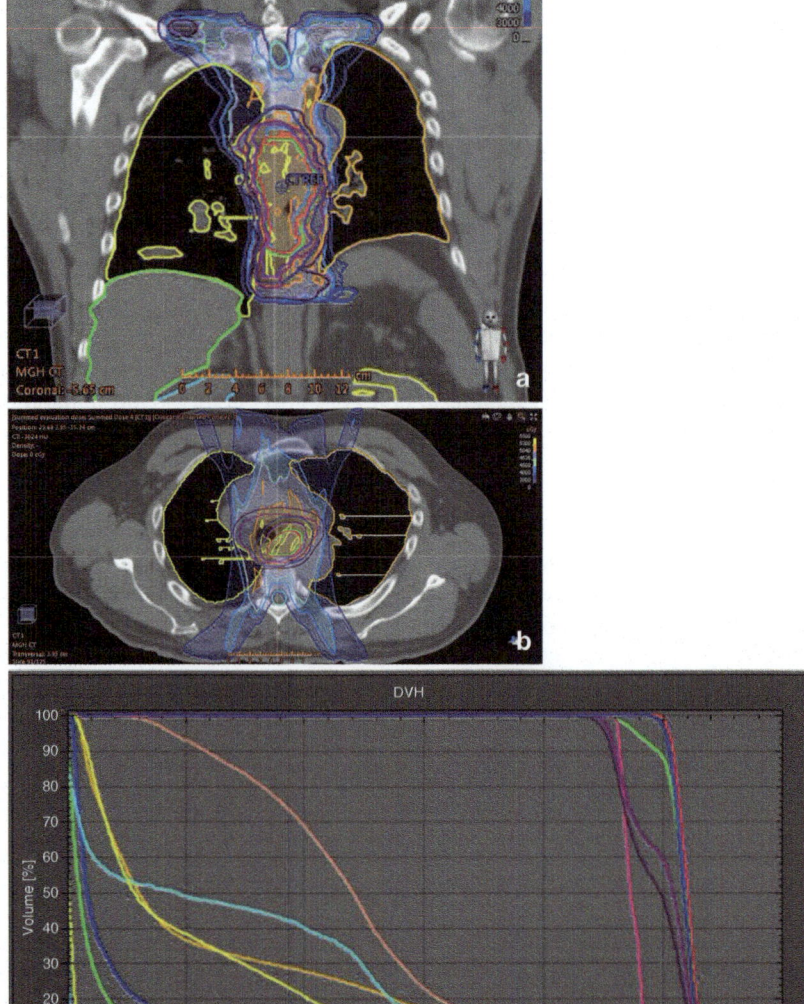

Fig. 12.1 IMRT plan for T3N0 thoracic esophageal squamous cell carcinoma. Patient planned for concurrent neoadjuvant chemoradiation therapy (carboplatin/paclitaxel) in anticipation of surgical resection. Treatment prescription for 45 Gy in 1.8 Gy fractions to CTV with 5.4 Gy in 1.8 Gy fraction boost to GTV. (**a**) Coronal slice of treatment plan with isodose lines. (**b**) Axial slice of treatment plan with isodose lines. (**c**) DVH histogram. CTV 4500 dark purple (average 4981 cGy), CTV 5040 light purple (average 5195 cGy), GTV red (average 5206 cGy), heart pink (average 2480 cGy), left lung orange (average 1277 cGy), right lung yellow (average 1136 cGy), spinal cord teal (average 1321 cGy)

planning (mean heart dose 22.9 vs. 28.2 Gy; V30 24.8% vs. 61%) [47]. Furthermore, advances in radiation delivery techniques including planning arc therapy [48, 49], 4D planning [50], and personalized risk assessment [51] may further aid in target delineation and minimizing treatment-associated toxicities.

Treatment Response

A complete pathologic response following neoadjuvant therapy for esophageal cancer is an important prognostic factor observed in multiple studies [2, 26, 31, 52], and post treatment pathologic stage is highly significant for survival with combined modality therapy [53]. An estimated 20–60% of patients with complete response to neoadjuvant therapy have residual disease on surgical resection or pathologic review [54].

PET scans following preoperative chemoradiation have shown mixed results in regard to predicting histopathologic response and survival outcomes for patients with locally advanced esophageal cancer [55–60]. CALGB 80803 is an ongoing phase II trial assessing PET response to guide treatment in locally advanced esophageal cancer. Here, patients are randomized to FOLFOX6 (three cycles) or carboplatin/paclitaxel (two cycles), and treatment response is assessed by interval PET. Patients that demonstrate an imaging response (>35% decrease in SUVmax) continue on the same chemotherapy regimen in anticipation of planned radiotherapy and surgery. Patients without favorable response are crossed over to the alternative chemotherapy in anticipation of further treatment.

Conclusions

A multidisciplinary approach in the initial evaluation and management of early-stage thoracic esophageal cancer is key to an appropriate treatment strategy. Treatment options include clinical trial enrollment for eligible and interested patients, concurrent chemoradiation in anticipation of surgical resection, definitive chemoradiation, and in select cases esophagectomy followed by chemoradiation. Continued improvements in the realms of diagnostic imaging and treatment assessment, molecular profiling, chemotherapy, minimally invasive surgical techniques, and improved radiation planning and delivery systems will aid in the goal of improved outcomes in the treatment of esophageal malignancies.

References

1. Ellis FH Jr, Gibb SP, Watkins E Jr. Esophagogastrectomy. A safe, widely applicable, and expeditious form of palliation for patients with carcinoma of the esophagus and cardia. Ann Surg. 1983;198(4):531–40.
2. Urba SG, Orringer MB, Turrisi A, Iannettoni M, Forastiere A, Strawderman M. Randomized trial of preoperative chemoradiation versus surgery alone in patients with locoregional esophageal carcinoma. J Clin Oncol. 2001;19(2):305–13.

3. Rao YG, Pal S, Pande GK, Sahni P, Chattopadhyay TK. Transhiatal esophagectomy for benign and malignant conditions. Am J Surg. 2002;184(2):136–42.
4. Chang AC, Ji H, Birkmeyer NJ, Orringer MB, Birkmeyer JD. Outcomes after transhiatal and transthoracic esophagectomy for cancer. Ann Thorac Surg. 2008;85(2):424–9. https://doi.org/10.1016/j.athoracsur.2007.10.007.
5. van Sandick JW, van Lanschot JJ, ten Kate FJ, Tijssen JG, Obertop H. Indicators of prognosis after transhiatal esophageal resection without thoracotomy for cancer. J Am Coll Surg. 2002;194(1):28–36.
6. Griffin SM, Shaw IH, Dresner SM. Early complications after Ivor Lewis subtotal esophagectomy with two-field lymphadenectomy: risk factors and management. J Am Coll Surg. 2002;194(3):285–97.
7. Hulscher JB, Tijssen JG, Obertop H, van Lanschot JJ. Transthoracic versus transhiatal resection for carcinoma of the esophagus: a meta-analysis. Ann Thorac Surg. 2001;72(1):306–13.
8. Urschel JD. Esophagogastrostomy anastomotic leaks complicating esophagectomy: a review. Am J Surg. 1995;169(6):634–40.
9. Patil PK, Patel SG, Mistry RC, Deshpande RK, Desai PB. Cancer of the esophagus: esophagogastric anastomotic leak--a retrospective study of predisposing factors. J Surg Oncol. 1992;49(3):163–7.
10. Whooley BP, Law S, Alexandrou A, Murthy SC, Wong J. Critical appraisal of the significance of intrathoracic anastomotic leakage after esophagectomy for cancer. Am J Surg. 2001;181(3):198–203.
11. Swanson SJ, Batirel HF, Bueno R, Jaklitsch MT, Lukanich JM, Allred E, Mentzer SJ, Sugarbaker DJ. Transthoracic esophagectomy with radical mediastinal and abdominal lymph node dissection and cervical esophagogastrostomy for esophageal carcinoma. Ann Thorac Surg. 2001;72(6):1918–24. discussion 1924-1915
12. Cooper JS, Guo MD, Herskovic A, Macdonald JS, Martenson JA Jr, Al-Sarraf M, Byhardt R, Russell AH, Beitler JJ, Spencer S, Asbell SO, Graham MV, Leichman LL. Chemoradiotherapy of locally advanced esophageal cancer: long-term follow-up of a prospective randomized trial (RTOG 85-01). Radiation Therapy Oncology Group. JAMA. 1999;281(17):1623–7.
13. Earlam R, Cunha-Melo JR. Oesophageal squamous cell carcinoma: I. A critical review of surgery. Br J Surg. 1980;67(6):381–90.
14. Earlam R, Cunha-Melo JR. Oesophogeal squamous cell carcinoms: II. A critical view of radiotherapy. Br J Surg. 1980;67(7):457–61.
15. Kelsen DP, Ginsberg R, Pajak TF, Sheahan DG, Gunderson L, Mortimer J, Estes N, Haller DG, Ajani J, Kocha W, Minsky BD, Roth JA. Chemotherapy followed by surgery compared with surgery alone for localized esophageal cancer. N Engl J Med. 1998;339(27):1979–84. https://doi.org/10.1056/NEJM199812313392704.
16. Law S, Fok M, Chow S, Chu KM, Wong J. Preoperative chemotherapy versus surgical therapy alone for squamous cell carcinoma of the esophagus: a prospective randomized trial. J Thorac Cardiovasc Surg. 1997;114(2):210–7.
17. Oppedijk V, van der Gaast A, van Lanschot JJ, van Hagen P, van Os R, van Rij CM, van der Sangen MJ, Beukema JC, Rutten H, Spruit PH, Reinders JG, Richel DJ, van Berge Henegouwen MI, Hulshof MC. Patterns of recurrence after surgery alone versus preoperative chemoradiotherapy and surgery in the CROSS trials. J Clin Oncol. 2014;32(5):385–91. https://doi.org/10.1200/JCO.2013.51.2186.
18. Harrison LE. Is esophageal cancer a surgical disease? J Surg Oncol. 2000;75(4):227–31.
19. Launois B, Delarue D, Campion JP, Kerbaol M. Preoperative radiotherapy for carcinoma of the esophagus. Surg Gynecol Obstet. 1981;153(5):690–2.
20. Gignoux M, Roussel A, Paillot B, Gillet M, Schlag P, Favre JP, Dalesio O, Buyse M, Duez N. The value of preoperative radiotherapy in esophageal cancer: results of a study of the E.O.R.T.C. World J Surg. 1987;11(4):426–32.
21. Arnott SJ, Duncan W, Gignoux M, Girling DJ, Hansen HS, Launois B, Nygaard K, Parmar MK, Roussel A, Spiliopoulos G, Stewart LA, Tierney JF, Mei W, Rugang Z. Preoperative

radiotherapy in esophageal carcinoma: a meta-analysis using individual patient data (Oesophageal Cancer Collaborative Group). Int J Radiat Oncol Biol Phys. 1998;41(3):579–83.

22. Teniere P, Hay JM, Fingerhut A, Fagniez PL. Postoperative radiation therapy does not increase survival after curative resection for squamous cell carcinoma of the middle and lower esophagus as shown by a multicenter controlled trial. French University Association for Surgical Research. Surg Gynecol Obstet. 1991;173(2):123–30.

23. Fok M, Sham JS, Choy D, Cheng SW, Wong J. Postoperative radiotherapy for carcinoma of the esophagus: a prospective, randomized controlled study. Surgery. 1993;113(2):138–47.

24. Kelsen DP, Winter KA, Gunderson LL, Mortimer J, Estes NC, Haller DG, Ajani JA, Kocha W, Minsky BD, Roth JA, Willett CG. Long-term results of RTOG trial 8911 (USA intergroup 113): a random assignment trial comparison of chemotherapy followed by surgery compared with surgery alone for esophageal cancer. J Clin Oncol. 2007;25(24):3719–25. https://doi.org/10.1200/JCO.2006.10.4760.

25. Group MRCOCW. Surgical resection with or without preoperative chemotherapy in oesophageal cancer: a randomised controlled trial. Lancet. 2002;359(9319):1727–33. https://doi.org/10.1016/S0140-6736(02)08651-8.

26. Ancona E, Ruol A, Santi S, Merigliano S, Sileni VC, Koussis H, Zaninotto G, Bonavina L, Peracchia A. Only pathologic complete response to neoadjuvant chemotherapy improves significantly the long term survival of patients with resectable esophageal squamous cell carcinoma: final report of a randomized, controlled trial of preoperative chemotherapy versus surgery alone. Cancer. 2001;91(11):2165–74.

27. Gebski V, Burmeister B, Smithers BM, Foo K, Zalcberg J, Simes J. Survival benefits from neoadjuvant chemoradiotherapy or chemotherapy in oesophageal carcinoma: a meta-analysis. Lancet Oncol. 2007;8(3):226–34. https://doi.org/10.1016/S1470-2045(07)70039-6.

28. Sjoquist KM, Burmeister BH, Smithers BM, Zalcberg JR, Simes RJ, Barbour A, Gebski V. Survival after neoadjuvant chemotherapy or chemoradiotherapy for resectable oesophageal carcinoma: an updated meta-analysis. Lancet Oncol. 2011;12(7):681–92. https://doi.org/10.1016/S1470-2045(11)70142-5.

29. Le Prise E, Etienne PL, Meunier B, Maddern G, Ben Hassel M, Gedouin D, Boutin D, Campion JP, Launois B. A randomized study of chemotherapy, radiation therapy, and surgery versus surgery for localized squamous cell carcinoma of the esophagus. Cancer. 1994;73(7):1779–84.

30. Bosset JF, Gignoux M, Triboulet JP, Tiret E, Mantion G, Elias D, Lozach P, Ollier JC, Pavy JJ, Mercier M, Sahmoud T. Chemoradiotherapy followed by surgery compared with surgery alone in squamous-cell cancer of the esophagus. N Engl J Med. 1997;337(3):161–7. https://doi.org/10.1056/NEJM199707173370304.

31. Burmeister BH, Smithers BM, Gebski V, Fitzgerald L, Simes RJ, Devitt P, Ackland S, Gotley DC, Joseph D, Millar J, North J, Walpole ET, Denham JW. Surgery alone versus chemoradiotherapy followed by surgery for resectable cancer of the oesophagus: a randomised controlled phase III trial. Lancet Oncol. 2005;6(9):659–68. https://doi.org/10.1016/S1470-2045(05)70288-6.

32. Tepper J, Krasna MJ, Niedzwiecki D, Hollis D, Reed CE, Goldberg R, Kiel K, Willett C, Sugarbaker D, Mayer R. Phase III trial of trimodality therapy with cisplatin, fluorouracil, radiotherapy, and surgery compared with surgery alone for esophageal cancer: CALGB 9781. J Clin Oncol. 2008;26(7):1086–92. https://doi.org/10.1200/JCO.2007.12.9593.

33. van Hagen P, Hulshof MC, van Lanschot JJ, Steyerberg EW, van Berge Henegouwen MI, Wijnhoven BP, Richel DJ, Nieuwenhuijzen GA, Hospers GA, Bonenkamp JJ, Cuesta MA, Blaisse RJ, Busch OR, ten Kate FJ, Creemers GJ, Punt CJ, Plukker JT, Verheul HM, Spillenaar Bilgen EJ, van Dekken H, van der Sangen MJ, Rozema T, Biermann K, Beukema JC, Piet AH, van Rij CM, Reinders JG, Tilanus HW, van der Gaast A. Preoperative chemoradiotherapy for esophageal or junctional cancer. N Engl J Med. 2012;366(22):2074–84. https://doi.org/10.1056/NEJMoa1112088.

34. Mariette C, Dahan L, Mornex F, Maillard E, Thomas PA, Meunier B, Boige V, Pezet D, Robb WB, Le Brun-Ly V, Bosset JF, Mabrut JY, Triboulet JP, Bedenne L, Seitz JF. Surgery alone versus chemoradiotherapy followed by surgery for stage I and II esophageal cancer: final analysis

of randomized controlled phase III trial FFCD 9901. J Clin Oncol. 2014;32(23):2416–22. https://doi.org/10.1200/JCO.2013.53.6532.

35. Shapiro J, van Lanschot JJ, Hulshof MC, Hagen PV, Henegouwen MI, Wijnhoven BP, Laarhoven HW, Nieuwenhuijzen, Hospers GA, Bonenkamp JJ, Cuesta MA, Blaisse RJ, Busch OR, Kate FJ, Creemers G-J, Punt CJ, Plukker JT, Verheul HM, Bilgen EJ, Dekken HV, Sangen MJ, Rozema T, Biermann K, Beukema J, Piet AH, Rij CM, Reinders JG, Tilanus HW, Steyerberg EW, Gaast AV. Neoadjuvant chemoradiotherapy plus surgery versus surgery alone for oesophageal or junctional cancer (CROSS): long-term results of a randomised controlled trial. Lancet Oncol. 16(9):1090–8. https://doi.org/10.1016/S1470-2045(15)00040-6.

36. Bedenne L, Michel P, Bouche O, Milan C, Mariette C, Conroy T, Pezet D, Roullet B, Seitz JF, Herr JP, Paillot B, Arveux P, Bonnetain F, Binquet C. Chemoradiation followed by surgery compared with chemoradiation alone in squamous cancer of the esophagus: FFCD 9102. J Clin Oncol. 2007;25(10):1160–8. https://doi.org/10.1200/JCO.2005.04.7118.

37. Stahl M, Stuschke M, Lehmann N, Meyer HJ, Walz MK, Seeber S, Klump B, Budach W, Teichmann R, Schmitt M, Schmitt G, Franke C, Wilke H. Chemoradiation with and without surgery in patients with locally advanced squamous cell carcinoma of the esophagus. J Clin Oncol. 2005;23(10):2310–7. https://doi.org/10.1200/JCO.2005.00.034.

38. Chiu PW, Chan AC, Leung SF, Leong HT, Kwong KH, Li MK, Au-Yeung AC, Chung SC, Ng EK. Multicenter prospective randomized trial comparing standard esophagectomy with chemoradiotherapy for treatment of squamous esophageal cancer: early results from the Chinese university research Group for Esophageal Cancer (CURE). J Gastrointest Surg. 2005;9(6):794–802.

39. Carstens H, Albertsson M, Friesland S, Adell G, Frykholm G, Wagenius G, Myrvold HE, Farago I, Stockeld D. A randomized trial of chemoradiotherapy versus surgery alone in patients with resectable esophageal cancer. J Clin Oncol. 2007;25(18S):205S: 4530.

40. Swisher S, Moughan J, Komaki R, Ajani J, Wu TT, Hofstetter W, Konski AA, Willett CG. Final results of RTOG 0246: a phase II study of selective surgical resection for locoregionally advanced esophageal cancer treated with a paclitaxel-based chemoradiation regimen. J Clin Oncol. 2013;31(4S):7.

41. Stahl M. Is there any role for surgery in the multidisciplinary treatment of esophageal cancer? Ann Oncol. 2010;21(Suppl 7):vii283–5. https://doi.org/10.1093/annonc/mdq294.

42. Wolf MC, Stahl M, Krause BJ, Bonavina L, Bruns C, Belka C, Zehentmayr F. Curative treatment of oesophageal carcinoma: current options and future developments. Radiat Oncol. 2011;6:55. https://doi.org/10.1186/1748-717X-6-55.

43. Minsky BD, Pajak TF, Ginsberg RJ, Pisansky TM, Martenson J, Komaki R, Okawara G, Rosenthal SA, Kelsen DP. INT 0123 (radiation therapy oncology group 94-05) phase III trial of combined-modality therapy for esophageal cancer: high-dose versus standard-dose radiation therapy. J Clin Oncol. 2002;20(5):1167–74.

44. Conroy T, Galais MP, Raoul JL, Bouche O, Gourgou-Bourgade S, Douillard JY, Etienne PL, Boige V, Martel-Lafay I, Michel P, Llacer-Moscardo C, Francois E, Crehange G, Abdelghani MB, Juzyna B, Bedenne L, Adenis A. Definitive chemoradiotherapy with FOLFOX versus fluorouracil and cisplatin in patients with oesophageal cancer (PRODIGE5/ACCORD17): final results of a randomised, phase 2/3 trial. Lancet Oncol. 2014;15(3):305–14. https://doi.org/10.1016/S1470-2045(14)70028-2.

45. Oetzel D, Schraube P, Hensley F, Sroka-Perez G, Menke M, Flentje M. Estimation of pneumonitis risk in three-dimensional treatment planning using dose-volume histogram analysis. Int J Radiat Oncol Biol Phys. 1995;33(2):455–60. https://doi.org/10.1016/0360-3016(95)00009-N.

46. Chandra A, Guerrero TM, Liu HH, Tucker SL, Liao Z, Wang X, Murshed H, Bonnen MD, Garg AK, Stevens CW, Chang JY, Jeter MD, Mohan R, Cox JD, Komaki R. Feasibility of using intensity-modulated radiotherapy to improve lung sparing in treatment planning for distal esophageal cancer. Radiother Oncol. 2005;77(3):247–53. https://doi.org/10.1016/j.radonc.2005.10.017.

47. Kole TP, Aghayere O, Kwah J, Yorke ED, Goodman KA. Comparison of heart and coronary artery doses associated with intensity-modulated radiotherapy versus three-dimensional conformal radiotherapy for distal esophageal cancer. Int J Radiat Oncol Biol Phys. 2012;83(5):1580–6. https://doi.org/10.1016/j.ijrobp.2011.10.053.
48. Lin CY, Huang WY, Jen YM, Chen CM, Su YF, Chao HL, Lin CS. Dosimetric and efficiency comparison of high-dose radiotherapy for esophageal cancer: volumetric modulated arc therapy versus fixed-field intensity-modulated radiotherapy. Dis Esophagus. 2014;27(6):585–90. https://doi.org/10.1111/dote.12144.
49. Yin Y, Chen J, Xing L, Dong X, Liu T, Lu J, Yu J. Applications of IMAT in cervical esophageal cancer radiotherapy: a comparison with fixed-field IMRT in dosimetry and implementation. J Appl Clin Med Phys. 2011;12(2):3343.
50. Patel AA, Wolfgang JA, Niemierko A, Hong TS, Yock T, Choi NC. Implications of respiratory motion as measured by four-dimensional computed tomography for radiation treatment planning of esophageal cancer. Int J Radiat Oncol Biol Phys. 2009;74(1):290–6. https://doi.org/10.1016/j.ijrobp.2008.12.060.
51. Vinogradskiy Y, Tucker SL, Bluett JB, Wages CA, Liao Z, Martel MK. Prescribing radiation dose to lung cancer patients based on personalized toxicity estimates. J Thorac Oncol. 2012;7(11):1676–82. https://doi.org/10.1097/JTO.0b013e318269410a.
52. Schneider PM, Baldus SE, Metzger R, Kocher M, Bongartz R, Bollschweiler E, Schaefer H, Thiele J, Dienes HP, Mueller RP, Hoelscher AH. Histomorphologic tumor regression and lymph node metastases determine prognosis following neoadjuvant radiochemotherapy for esophageal cancer: implications for response classification. Ann Surg. 2005;242(5):684–92.
53. Meredith KL, Weber JM, Turaga KK, Siegel EM, McLoughlin J, Hoffe S, Marcovalerio M, Shah N, Kelley S, Karl R. Pathologic response after neoadjuvant therapy is the major determinant of survival in patients with esophageal cancer. Ann Surg Oncol. 2010;17(4):1159–67. https://doi.org/10.1245/s10434-009-0862-1.
54. Vogel SB, Mendenhall WM, Sombeck MD, Marsh R, Woodward ER. Downstaging of esophageal cancer after preoperative radiation and chemotherapy. Ann Surg. 1995;221(6):685–93. discussion 693-685
55. Swisher SG, Erasmus J, Maish M, Correa AM, Macapinlac H, Ajani JA, Cox JD, Komaki RR, Hong D, Lee HK, Putnam JB Jr, Rice DC, Smythe WR, Thai L, Vaporciyan AA, Walsh GL, Wu TT, Roth JA. 2-Fluoro-2-deoxy-D-glucose positron emission tomography imaging is predictive of pathologic response and survival after preoperative chemoradiation in patients with esophageal carcinoma. Cancer. 2004;101(8):1776–85. https://doi.org/10.1002/cncr.20585.
56. Konski AA, Cheng JD, Goldberg M, Li T, Maurer A, Yu JQ, Haluszka O, Scott W, Meropol NJ, Cohen SJ, Freedman G, Weiner LM. Correlation of molecular response as measured by 18-FDG positron emission tomography with outcome after chemoradiotherapy in patients with esophageal carcinoma. Int J Radiat Oncol Biol Phys. 2007;69(2):358–63. https://doi.org/10.1016/j.ijrobp.2007.03.053.
57. Higuchi I, Yasuda T, Yano M, Doki Y, Miyata H, Tatsumi M, Fukunaga H, Takiguchi S, Fujiwara Y, Hatazawa J, Monden M. Lack of fludeoxyglucose F 18 uptake in posttreatment positron emission tomography as a significant predictor of survival after subsequent surgery in multimodality treatment for patients with locally advanced esophageal squamous cell carcinoma. J Thorac Cardiovasc Surg. 2008;136(1):205–212, 212 e201-203. https://doi.org/10.1016/j.jtcvs.2008.02.016.
58. Monjazeb AM, Riedlinger G, Aklilu M, Geisinger KR, Mishra G, Isom S, Clark P, Levine EA, Blackstock AW. Outcomes of patients with esophageal cancer staged with [(1)(8)F]fluorodeoxyglucose positron emission tomography (FDG-PET): can postchemoradiotherapy FDG-PET predict the utility of resection? J Clin Oncol. 2010;28(31):4714–21. https://doi.org/10.1200/JCO.2010.30.7702.

59. Downey RJ, Akhurst T, Ilson D, Ginsberg R, Bains MS, Gonen M, Koong H, Gollub M, Minsky BD, Zakowski M, Turnbull A, Larson SM, Rusch V. Whole body 18FDG-PET and the response of esophageal cancer to induction therapy: results of a prospective trial. J Clin Oncol. 2003;21(3):428–32.
60. Gillham CM, Lucey JA, Keogan M, Duffy GJ, Malik V, Raouf AA, O'Byrne K, Hollywood D, Muldoon C, Reynolds JV. (18)FDG uptake during induction chemoradiation for oesophageal cancer fails to predict histomorphological tumour response. Br J Cancer. 2006;95(9):1174–9. https://doi.org/10.1038/sj.bjc.6603412.

The Multidisciplinary Management of Early Distal Esophageal and Gastroesophageal Junction Cancer

13

Megan Greally and David H. Ilson

Introduction

Esophageal cancer is a highly lethal malignancy which occurs less frequently in the USA than in other geographic regions. It is estimated that it will account for 17,290 diagnoses and will be responsible for 15,850 deaths in the USA in 2018, making it the seventh leading cause of cancer-related death in American men [1]. Conversely, it is a major contributor to the cancer burden worldwide and is endemic in parts of East Asia where more than half of the approximately 500,000 cases per year worldwide develop [2]. High incidences are also observed in the Caspian littoral and the Transkei province in South Africa [3, 4]. It should be noted that this number does not fully take into account gastroesophageal or gastroesophageal junction (GEJ) tumors, which may variably be categorized as gastric cancers.

Squamous cell carcinomas (SCCs) and adenocarcinoma account for 98% of all cases of esophageal cancer. In the USA, adenocarcinomas account for 75% of cases following an increase of 4–10% per year in men since the mid-1970s. In contrast, there has been a steady decline in the number of cases of SCC which has been attributed to a decline in tobacco and alcohol consumption [5, 6]. In contrast, 90% of cases in Asia are SCC [7, 8]. Adenocarcinomas have increased in frequency due potentially to an increase in the incidence of gastroesophageal reflux disease (GERD) and obesity [9]. *Helicobacter pylori*, implicated in peptic ulcer disease and associated with an increased risk of gastric cancer, has not been linked with the development of esophageal cancer. Furthermore, infection with *H. pylori* may lead to a reduction in gastric acidity in association with atrophic gastritis leading to speculation that a decline in the prevalence of *H. pylori* infection may predispose to an

M. Greally · D. H. Ilson (✉)
Gastrointestinal Oncology Service, Department of Medicine, Memorial Sloan Kettering Cancer Center, New York, NY, USA
e-mail: ilsond@mskcc.org

© Springer Nature Switzerland AG 2020
N. F. Saba, B. F. El-Rayes (eds.), *Esophageal Cancer*,
https://doi.org/10.1007/978-3-030-29832-6_13

increase in GERD and therefore contribute to the increased incidence of GEJ adeno-carcinoma [10, 11]. SCCs classically occur in the proximal two-thirds of the esoph-agus, and adenocarcinomas arise in the distal third of the esophagus and GEJ.

Recent years have seen advances in the management of esophageal cancer which have led to clinically meaningful improvements in outcomes. While surgical resec-tion is the mainstay of treatment for locally advanced esophageal cancer, resulting in 5-year overall survival (OS) rates from 10 to 30–40% in various studies [12, 13], the addition of chemotherapy and/or radiotherapy are also recognized to be key in improving outcomes. Numerous studies—that have evaluated patients with both adenocarcinoma and SCC histologies and focused on tumors of the esophagus/GEJ and/or stomach—have demonstrated, as a whole, that pre- and post-operative strate-gies for locally advanced disease, including chemotherapy or chemoradiation, improve outcomes when added to surgery. This chapter focuses on the studies which have established pre- and post-operative therapy as standard of care in the treatment of localized esophageal cancer, which accounts for approximately 40–50% of patients with this diagnosis. Where relevant, we will note whether these studies primarily enrolled patients with esophageal/GEJ or gastric tumors. Evolving approaches and areas of clinical equipoise are also discussed.

Pre-operative Chemotherapy

Given that the risk of distant relapse is significant, pre-operative chemotherapy has been evaluated with the rationale that early systemic therapy might eradicate micro-metastatic disease.

Some of the earlier phase III trials evaluating pre- or peri-operative chemother-apy in esophagogastric adenocarcinomas have either been negative or demonstrated more marginal benefit. The North American Intergroup 113 trial randomized 440 patients with esophageal cancer to pre-operative 5-fluorouracil (5-FU)/cisplatin or immediate surgery [14]. No significant difference in survival was detected. About half of the patients had adenocarcinoma, and those with tumor extension 2 cm dis-tally beyond the GEJ were excluded. The MRC OE2 trial evaluated surgery with or without pre-operative cisplatin/5-FU. This study enrolled 802 patients and reported a modest improvement in 5-year OS with the addition of pre-operative therapy (23% vs. 17%, $p = 0.03$) to surgery [15]. Two-thirds of patients had adenocarcino-mas, and 75% had distal esophagus or gastric cardia tumors. Finally, the European EORTC 40954 trial evaluated pre-operative 5-FU/leucovorin and cisplatin in 144 patients with GEJ and gastric adenocarcinoma [16]. The study closed prematurely due to poor accrual, and while no significant difference in survival was detected, the power of this study was limited.

Data from the UK phase III MAGIC (Medical Research Council Adjuvant Gastric Infusional Chemotherapy) trial led to peri-operative chemotherapy being adopted as the principal approach in Europe [17]. This trial evaluated three cycles (9 weeks) each of pre- and post-operative ECF (epirubicin/cisplatin/5-FU) and sur-gery or surgery alone. Of 503 patients, 15% and 11% had GEJ and lower esophageal tumors, respectively. Peri-operative chemotherapy resulted in significant improvement in 5-year OS (36% vs. 23%, $p = 0.009$), establishing this regimen as a standard of care. Of note, the complete resection rate (R0) was relatively poor at 69.3% in patients who received pre-operative therapy and 66.4% in the surgery-alone group.

More recently, the French FFCD 9703 trial reported a similar degree of benefit to that seen with pre-operative chemotherapy in the MAGIC trial [18]. This study randomized 224 patients with esophagogastric adenocarcinoma to six cycles (18 weeks) of pre-operative 5-FU/cisplatin followed by surgery vs. surgery alone. A significant improvement in 5-year disease-free survival (DFS; 34% vs. 19%, $p = 0.003$) and OS (38% vs. 24%, $p = 0.02$) was detected. While cross-trial comparisons are made with caution, the survival benefit seen in this study is very similar to that observed with ECF in the MAGIC study, raising questions about the benefit of the anthracycline. The R0 resection rate was improved in patients who received pre-operative therapy compared to patients who underwent surgery alone (84% vs. 73%, $p = 0.04$).

The UK MRC OEO-5 study randomized 897 patients with esophageal and GEJ adenocarcinomas to pre-operative chemotherapy with 6 weeks of 5-FU/cisplatin or 12 weeks of ECX (epirubicin/cisplatin/capecitabine) [19]. While an improved pathologic complete response (pCR) was observed in the ECX group vs. the 5-FU/cisplatin group (11% vs. 3%), there was no difference in median DFS (14.4 months vs. 11.6 months, $p = 0.051$) or OS (26.1 months vs. 23.4 months, $p = 0.19$) between groups. In addition, the R0 resection rates were poor, 66% in the patients who received ECX and 59% in the patients who received 5-FU/cisplatin.

These results also challenge the convention that anthracycline provides additional benefit in this setting. In addition, this study raises uncertainty regarding the optimal duration of neoadjuvant therapy as this study suggests that 6 weeks of pre-operative chemotherapy conveys the same survival benefit as the 12 weeks of therapy administered in the MAGIC and FFCD studies. While this may be counterintuitive based on the MAGIC and FFCD studies as well as other studies in gastric cancer that have administered 6–12 months of adjuvant chemotherapy, these results are not without precedent [20, 21]. A randomized phase II study by Ajani et al., discussed in more detail below, found no survival benefit for the addition of four cycles of induction 5-FU/oxaliplatin before pre-operative chemoradiation for 5 weeks with 5-FU/oxaliplatin [22]. Furthermore, the CROSS study (which is discussed later) also found an absolute improvement in OS in the range of 10–15% as seen in other positive phase III studies discussed here, despite only receiving 5 weeks of carboplatin/paclitaxel [23, 24]. In addition, only 40–50% of patients in the MAGIC and FFCD studies received or completed adjuvant therapy following surgery indicating that patients obtain benefit from chemotherapy at durations significantly less than 6 months. Results from the CRITICS study (presented in abstract form), which will be discussed later, underline further the difficulty in administering adjuvant therapy [25]. These data suggest, given the lack of a biological rationale to split systemic therapy to before and after surgery, that future clinical trials should focus on evaluating pre-operative approaches.

The recently published STO3 trial from the UK evaluated the addition of the anti-vascular endothelial growth factor A (VEGF-A) antibody, bevacizumab, to three cycles each of pre- and post-operative chemotherapy with ECX in patients with operable distal esophagus, GEJ, and gastric cancers [26]. Patients had rigorous staging with endoscopic ultrasound (EUS), CT, and laparoscopic staging. Of 1063 patients enrolled, the majority had cancers of the distal esophagus (13–14%) or GEJ (50–51%). Bevacizumab in combination with ECX did not improve outcomes. Three-year OS was 50.3% in the chemotherapy-alone group vs. 48.1% in the chemotherapy plus bevacizumab group (HR 1.08, 95% CI 0.91–1.29, $p = 0.36$). The rate of anastomotic leak was higher in the patients who received bevacizumab. Of note, rates of R0 resection were relatively low (61% vs. 64%) with distal gastric cancers having a high R0 resection rate (87%) and distal esophageal and Siewert type I tumors having the lowest rate (66% and 61%, respectively). Preliminary results of the FLOT4-AIO phase III trial were recently presented in abstract form [27]. This study randomized 716 patients with resectable gastric or GEJ adenocarcinoma to peri-operative FLOT (5-FU/oxaliplatin/docetaxel) or physician's choice of ECF or ECX. Over 80% had T3/4 disease, and 79.5% were node positive, while 56% had GEJ adenocarcinoma. Forty-four percent of patients had distal gastric cancers. FLOT was superior to ECF/ECX in all efficacy endpoints including curative resection rates (84% vs. 77%, $p = 0.011$), progression-free survival (PFS; 30 vs. 18 months, hazard ratio [HR] 0.75, $p = 0.004$), and OS (median OS 50 vs. 35 months; 5-year OS 45% vs. 36%, HR 0.77, $p = 0.012$). Benefit was seen across all subgroups, and while the rate of adverse events was similar between groups, there was more grade 3/4 nausea and vomiting with ECF/ECX and more grade 3/4 neutropenia with FLOT. Thus, while there is no benefit to addition of an anthracycline to pre-operative systemic therapy, there appears to be benefit for a docetaxel-containing three-drug regimen. Only half of patients completed all planned chemotherapy (largely due to failure to deliver post-operative chemotherapy), again highlighting the difficulty in administering adjuvant therapy and suggesting that future clinical trials should focus on evaluating pre-operative approaches. The data for pre-operative chemotherapy is summarized in Table 13.1.

Finally, a meta-analysis of ten randomized studies evaluating pre-operative chemotherapy for esophageal and GEJ cancers demonstrated a 13% decreased risk of all-cause mortality in patients with adenocarcinoma compared to surgery alone (HR 0.87, 95% CI 0.79–0.96, $p < 0.005$) [28]. There was a non-significant trend toward benefit for pre-operative therapy in patients with SCC (HR 0.92, 95% CI 0.81–1.04, $p = 0.18$). There was no significant difference in the rate of complete (R0) resections with neoadjuvant therapy (relative risk [RR] 1.11) or in the risk of distant recurrence (RR 0.94). The MAGIC and EORTC 40954 trials were excluded from this analysis as outcomes were not stratified by tumor location (gastric vs. GEJ tumors).

Pre-operative Chemoradiation

The Radiation Therapy Oncology Group (RTOG) 85-01 trial was a landmark phase III study which established the superiority of chemoradiation over radiation alone [29]. Patients with locoregional thoracic esophageal carcinoma were randomized to

Table 13.1 Results of phase III pre- or peri-operative chemotherapy trials in esophageal/GEJ cancer

Treatment	Histology	No. of patients	R0 resection rate	Pathologic complete response rate	Survival Median (months)	Overall	Local failure*	Reference
Peri-op ECF + surgery	Adeno	250	69%	0%	24	5-year 36%	14%	Cunningham et al. [17]
Surgery		253	66%	N/A	20	5-year 23%	21%	
Peri-op ECF + bev + surgery	Adeno	530	61%	11%	NS	3-year 48.1%	NS	Cunningham et al. [26]
Peri-op ECF + surgery	Adeno	533	64%	8%	NS	3-year 50.3%	NS	
Peri-op 5-FU/Cis + surgery	Adeno	109	87%	NS	NS	5-year 38%	24%	Ychou et al. [18]
Surgery		110	74%	N/A	NS	5-year 24%	26%	
Pre-op ECX + surgery	Adeno	446	66%	11%	26.1	3-year 42%	NS	Alderson et al. [19]
Pre-op 5-FU/Cis + surgery		451	59%	3%	23.4	3-year 39%	NS	
Peri-op FLOT + surgery	Adeno	356	84%	NS	50	3-year 45%	NS	Al-Batran et al. [27]
Peri-op ECF/ECX + surgery		360	77%	NS	35	3-year 36%	NS	
Peri-op 5-FU/Cis + surgery	Adeno (54%) + SCC	213	62%	2.5%	14.9	3-year 23%	32%	Kelsen et al. [14]
Surgery		227	59%	N/A	16.1	3-year 26%	31%	
Pre-op 5-FU/Cis + surgery	Adeno (66%) + SCC	400	60%	NS	16.8	5-year 23%	19%	Medical Research Council [70], Allum et al. [15]
Surgery		402	54%	N/A	13.3	5-year 17%	17%	

Adeno adenocarcinoma; Cis cisplatin; ECF epirubicin, cisplatin, 5-fluorouracil; ECX epirubicin, cisplatin, capecitabine; N/A not applicable; NS not stated radiation with 64 Gy in 32 fractions over 6.5 weeks or cisplatin and infusional 5-FU during weeks 1 and 5 concurrent with radiation 50 Gy in 25 fractions over 5 weeks. The chemoradiotherapy group also received two further cycles of chemotherapy after completion of radiation. Patients did not undergo surgery in this study. The trial closed prematurely after 121 patients had been accrued, when an interim analysis demonstrated improved median OS with chemoradiation compared to radiation alone (12.5 months vs. 8.9 months). Two-year and 5-year survival were also improved in the chemoradiation arm (38% vs. 10% and 27% versus 0%, respectively) compared to the radiation-alone arm [30]. While 90% of patients on this study had SCC, long-term survival was also demonstrated in the small minority of patients with adenocarcinoma with 13% of patients alive at 5 years. In addition to a survival benefit, disease recurrence was significantly reduced by the addition of chemotherapy to radiation. At 1 year, the rate of persistent or recurrent disease was 62% in patients who received radiation versus 44% in the chemoradiation arm, still an unacceptably high rate of local failure suggesting that surgery should continue to have a role in the treatment paradigm. Distant recurrence rates were 38% and 22%, respectively. Based on this seminal study, chemoradiation became the standard nonoperative management of patients with locally advanced esophageal SCC.

Since then, several randomized trials have evaluated pre-operative chemoradiation vs. surgery alone in esophageal cancer. Of six contemporary randomized studies [23, 31–35] which compared pre-operative chemoradiation followed by surgery to surgery alone, three have demonstrated a survival benefit to this approach. The results are outlined in Table 13.2.

The Dutch CROSS trial was a well-conducted phase III study which enrolled 366 patients with esophageal tumors, 75% of whom had adenocarcinoma. Over 80% had T3/4 tumors and 65% were node positive by EUS [23]. Pre-operative radiation at a dose of 41.4 Gy concurrent with weekly carboplatin/paclitaxel for 5 weeks was compared to surgery alone and resulted in a higher R0 resection rate (92% vs. 67%, $p < 0.001$), a pCR rate of 29% (23% for adenocarcinoma; 49% for SCC), and improved median OS (49.4 vs. 24.0 months, $p = 0.003$).The 3-year OS rate was 58% vs. 44%, and the survival benefit persisted with longer (median 84 months) follow-up (5-year OS 47% vs. 33%, HR 0.67). Pre-operative therapy was relatively well-tolerated, with mostly grade 3 toxicities noted in only 20% of patients. There was no increased post-operative mortality with the addition of chemoradiation. Patients with SCC appeared to derive greater benefit than those with adenocarcinoma (univariate HR for death 0.45 vs. 0.73). However, long-term follow-up has confirmed a clinically relevant OS benefit for patients with both adenocarcinoma and SCC histologies and a 9% reduction in the occurrence of distant metastases in patients treated with chemoradiation (39% vs. 48%, HR 0.63, $p = 0.0040$) [24]. This regimen has become a standard of care and the reference regimen for most clinical trials.

Carboplatin/paclitaxel is well-tolerated, convenient to administer, and associated with the highest pCR rate for SCC (49%) to date in a phase III trial. The pCR rate of 23% for adenocarcinoma compares favorably to other studies. However, it remains unclear if carboplatin/paclitaxel is the optimal regimen, relative to standard 5-FU/cisplatin used in other trials, to combine with radiotherapy in the pre-operative

Table 13.2 Results of phase III pre-operative chemoradiation trials in esophageal/GEJ cancer

Treatment	Histology	No. of patient	R0 resection rate	Pathologic complete response rate	Survival Median	Overall	Local failure	Reference
Pre-op CRT	Adeno (76%)	50	45%	24%	16.9 months	3-year 30%	19%	Urba et al. [33]
Surgery	+ SCC	50	45%	N/A	17.6 months	3-year 16%	42%	
Pre-op CRT	Adeno	58	NS	25%	**16 months**	3-year **32%**	NS	Walsh et al. [34]
Surgery		55		N/A	**11 months**	3-year **6%**		
Pre-op CRT	SCC	143	81%	26%	18.6 months	5-year 26%	NS	Bosset et al. [31]
Surgery		139	69%	N/A	18.6 months	5-year 26%		
Pre-op CRT	Adeno (63%)	128	**80%**	9%	22.2 months	NS	15%	Burmeister et al. [32]
Surgery	+ SCC + others	128	**59%**	N/A	19.3 months		26%	
Pre-op CRT	Adeno (75%)	30	NS	40%	**4.5 years**	5-year **39%**	NS	Tepper et al. [35]
Surgery	+ SCC	26		N/A	**1.8 years**	5-year **16%**		
Pre-op CRT	Adeno (74%)	178	**92%**	29%	**49.4 months**	5-year **47%**	NS	Van Hagen et al. [23], Shapiro et al. [24]
Surgery	+ SCC	188	**69%**	N/A	**24.0 months**	5-year **33%**		

Adeno adenocarcinoma, *CR*, *NS* not stated, *Pre-op CRT* pre-operative chemoradiation setting. The Cancer and Leukemia Group B (CALGB) 80803 study provides some insight into the relative merits of carboplatin/paclitaxel versus a 5-FU plus platinum regimen [36]. This study randomized 257 patients with esophageal and GEJ adenocarcinoma, to receive induction modified FOLFOX6 (infusional 5-FU/leucovorin/oxaliplatin) or carboplatin/paclitaxel for 5–6 weeks followed by a [^{18}F]2-fluorodeoxy-D-glucose positron emission tomography (FDG-PET) scan. Patients who were PET responders continued with the same regimen during subsequent concurrent chemoradiation, and patients who were PET non-responders crossed to the other chemotherapy regimen with radiation prior to surgery. Preliminary results of this study are discussed in more detail below. The pCR rate in the patients who were PET responders to induction FOLFOX who went on to receive the same regimen with radiotherapy was 37.5% compared to a 12.5% pCR rate in patients who were PET responders to induction carboplatin/paclitaxel and who received this regimen with radiation. Both treatments were well-tolerated. While the study was not designed to detect a difference in outcome between induction regimens, these results are hypothesis-generating. We await survival data from this study.

In contrast, the NEOSCOPE phase II trial enrolled patients with ≥T3 and/or ≥N1 esophageal or Siewert 1/2 GEJ adenocarcinoma to receive two cycles of induction capecitabine/oxaliplatin, and subsequently patients were randomized to preoperative capecitabine/oxaliplatin with radiation or carboplatin/paclitaxel with radiation [37]. Eighty-five patients were enrolled in this study. Of 77 patients who underwent surgery, 12/41 (29.3%) who received carboplatin/paclitaxel achieved pCR vs. 4/36 (11.1%) of those who received capecitabine/oxaliplatin. However, the trial was not powered to detect a difference in pCR between arms. Of note, the neutropenia rate during chemoradiation was significantly higher in the carboplatin/paclitaxel arm (21.4% vs. 2.6%, $p = 0.01$). This did not translate into an increased risk of mortality. There continues to be clinical equipoise regarding the preferred chemotherapy regimen to combine with radiation.

Many other randomized trials completed in this setting are associated with methodological concerns (such as the lack of meticulous pre-treatment staging with EUS or laparoscopy) and enrolled significantly smaller numbers of patients than randomized pre-operative chemotherapy trials (e.g., the positive CALGB 9781 study enrolled only 56 patients), and debate continues regarding their interpretation. While the results of these trials are conflicting, cumulatively, they demonstrate higher rates of complete resection and decreased local recurrence rates. A benefit for pre-operative chemoradiation is also supported by the previously discussed meta-analysis, in which 13 randomized trials of chemoradiation prior to surgery (including the 5 trials discussed above) were analyzed [28]. Pre-operative chemoradiation was associated with a decreased risk of all-cause mortality of 25% (HR 0.75, 95% CI 0.59–0.95, $p = 0.02$) in patients with adenocarcinoma histology and 20% (HR 0.80, 95% CI 0.68–0.93, $p = 0.004$) in patients with squamous histology compared to surgery alone.

Benefit for intensification of combined modality therapy with the addition of induction chemotherapy prior to pre-operative chemoradiation and surgery has been evaluated in a randomized phase II trial [22]. As discussed above, patients received weekly oxaliplatin/5-FU (96 h infusion dosed at 250 mg/m^2/day) for 5 weeks with 50.4 Gy radiation with or without four cycles of induction chemotherapy with oxaliplatin/5-FU every 2 weeks prior to chemoradiation. Of 120 patients treated, 97% had adenocarcinoma and 97% had GEJ tumors. There was no significant difference in the pCR rate, the primary endpoint (26% in the induction arm vs. 11% in the chemoradiation alone arm, $p = 0.094$), or OS between groups (43.6 vs. 45.6 months, $p = 0.69$).

The role of adjuvant chemotherapy in patients who have received pre-operative chemoradiation and curative-intent surgery has also been evaluated in a recent propensity score-matched analysis [38]. Over 10,000 patients with ≥T2 or node-positive adenocarcinoma of the distal esophagus or gastric cardia were identified from the US National Cancer Database. A total of 732 propensity score-matched patients who received post-operative chemotherapy were compared to 3660 patients who underwent observation alone. The 5-year OS was improved in the patients who received adjuvant therapy (38% vs. 34%), suggesting a potential benefit for post-operative chemotherapy. However, given the small survival benefit coupled with the recognized difficulty in administering adjuvant therapy after surgery and the potential selection bias of patients capable of receiving adjuvant therapy, these results are hypothesis-generating rather than practice-changing.

Pre-operative Chemoradiation for Early-Stage Disease

The majority of patients enrolled in the above studies had locally advanced disease (currently defined as uT3–4, node-positive tumors by EUS staging), and the management of patients with earlier stage disease is less well defined.

The French FFCD 9901 study addressed this issue. This trial randomized 195 patients with early-stage cT1-2N$_{any}$ or cT3N0 tumors to pre-operative 5-FU/cisplatin (2 cycles of infusional 5-FU on days 1–4 and 29–32 and cisplatin on days 1 or 2 of each cycle) and radiation (45 Gy) followed by surgery vs. surgery alone [39]. A majority of patients (72%) had SCCs, and 24% and 74%, respectively, had cT1 and cN0 tumors. The R0 resection rate in the surgery-alone arm was a remarkable 93%, and this was not enhanced with pre-operative chemoradiation. Similarly, median DFS and OS (47.5% vs. 53%, HR 0.99) were not significantly different between study arms at a median follow-up of 94 months. There was no benefit across subgroups analyzed. However, in-hospital post-operative mortality was significantly increased in the chemoradiation arm (11.1% versus 3.4%, $p = 0.049$).

Surprisingly, despite the lack of improvement in R0 resection rates, locoregional recurrence was reduced in the chemoradiation arm (22.1% versus 28.9%, $p = 0.02$). However, the rate of distant recurrence was not significantly different between both arms (22.5% vs. 28.9%, $p = 0.31$). Furthermore, the unexpectedly high post-operative mortality in the chemoradiation arm as compared with 4% in both treatment arms of the CROSS study might have obscured a small survival benefit from chemoradiation.

However, these results are consistent with other published data and in keeping with the current guidelines from the National Comprehensive Cancer Network which recommend upfront surgery for patients with cT1N0 tumors. An accepted approach—discussed below—is definitive chemoradiation without surgery for patients with SCC who achieve a clinical complete response.

Pre-operative Chemoradiation Versus Chemotherapy

Pre-operative chemoradiation has been compared to pre-operative chemotherapy in a number of studies. The German POET (Pre-operative Chemotherapy or Radiochemotherapy in Esophagogastric Adenocarcinoma Trial) study randomized 119 patients with GEJ adenocarcinomas to 16 weeks of infusional 5-FU with leucovorin and cisplatin followed by surgery or 12 weeks of infusional 5-FU with leucovorin and cisplatin followed by chemoradiation with cisplatin/etoposide and then surgery and suggested possible superiority of chemoradiation over chemotherapy [40]. The trial closed prematurely due to poor accrual, limiting its power to detect a difference between the treatment groups. However, patients who received pre-operative chemoradiation had a higher pCR rate (15.6% vs. 2%, $p = 0.03$) and node-negative status (ypN0 64.4% vs. 36.7%, $p = 0.01$) than those who received pre-operative chemotherapy alone. There was a trend toward an improvement in local control (76.5% vs. 59%, $p = 0.06$) and 3-year OS (47.4% vs. 27.7%, $p = 0.07$) for the chemoradiation group.

The meta-analysis by Sjoquist et al. discussed above also reported a nonsignificant trend toward improved outcomes with pre-operative chemoradiation over chemotherapy where the HR for all-cause mortality was 0.88 (95% CI 0.76–1.01, $p = 0.07$) in favor of chemoradiation [28].

Potentially, the most compelling justification favoring pre-operative chemoradiation over chemotherapy alone is the suggestion of an improvement in R0 resection rates for tumors that involve the GEJ. The R0 resection rates in the 1400 patients treated on the contemporary MAGIC and OEO-5 studies were less than 70%, and importantly, in the OEO-5 study, the majority of patients were rigorously assessed to be surgical candidates with EUS and FDG-PET imaging. In contrast, patients who received pre-operative chemoradiation in the CROSS study had R0 resection rates exceeding 90%.

Use of PET Imaging to Guide Pre-operative Therapy

FDG-PET imaging is an increasingly well-defined tool to assess response to therapy. A number of studies have shown that the degree of response as detected by PET following pre-operative chemoradiation [41, 42] or chemotherapy [43, 44] correlates highly with pathologic response at surgery and with patient survival.

In the German MUNICON trial, patients with locally advanced GEJ adenocarcinomas who had a suboptimal response to 2 weeks of induction 5-FU/cisplatin, as determined by serial PET imaging, had treatment discontinued and underwent surgery. Patients who had a metabolic response by PET (defined as ≥35% reduction in standard uptake value between baseline and repeat scan) continued with an additional 12 weeks of chemotherapy prior to surgery [45].

Patients who were PET responders had a significantly improved R0 resection rate (96% vs. 74%, $p = 0.002$), pathologic response rate (58% vs. 0%, $p = 0.001$), median event-free survival (29.7 vs. 14.1 months, $p = 0.002$), and median OS (not reached vs. 25.8 months, $p = 0.015$) compared to patients who were PET non-responders. Of note, outcomes for patients who were PET non-responders and underwent immediate surgery were similar to outcomes of such patients in an earlier trial who completed 3 months of pre-operative chemotherapy [43], indicating that outcomes were not compromised by immediate surgery. These results therefore support early discontinuation of inactive pre-operative chemotherapy in PET non-responder patients.

Subsequently, MUNICON-2 evaluated "salvage" chemoradiation with cisplatin prior to surgery in patients who were PET non-responders to pre-operative cisplatin/5-FU [46]. Of 56 patients enrolled, 23 were defined as PET non-responders. While histopathologic responses were seen in the PET non-responders, they were found to have inferior 2-year PFS (64% vs. 33%, $p = 0.035$) and a trend toward inferior 2-year OS (71% vs. 42%, $p = 0.10$). These results underline the unfavorable biology of patients who are PET non-responders but do not out rule the possibility that these patients can receive effective salvage therapy. However, in this study, cisplatin was administered with radiation despite having been associated with suboptimal outcomes by PET when administered with 5-FU as induction therapy.

The use of PET assessment as a strategy to tailor subsequent chemotherapy during concurrent radiation has been explored. Long-term DFS has been reported in patients who had progression on PET imaging after induction chemotherapy and were changed to alternative chemotherapy during subsequent chemoradiation [47]. A subsequent retrospective review of 201 patients with esophageal and GEJ adenocarcinomas where treatment was changed to alternative chemotherapy during radiation for some PET non-responders was undertaken [48]. These data suggested that improvements in pCR rate and PFS are achievable in PET non-responder patients whose treatment is switched. A trend toward improvement in OS was observed.

As described above, this concept was directly studied in the CALGB 80803 trial. Preliminary results presented in abstract form indicated improvement in the pCR rate in PET non-responders who changed chemotherapy to 17% (carboplatin/paclitaxel switched to mFOLFOX6) and 19% (mFOLFOX6 switched to carboplatin/paclitaxel) [36], when compared to a historical rate of 3% in the retrospective analysis discussed above. Survival data are awaited. The study met its primary endpoint and suggests that early response assessment using PET could be incorporated into future studies aiming to identify more effective regimens for treatment of esophageal and GEJ cancers.

Definitive Chemoradiation

Direct comparisons of chemoradiation vs. surgery in resectable esophageal carcinoma are lacking. Two randomized European studies have compared definitive chemoradiation with chemoradiation followed by surgery and have provided data to support a non-surgical approach in select patients [49, 50]. Despite improvement in local control with surgery, neither trial demonstrated improved survival with trimodality therapy. The populations enrolled were predominantly patients with SCC histology. Therefore, definitive chemoradiation is a reasonable approach in patients with SCC who obtain an endoscopic complete response and who are not surgical candidates.

One of these studies (FFCD 9102) also provides some data with regard to whether patients who do not respond to initial chemoradiation with cisplatin/5-FU benefit from subsequent surgery. In this study, patients with potentially resectable T3, N0–1 esophageal SCC (89%) or adenocarcinoma (11%) received induction chemoradiotherapy with either 46 Gy in 4.5 weeks or split course 2 × 15 Gy (days 1–5 and 22–26) radiation concurrent with two cycles of 5-FU/ cisplatin. Only patients with at least a partial response were randomized to surgery vs. further chemoradiation [three further cycles of chemotherapy with either 20 Gy or 15 Gy (split course) radiation]. Of the 451 registered patients, 192 were not randomized to further protocol therapy, due to poor response, medical contraindications, or patient refusal [51]. Of these 192 non-randomized patients, 112 underwent subsequent surgery with 80 undergoing R0 resections. The median OS for the patients who underwent surgery was significantly superior to patients who did not (17.0 vs. 5.5 months, $p < 0.0001$) and was comparable to the median OS of the patients who were randomized (18.9 months, $p = 0.40$). While this analysis has clear limitations and must be interpreted cautiously, it does suggest that salvage esophagectomy may be beneficial for a subset of patients who do not respond to initial chemoradiation.

FOLFOX also appears to be a comparable option to 5-FU/cisplatin based on the French PRODIGE5/ACCORD17 study, which randomized 267 patients to either regimen with radiation as definitive therapy [52]. Similar to the studies above, 85% of patients had SCC. Survival and toxicities were comparable in both arms.

Patients with adenocarcinoma have lower rates of pCR after chemoradiation, and there are no randomized data demonstrating that definitive chemoradiation is comparable to chemoradiation and surgery. In patients where the operative risk is estimated to be substantial and given the high morbidity and mortality associated with esophagectomy, one option is to closely monitor those patients who obtain a clinical complete response to pre-operative chemoradiation with follow-up endoscopy and imaging. A salvage esophagectomy can be considered in those patients who develop locoregional relapse with no evidence of distant progression. A potential drawback to this approach is that operative morbidity and mortality may significantly increase when surgery is delayed beyond 6–8 weeks following completion of chemoradiation. However, three studies have reported no significant deterioration in outcomes in patients who underwent delayed surgery with salvage esophagectomy [53–55].

A study from MD Anderson Cancer Center reported outcomes in 65 patients with esophageal adenocarcinoma who underwent salvage esophagectomies a median of 216 days following chemoradiation [53]. When compared to matched patients who underwent planned esophagectomy after chemoradiation, postoperative complications and survival did not appear to be different between groups. A French retrospective review also examined this approach in 848 patients, 540 of whom underwent esophagectomy following pre-operative chemoradiation and 308 who underwent salvage surgery after chemoradiation for either persistent (234 patients) or recurrent (74 patients) disease [54]. While the rate of anastomotic leak and surgical infection were increased in the salvage group, in-hospital mortality was similar and relatively high in both groups (8.4% versus 9.3%, $p = 0.688$). Three-year DFS (39.2% versus 32.8%, $p = 0.232$) and OS (43.3% versus 40.1%, $p = 0.542$) were also comparable between groups.

Finally, the RTOG 0246 study evaluated induction chemotherapy with 5-FU/cisplatin/paclitaxel and chemoradiation with 5-FU/cisplatin in 43 patients with locally advanced esophageal cancer. Surgery was reserved for patients with locally persistent/recurrent disease [55]. While this trial did not meet its primary endpoint of improving 1-year survival to 77.5%, it did suggest that post-operative mortality was not increased by delaying surgery.

Based on the above data, definitive chemoradiation may be considered for selected patients at institutions with significant multidisciplinary experience in this strategy. Decisions regarding surgery versus chemoradiation should be made with a fully informed patient.

Addition of the anti-epidermal growth factor receptor (EGFR) antibody, cetuximab, to definitive chemoradiation was not associated with an improvement in outcomes in two phase III studies. The UK SCOPE-1 study enrolled 258 patients, 73% of whom had SCC histology and 60% had stage III disease, who were randomized to capecitabine/cisplatin and radiation with or without cetuximab [56]. The primary endpoint of being treatment failure-free at 24 weeks was lower in the cetuximab arm vs. the standard arm (66.4% vs. 76.9%). Patients in the cetuximab arm also had inferior OS (22.1 vs. 25.4 months, HR 1.45, $p = 0.035$), were less likely to complete standard chemoradiation, and also had higher rates of dermatologic and metabolic toxicities. More recently, the RTOG 0436 study was presented in abstract form [57]. This study evaluated cisplatin/paclitaxel and radiation with or without cetuximab in the non-operative setting for locally advanced esophageal adenocarcinomas and SCCs. There was no difference in outcomes between both arms, confirming a lack of benefit for cetuximab combined with chemoradiation.

Post-operative Chemoradiation

In the USA, post-operative chemoradiation is a standard of care for GEJ and gastric cancers following upfront resection, in large part due to results of the influential Intergroup 116 trial [58].

This trial randomized 556 patients (20% had tumors that involved the GEJ) with resected stage $\geq$ IB disease to adjuvant chemoradiation with bolus 5-FU/leucovorin or observation alone. The 3-year relapse-free survival (RFS; 48% vs. 31%, $p < 0.001$) and 3-year OS (51% vs. 40%, $p = 0.005$) were significantly improved in patients who received chemoradiation. However, many patients in this trial underwent inadequate surgical resections—54% had less than a D1 or D2 lymph node resection. This trial is often criticized because the radiation administered potentially compensated for inadequate surgery given that the greatest impact of chemoradiation was a reduction in the rates of local recurrence. Radiotherapy may not provide meaningful benefit in the setting where optimal D1 or D2 surgical resection is undertaken.

Based on these results, the CALGB 80101 trial investigated the role of more intensive chemotherapy with ECF in 546 patients with gastric cancer (30% of whom had tumors involving the GEJ and proximal stomach) [59]. Patients were randomized to bolus 5-FU/leucovorin preceding and following chemoradiation with infusional 5-FU or ECF before and after chemoradiation with infusional 5-FU. There was no improvement in 5-year DFS (44% vs. 44%, $p = 0.69$) or OS (39% vs. 37%, $p = 0.94$) with the addition of an anthracycline and platinum/5-FU. These results suggest that chemoradiation with 5-FU alone remains a standard of care in the adjuvant setting. While pre- and post-operative ECF without radiation is a standard treatment option, data does not support the use of ECF solely as an adjuvant treatment regimen.

The Dutch CRITICS trial compared peri-operative ECX or EOX (epirubicin, oxaliplatin, capecitabine) to pre-operative ECX or EOX and adjuvant chemoradiation with capecitabine in patients with gastric and GEJ (17% of patients) adenocarcinoma. These results have been presented in abstract form and demonstrated no difference in PFS or 5-year OS (40.8% vs. 40.9%) for either treatment arm. Although subgroup analyses are planned, the nearly superimposable Kaplan-Meier survival curves confirm, for now at least, that patients who have received pre-operative chemotherapy should not receive adjuvant chemoradiation in a standard fashion [25]. These results are summarized in Table 13.3.

In general, adjuvant therapy should be reserved for patients with resected node-positive or T3/4 disease who did not undergo pre-operative therapy. Only approximately 50–60% of patients in the Intergroup 116, CALGB, and CRITICS studies completed all planned treatment, providing strong rationale for the administration of pre-operative therapy. The above studies are outlined in Table 13.3.

Post-operative Chemotherapy

Two large phase III East Asian trials have demonstrated a survival benefit for post-operative chemotherapy alone in patients with gastric carcinoma.

The Japanese ACTS-GC (Adjuvant Chemotherapy Trial of TS-1 for Gastric Cancer) study randomized 1059 patients with stage II/III gastric cancer who had undergone D2 resection to 1 year of adjuvant S-1 or observation [60]. There was a significant improvement in 5-year RFS (65.4% vs. 53.1%, HR 0.65, 95% CI 0.54–0.79) and OS (71.7% vs. 61.1%, HR 0.67, 95% CI 0.54–0.83) compared to observation alone. A benefit was seen across all subgroups.

The CLASSIC trial (Capecitabine and Oxaliplatin Adjuvant Study in Stomach Cancer) enrolled 1035 East Asian patients following D2 resection for stage II–IIIB gastric carcinoma [61]. Patients were randomized to adjuvant capecitabine and oxaliplatin for 6 months or observation. Five-year DFS (68% vs. 53%, HR 0.58,

Table 13.3 Results of significant phase III trials of post-operative chemoradiation in GEJ/gastric adenocarcinoma

Treatment	No. of patients	Disease-free survival Median	Overall	Overall survival Median	Overall	Local failure*	Reference
Surgery	275	**19 months**	3-year 31%	**27 months**	3-year 41%	29%	MacDonald et al. [58]
Post-op 5-FU/LV → 5-FU/RT → 5-FU/LV	281	**30 months**	3-year 48%	**36 months**	3-year 50%	19%	
Post-op 5-FU/LV → 5-FU/RT → 5-FU/LV	280	30 months	5-year 39%	36.6 months	5-year 44%	NS	Fuchs et al. [59]
Post-op ECF → 5-FU/RT → ECF	266	28 months	5-year 37%	37.8 months	5-year 44%	NS	
ECX/EOX → surgery → ECX/EOX	393	27.6 months	5-year 38.5%	42 months	5-year 40.8%	NS	Verheij et al. [25]
ECX/EOX → surgery → chemoRT	395	30 months	5-year 39.5%	39.6 months	5-year 40.9%	NS	

Adeno adenocarcinoma, *ECF* epirubicin/cisplatin/infusional 5-fluorouracil, *ECX* epirubicin/cisplatin/capecitabine, *EOX* epirubicin/oxaliplatin/capecitabine, *LV* leucovorin, *NS* not stated, *RT* radiotherapy

$p < 0.0001$) and OS (78% vs. 69%, HR 0.66, $p = 0.0015$) were improved in patients who received chemotherapy.

Given that most East Asian patients have distal gastric tumors and both studies included only a very small minority of patients with GEJ tumors, it is unclear whether these data can be extrapolated to the patient population discussed here.

Currently, it remains unclear whether post-operative chemotherapy in patients with resected esophageal SCC improves outcomes. Two Japanese studies randomized patients with esophageal SCC to receive cisplatin/vindesine [62] or 5-FU/cisplatin (JCOG 9204) [63], respectively. While adjuvant cisplatin/vindesine was not associated with a survival benefit, an unplanned subset analysis of JCOG 9204 demonstrated a survival benefit for patients with lymph node involvement (5-year DFS 52% vs. 38%).

The possible benefit of post-operative therapy suggested by the above trial led to the JCOG 9907 study which randomized 330 patients with esophageal SCC to surgery and two cycles of either pre- or post-operative 5-FU/cisplatin [64]. Pre-operative chemotherapy improved 5-year OS (55% vs. 43%, $p = 0.04$) compared to post-operative therapy. However, only 58% of the patients randomized to post-operative therapy received any treatment, and 23% of the patients randomized to this arm of the study had pN0 disease and did not receive post-operative therapy per protocol, based on prior data that adjuvant therapy only benefited patients with lymph node positivity. In addition, pre-operative chemotherapy was associated with

Table 13.4 Results of phase III post-operative chemotherapy trials in esophageal and gastric cancer

Treatment	Histology	No. of patients	Survival Median	Overall	Local failure[a]	Reference
Surgery	Adeno (gastric)	530	NR	5-year **61%**	2.8%	Sakuramoto et al. [20], Sasako et al. [60]
Surgery +S-1		529	NR	5-year **72%**	1.3%	
Surgery	Adeno (gastric)	515	NR[+]	5-year **78%**	44%	Bang et al. [21, 61]
Surgery + Capeox		520	NR[+]	5-year **69%**	21%	
Surgery	SCC	100	NS	5-year 45%	30%	Ando et al. [62]
Surgery + cisplatin/ vindesine		105	NS	5-year 48%	30%	
Surgery	SCC	122	NS	5-year 52%	**46%**	Ando et al. [63]
Surgery +5-FU/ cisplatin		120	NS	5-year 61%	**8%**	
5-FU/cisplatin + surgery	SCC	164	NS	**5-year 55%**	NS	Ando et al. [64]
Surgery +5-FU/ cisplatin		166	NS	**5-year 43%**	NS	

Capeox, capecitabine/oxaliplatin, *CR* complete response, *N/A* not applicable, *NR* not reached, *NS* not stated, S-1 tegafur/gimeracil/oteracil
Numbers in **bold** indicate statistically significant differences
[a]Local failure with or without distant recurrence

a survival benefit only in N0 patients, contrasting with the JCOG 9204 study which reported a benefit only in N1 patients.

The above results are summarized in Table 13.4.

Future Directions

Potential for progress in this disease may lie in enhancing our understanding of and ability to exploit the molecular biology of esophageal tumors. A comprehensive molecular evaluation of 295 primary gastric adenocarcinomas as part of The Cancer Genome Atlas (TCGA) project identified four molecular subtypes of gastric cancer [65]. The chromosomal instability subtype was most common, occurring in 50% of gastric tumors but nearly 95% of esophageal and GEJ adenocarcinomas. Focal amplifications of receptor tyrosine kinases, and mutations in such genes as TP53, ARID1A, SMAD4, and CDKN2A occur commonly in this subtype. A more recent study by the TCGA research network has demonstrated that the histologic subtypes of esophageal adenocarcinoma and SCC are distinct in their molecular characteristics [66]. SCCs showed frequent genomic amplifications of CCDN1 and SOX2 and/ or TP63, while ERBB2, VEGFA, and GATA4 and GATA6 were commonly amplified in adenocarcinomas. In addition to ERBB2, other potential targetable amplifications identified in adenocarcinomas were EGFR, IGF1R, RAS, VEGFA, and cell cycle pathway amplifications. In addition, in this study, esophageal and GEJ adenocarcinomas strongly resembled the chromosomally unstable variant of gastric adenocarcinoma but had a higher frequency of DNA hypermethylation.

This data suggests that adenocarcinomas and SCCs should not be considered a single entity and clinical trials evaluating neoadjuvant, adjuvant, or systemic therapies should avoid enrolling patients with both histologies. Furthermore, the emergence of a more rational categorization of esophageal tumors may provide a framework to develop new therapies.

As discussed in previous sections, the addition of anti-VEGFA antibodies (bevacizumab) and anti-EGFR antibodies to peri-operative chemotherapy and definitive chemoradiation, respectively, has not led to an improvement in outcomes. Her2-directed therapy in combination with pre-operative and adjuvant therapy is also being evaluated. The RTOG 1010 study (NCT01196390) enrolled 591 patients with Her2-positive ≥T2 or node-positive adenocarcinoma of the esophagus or GEJ. Patients received trastuzumab during pre-operative chemoradiation with carboplatin/paclitaxel and for an additional 9 months after surgery. Results from this study are pending.

Novel treatments that target specific molecular alterations in esophageal cancer continue to be evaluated. Evaluation of anti-EGFR therapy in the metastatic setting has shown no benefit, and in the UK Gefitinib for Oesophageal Cancer Progressing After Chemotherapy (COG) trial, the use of gefitinib as second-line therapy did not improve OS over best supportive care in an unselected population [67]. A subsequent prespecified molecular analysis was performed which demonstrated [68] that EGFR copy number gain (CNG), as assessed by fluorescence in situ hybridization (FISH), appears to identify a subgroup of patients with esophageal cancer who may benefit from gefitinib as second-line therapy [69]. Patients with EGFR CNG had improved response rates and OS. However, this finding requires validation in other trials.

Another recent study evaluated rilotumumab, which selectively targets the ligand of the MET receptor, hepatocyte growth factor, in combination with ECX in patients with advanced MET-positive gastric or GEJ adenocarcinoma. There was no improvement in outcomes with the addition of this therapy to first-line chemotherapy in the metastatic setting.

Immune checkpoint inhibitors (pembrolizumab and nivolumab) have shown benefit in the chemorefractory setting and are now being evaluated in earlier-stage disease. The CheckMate 577 study (NCT02743494) is evaluating adjuvant nivolumab vs. placebo following pre-operative chemoradiotherapy and surgery in 760 patients with esophageal and GEJ cancer.

Finally, comparative studies of peri-operative chemotherapy vs. chemoradiation are ongoing. The ESOPEC study (NCT 92509286) is comparing chemoradiation with carboplatin/paclitaxel as per CROSS to FLOT and is recruiting 438 patients with ≥T2 or node-positive esophageal adenocarcinoma. The Neo-AEGIS trial (NCT01726452) is recruiting 594 patients with ≥T2 or node-positive disease and randomizing patients to the CROSS approach or peri-operative chemo with ECF/

ECX, and finally TOPGEAR (NCT01924819) is enrolling 752 patients with esophageal, GEJ, or gastric cancers who will receive peri-operative ECF or two cycles of ECF followed by chemoradiation with either infusional 5-FU or capecitabine and then three further cycles of ECF after surgery. Interpretation of Neo-AEGIS and TOPGEAR will be difficult in light of recent data showing superiority of FLOT over ECF/ECX and OEO-5 showing no benefit for ECX above two cycles of 5-FU/cisplatin. However, these trials have been amended to allow substitution of FLOT for the ECX or ECX regimen.

Conclusions

Esophageal cancer continues to be a significant worldwide health problem, and esophageal adenocarcinoma is becoming an epidemic in Western countries. The treatment of locally advanced esophageal carcinoma has evolved considerably over the last 15 years, and based on multiple phase III trials, it is recognized that multimodal therapy improves outcomes. Several trials have demonstrated a survival benefit for the addition of pre-operative chemoradiation to surgery in patients with esophageal and GEJ tumors. The use of PET imaging to guide the choice of chemotherapy with radiation appears to be a promising strategy. While peri-operative chemotherapy is an alternative treatment option for GEJ adenocarcinomas, it is unclear if chemotherapy improves local control over surgery alone, and recent studies have shown suboptimal R0 resection rates of 70% with this approach. Definitive chemoradiation is the standard of care in patients who are not surgical candidates, and in addition, it is an acceptable approach for patients with SCC who obtain a clinical complete response.

Adjuvant chemoradiation is a validated treatment option in patients with resected esophageal or GEJ adenocarcinoma. While adjuvant chemotherapy alone is associated with improved outcomes in East Asian studies, it is unclear if these data can be extrapolated to patients with GEJ tumors. There remains no proven benefit for adjuvant chemotherapy in patients with resected SCC.

References

1. Siegel RL, Miller KD, Jemal A. Cancer statistics, 2018. CA Cancer J Clin. 2018;68:7–30.
2. Ferlay J, Soerjomataram I, Dikshit R, Eser S, Mathers C, Rebelo M, Parkin DM, Forman D, Bray F. Cancer incidence and mortality worldwide: sources, methods and major patterns in GLOBOCAN 2012. Int J Cancer. 2015;136:E359–86.
3. Kmet J, Mahboubi E. Esophageal cancer in the Caspian littoral of Iran: initial studies. Science. 1972;175:846–53.
4. McGlashan ND. Oesophageal cancer and alcoholic spirits in central Africa. Gut. 1969;10:643–50.
5. Crew KD, Neugut AI. Epidemiology of upper gastrointestinal malignancies. Semin Oncol. 2004;31:450–64.
6. Devesa SS, Fraumeni JF Jr. The rising incidence of gastric cardia cancer. J Natl Cancer Inst. 1999;91:747–9.

7. Gholipour C, Shalchi RA, Abbasi M. A histopathological study of esophageal cancer on the western side of the Caspian littoral from 1994 to 2003. Dis Esophagus. 2008;21:322–7.
8. Tran GD, Sun XD, Abnet CC, Fan JH, Dawsey SM, Dong ZW, Mark SD, Qiao YL, Taylor PR. Prospective study of risk factors for esophageal and gastric cancers in the Linxian general population trial cohort in China. Int J Cancer. 2005;113:456–63.
9. Hampel H, Abraham NS, El-Serag HB. Meta-analysis: obesity and the risk for gastroesophageal reflux disease and its complications. Ann Intern Med. 2005;143:199–211.
10. Xia HH, Talley NJ. Helicobacter pylori infection, reflux esophagitis, and atrophic gastritis: an unexplored triangle. Am J Gastroenterol. 1998;93:394–400.
11. Ye W, Held M, Lagergren J, Engstrand L, Blot WJ, McLaughlin JK, Nyren O. Helicobacter pylori infection and gastric atrophy: risk of adenocarcinoma and squamous-cell carcinoma of the esophagus and adenocarcinoma of the gastric cardia. J Natl Cancer Inst. 2004;96:388–96.
12. Muller JM, Erasmi H, Stelzner M, Zieren U, Pichlmaier H. Surgical therapy of oesophageal carcinoma. Br J Surg. 1990;77:845–57.
13. Hulscher JB, van Sandick JW, de Boer AG, Wijnhoven BP, Tijssen JG, Fockens P, Stalmeier PF, ten Kate FJ, van Dekken H, Obertop H, Tilanus HW, van Lanschot JJ. Extended transthoracic resection compared with limited transhiatal resection for adenocarcinoma of the esophagus. N Engl J Med. 2002;347:1662–9.
14. Kelsen DP, Ginsberg R, Pajak TF, Sheahan DG, Gunderson L, Mortimer J, Estes N, Haller DG, Ajani J, Kocha W, Minsky BD, Roth JA. Chemotherapy followed by surgery compared with surgery alone for localized esophageal cancer. N Engl J Med. 1998;339:1979–84.
15. Allum WH, Stenning SP, Bancewicz J, Clark PI, Langley RE. Long-term results of a randomized trial of surgery with or without preoperative chemotherapy in esophageal cancer. J Clin Oncol. 2009;27:5062–7.
16. Schuhmacher C, Gretschel S, Lordick F, Reichardt P, Hohenberger W, Eisenberger CF, Haag C, Mauer ME, Hasan B, Welch J, Ott K, Hoelscher A, Schneider PM, Bechstein W, Wilke H, Lutz MP, Nordlinger B, Van Cutsem E, Siewert JR, Schlag PM. Neoadjuvant chemotherapy compared with surgery alone for locally advanced cancer of the stomach and cardia: European organisation for research and treatment of cancer randomized trial 40954. J Clin Oncol. 2010;28:5210–8.
17. Cunningham D, Allum WH, Stenning SP, Thompson JN, Van de Velde CJ, Nicolson M, Scarffe JH, Lofts FJ, Falk SJ, Iveson TJ, Smith DB, Langley RE, Verma M, Weeden S, Chua YJ, Participants MT. Perioperative chemotherapy versus surgery alone for resectable gastroesophageal cancer. N Engl J Med. 2006;355:11–20.
18. Ychou M, Boige V, Pignon JP, Conroy T, Bouche O, Lebreton G, Ducourtieux M, Bedenne L, Fabre JM, Saint-Aubert B, Geneve J, Lasser P, Rougier P. Perioperative chemotherapy compared with surgery alone for resectable gastroesophageal adenocarcinoma: an FNCLCC and FFCD multicenter phase III trial. J Clin Oncol. 2011;29:1715–21.
19. Alderson D, Cunningham D, Nankivell M, Blazeby JM, Griffin SM, Crellin A, Grabsch HI, Langer R, Pritchard S, Okines A, Krysztopik R, Coxon F, Thompson J, Falk S, Robb C, Stenning S, Langley RE. Neoadjuvant cisplatin and fluorouracil versus epirubicin, cisplatin, and capecitabine followed by resection in patients with oesophageal adenocarcinoma (UK MRC OE05): an open-label, randomised phase 3 trial. Lancet Oncol. 2017;18:1249–60.
20. Sakuramoto S, Sasako M, Yamaguchi T, Kinoshita T, Fujii M, Nashimoto A, Furukawa H, Nakajima T, Ohashi Y, Imamura H, Higashino M, Yamamura Y, Kurita A, Arai K, Group A-G. Adjuvant chemotherapy for gastric cancer with S-1, an oral fluoropyrimidine. N Engl J Med. 2007;357:1810–20.
21. Bang YJ, Kim YW, Yang HK, Chung HC, Park YK, Lee KH, Lee KW, Kim YH, Noh SI, Cho JY, Mok YJ, Kim YH, Ji J, Yeh TS, Button P, Sirzen F, Noh SH, investigators Ct. Adjuvant capecitabine and oxaliplatin for gastric cancer after D2 gastrectomy (CLASSIC): a phase 3 open-label, randomised controlled trial. Lancet. 2012;379:315–21.
22. Ajani JA, Xiao L, Roth JA, Hofstetter WL, Walsh G, Komaki R, Liao Z, Rice DC, Vaporciyan AA, Maru DM, Lee JH, Bhutani MS, Eid A, Yao JC, Phan AP, Halpin A, Suzuki A, Taketa T, Thall PF, Swisher SG. A phase II randomized trial of induction chemotherapy versus no

induction chemotherapy followed by preoperative chemoradiation in patients with esophageal cancer. Ann Oncol. 2013;24:2844–9.

23. van Hagen P, Hulshof MC, van Lanschot JJ, Steyerberg EW, van Berge Henegouwen MI, Wijnhoven BP, Richel DJ, Nieuwenhuijzen GA, Hospers GA, Bonenkamp JJ, Cuesta MA, Blaisse RJ, Busch OR, ten Kate FJ, Creemers GJ, Punt CJ, Plukker JT, Verheul HM, Spillenaar Bilgen EJ, van Dekken H, van der Sangen MJ, Rozema T, Biermann K, Beukema JC, Piet AH, van Rij CM, Reinders JG, Tilanus HW, van der Gaast A, Group C. Preoperative chemoradiotherapy for esophageal or junctional cancer. N Engl J Med. 2012;366:2074–84.

24. Shapiro J, van Lanschot JJB, Hulshof M, van Hagen P, van Berge Henegouwen MI, BPL W, van Laarhoven HWM, Nieuwenhuijzen GAP, Hospers GAP, Bonenkamp JJ, Cuesta MA, Blaisse RJB, Busch ORC, Ten Kate FJW, Creemers GM, Punt CJA, Plukker JTM, Verheul HMW, Bilgen EJS, van Dekken H, van der Sangen MJC, Rozema T, Biermann K, Beukema JC, Piet AHM, van Rij CM, Reinders JG, Tilanus HW, Steyerberg EW, van der Gaast A, group Cs. Neoadjuvant chemoradiotherapy plus surgery versus surgery alone for oesophageal or junctional cancer (CROSS): long-term results of a randomised controlled trial. Lancet Oncol. 2015;16:1090–8.

25. Verheij M, Jansen EP, Cats A, van Grieken NC, Aaronson N, Boot H, Lind PA, Meershook-Klein Kranenberg E, Nordsmark M, Putter H, Trip AK, van Sandick JW, Sikorska K, van Tinteren H, Van de Velde CJ. A multicenter randomized phase III trial of neo-adjuvant chemotherapy followed by surgery and chemotherapy or by surgery and chemoradiotherapy in resectable gastric cancer: first results from the CRITICS study. J Clin Oncol. 2016;34:4000.

26. Cunningham D, Stenning SP, Smyth EC, Okines AF, Allum WH, Rowley S, Stevenson L, Grabsch HI, Alderson D, Crosby T, Griffin SM, Mansoor W, Coxon FY, Falk SJ, Darby S, Sumpter KA, Blazeby JM, Langley RE. Peri-operative chemotherapy with or without bevacizumab in operable oesophagogastric adenocarcinoma (UK Medical Research Council ST03): primary analysis results of a multicentre, open-label, randomised phase 2-3 trial. Lancet Oncol. 2017;18:357–70.

27. Al-Batran S-E, Homann N, Schmalenberg H, Kopp H-G, Haag GM, Luley KB, Schmiegel WH, Folprecht G, Probst S, Prasnikar N, Thuss-Patience PC, Fischbach W, Trojan J, Koenigsmann M, Pauligk C, Goetze TO, Jaeger E, Meiler J, Schuler MH, Hofheinz R. Perioperative chemotherapy with docetaxel, oxaliplatin, and fluorouracil/leucovorin (FLOT) versus epirubicin, cisplatin, and fluorouracil or capecitabine (ECF/ECX) for resectable gastric or gastroesophageal junction (GEJ) adenocarcinoma (FLOT4-AIO): a multicenter, randomized phase 3 trial. J Clin Oncol. 2017;35:4004.

28. Sjoquist KM, Burmeister BH, Smithers BM, Zalcberg JR, Simes RJ, Barbour A, Gebski V, Australasian Gastro-Intestinal Trials G. Survival after neoadjuvant chemotherapy or chemoradiotherapy for resectable oesophageal carcinoma: an updated meta-analysis. Lancet Oncol. 2011;12:681–92.

29. Herskovic A, Martz K, al-Sarraf M, Leichman L, Brindle J, Vaitkevicius V, Cooper J, Byhardt R, Davis L, Emami B. Combined chemotherapy and radiotherapy compared with radiotherapy alone in patients with cancer of the esophagus. N Engl J Med. 1992;326:1593–8.

30. Cooper JS, Guo MD, Herskovic A, Macdonald JS, Martenson JA Jr, Al-Sarraf M, Byhardt R, Russell AH, Beitler JJ, Spencer S, Asbell SO, Graham MV, Leichman LL. Chemoradiotherapy of locally advanced esophageal cancer: long-term follow-up of a prospective randomized trial (RTOG 85-01). Radiation Therapy Oncology Group. JAMA. 1999;281:1623–7.

31. Bosset JF, Gignoux M, Triboulet JP, Tiret E, Mantion G, Elias D, Lozach P, Ollier JC, Pavy JJ, Mercier M, Sahmoud T. Chemoradiotherapy followed by surgery compared with surgery alone in squamous-cell cancer of the esophagus. N Engl J Med. 1997;337:161–7.

32. Burmeister BH, Smithers BM, Gebski V, Fitzgerald L, Simes RJ, Devitt P, Ackland S, Gotley DC, Joseph D, Millar J, North J, Walpole ET, Denham JW, Trans-Tasman Radiation Oncology G, Australasian Gastro-Intestinal Trials G. Surgery alone versus chemoradiotherapy followed by surgery for resectable cancer of the oesophagus: a randomised controlled phase III trial. Lancet Oncol. 2005;6:659–68.

33. Urba SG, Orringer MB, Turrisi A, Iannettoni M, Forastiere A, Strawderman M. Randomized trial of preoperative chemoradiation versus surgery alone in patients with locoregional esophageal carcinoma. J Clin Oncol. 2001;19:305–13.
34. Walsh TN, Noonan N, Hollywood D, Kelly A, Keeling N, Hennessy TP. A comparison of multimodal therapy and surgery for esophageal adenocarcinoma. N Engl J Med. 1996;335:462–7.
35. Tepper J, Krasna MJ, Niedzwiecki D, Hollis D, Reed CE, Goldberg R, Kiel K, Willett C, Sugarbaker D, Mayer R. Phase III trial of trimodality therapy with cisplatin, fluorouracil, radiotherapy, and surgery compared with surgery alone for esophageal cancer: CALGB 9781. J Clin Oncol. 2008;26:1086–92.
36. Goodman K, Niedzwiecki D, Hall N, Bekaii-Saab TS, Ye X, Meyers MO, Mitchell-Richards K, Boffa DJ, Frankel WL, Venook AP, Hochster HS, Crane CH, O'Reilly EM, Ilson DH. Initial results of CALGB 80803 (Alliance): a randomized phase II trial of PET scan-directed combined modality therapy for esophageal cancer. J Clin Oncol. 2017;35:1.
37. Mukherjee S, Hurt CN, Gwynne S, Sebag-Montefiore D, Radhakrishna G, Gollins S, Hawkins M, Grabsch HI, Jones G, Falk S, Sharma R, Bateman A, Roy R, Ray R, Canham J, Griffiths G, Maughan T, Crosby T. NEOSCOPE: a randomised phase II study of induction chemotherapy followed by oxaliplatin/capecitabine or carboplatin/paclitaxel based pre-operative chemoradiation for resectable oesophageal adenocarcinoma. Eur J Cancer. 2017;74:38–46.
38. Mokdad AA, Yopp AC, Polanco PM, Mansour JC, Reznik SI, Heitjan DF, Choti MA, Minter RR, Wang SC, Porembka MR. Adjuvant chemotherapy vs postoperative observation following preoperative chemoradiotherapy and resection in gastroesophageal cancer: a propensity score-matched analysis. JAMA Oncol. 2018;4:31–8.
39. Mariette C, Dahan L, Mornex F, Maillard E, Thomas PA, Meunier B, Boige V, Pezet D, Robb WB, Le Brun-Ly V, Bosset JF, Mabrut JY, Triboulet JP, Bedenne L, Seitz JF. Surgery alone versus chemoradiotherapy followed by surgery for stage I and II esophageal cancer: final analysis of randomized controlled phase III trial FFCD 9901. J Clin Oncol. 2014;32:2416–22.
40. Stahl M, Walz MK, Stuschke M, Lehmann N, Meyer HJ, Riera-Knorrenschild J, Langer P, Engenhart-Cabillic R, Bitzer M, Konigsrainer A, Budach W, Wilke H. Phase III comparison of preoperative chemotherapy compared with chemoradiotherapy in patients with locally advanced adenocarcinoma of the esophagogastric junction. J Clin Oncol. 2009;27:851–6.
41. Downey RJ, Akhurst T, Ilson D, Ginsberg R, Bains MS, Gonen M, Koong H, Gollub M, Minsky BD, Zakowski M, Turnbull A, Larson SM, Rusch V. Whole body 18FDG-PET and the response of esophageal cancer to induction therapy: results of a prospective trial. J Clin Oncol. 2003;21:428–32.
42. Flamen P, Van Cutsem E, Lerut A, Cambier JP, Haustermans K, Bormans G, De Leyn P, Van Raemdonck D, De Wever W, Ectors N, Maes A, Mortelmans L. Positron emission tomography for assessment of the response to induction radiochemotherapy in locally advanced oesophageal cancer. Ann Oncol. 2002;13:361–8.
43. Ott K, Weber WA, Lordick F, Becker K, Busch R, Herrmann K, Wieder H, Fink U, Schwaiger M, Siewert JR. Metabolic imaging predicts response, survival, and recurrence in adenocarcinomas of the esophagogastric junction. J Clin Oncol. 2006;24:4692–8.
44. Weber WA, Ott K, Becker K, Dittler HJ, Helmberger H, Avril NE, Meisetschlager G, Busch R, Siewert JR, Schwaiger M, Fink U. Prediction of response to preoperative chemotherapy in adenocarcinomas of the esophagogastric junction by metabolic imaging. J Clin Oncol. 2001;19:3058–65.
45. Lordick F, Ott K, Krause BJ, Weber WA, Becker K, Stein HJ, Lorenzen S, Schuster T, Wieder H, Herrmann K, Bredenkamp R, Hofler H, Fink U, Peschel C, Schwaiger M, Siewert JR. PET to assess early metabolic response and to guide treatment of adenocarcinoma of the oesophagogastric junction: the MUNICON phase II trial. Lancet Oncol. 2007;8:797–805.
46. zum Buschenfelde CM, Herrmann K, Schuster T, Geinitz H, Langer R, Becker K, Ott K, Ebert M, Zimmermann F, Friess H, Schwaiger M, Peschel C, Lordick F, Krause BJ. (18)F-FDG PET-guided salvage neoadjuvant radiochemotherapy of adenocarcinoma of the esophagogastric junction: the MUNICON II trial. J Nucl Med. 2011;52:1189–96.

47. Ilson DH, Minsky BD, Ku GY, Rusch V, Rizk N, Shah M, Kelsen DP, Capanu M, Tang L, Campbell J, Bains M. Phase 2 trial of induction and concurrent chemoradiotherapy with weekly irinotecan and cisplatin followed by surgery for esophageal cancer. Cancer. 2012;118:2820–7.

48. Ku GY, Kriplani A, Janjigian YY, Kelsen DP, Rusch VW, Bains M, Chou J, Capanu M, Wu AJ, Goodman KA, Ilson DH. Change in chemotherapy during concurrent radiation followed by surgery after a suboptimal positron emission tomography response to induction chemotherapy improves outcomes for locally advanced esophageal adenocarcinoma. Cancer. 2016;122:2083–90.

49. Stahl M, Stuschke M, Lehmann N, Meyer HJ, Walz MK, Seeber S, Klump B, Budach W, Teichmann R, Schmitt M, Schmitt G, Franke C, Wilke H. Chemoradiation with and without surgery in patients with locally advanced squamous cell carcinoma of the esophagus. J Clin Oncol. 2005;23:2310–7.

50. Bedenne L, Michel P, Bouche O, Milan C, Mariette C, Conroy T, Pezet D, Roullet B, Seitz J-F, Herr J-P, Paillot B, Arveux P, Bonnetain F, Binquet C. Chemoradiation followed by surgery compared with chemoradiation alone in squamous cancer of the esophagus: FFCD 9102. J Clin Oncol. 2007;25:1160–8.

51. Vincent J, Mariette C, Pezet D, Huet E, Bonnetain F, Bouche O, Conroy T, Roullet B, Seitz JF, Herr JP, Di Fiore F, Jouve JL, Bedenne L, Federation Francophone de Cancerologie D. Early surgery for failure after chemoradiation in operable thoracic oesophageal cancer. Analysis of the non-randomised patients in FFCD 9102 phase III trial: chemoradiation followed by surgery versus chemoradiation alone. Eur J Cancer. 2015;51:1683–93.

52. Conroy T, Galais MP, Raoul JL, Bouche O, Gourgou-Bourgade S, Douillard JY, Etienne PL, Boige V, Martel-Lafay I, Michel P, Llacer-Moscardo C, Francois E, Crehange G, Abdelghani MB, Juzyna B, Bedenne L, Adenis A. Federation Francophone de Cancerologie D, Group U-G: Definitive chemoradiotherapy with FOLFOX versus fluorouracil and cisplatin in patients with oesophageal cancer (PRODIGE5/ACCORD17): final results of a randomised, phase 2/3 trial. Lancet Oncol. 2014;15:305–14.

53. Marks JL, Hofstetter W, Correa AM, Mehran RJ, Rice D, Roth J, Walsh G, Vaporciyan A, Erasmus J, Chang J, Maru D, Lee JH, Lee J, Ajani JA, Swisher SG. Salvage esophagectomy after failed definitive chemoradiation for esophageal adenocarcinoma. Ann Thorac Surg. 2012;94:1126–32; discussion 1132-3.

54. Markar S, Gronnier C, Duhamel A, Pasquer A, Thereaux J, du Rieu MC, Lefevre JH, Turner K, Luc G, Mariette C. Salvage surgery after chemoradiotherapy in the management of esophageal cancer: is it a viable therapeutic option? J Clin Oncol. 2015;33:3866–73.

55. Swisher SG, Winter KA, Komaki RU, Ajani JA, Wu TT, Hofstetter WL, Konski AA, Willett CG. A phase II study of a paclitaxel-based chemoradiation regimen with selective surgical salvage for resectable locoregionally advanced esophageal cancer: initial reporting of RTOG 0246. Int J Radiat Oncol Biol Phys. 2012;82:1967–72.

56. Crosby T, Hurt CN, Falk S, Gollins S, Mukherjee S, Staffurth J, Ray R, Bashir N, Bridgewater JA, Geh JI, Cunningham D, Blazeby J, Roy R, Maughan T, Griffiths G. Chemoradiotherapy with or without cetuximab in patients with oesophageal cancer (SCOPE1): a multicentre, phase 2/3 randomised trial. Lancet Oncol. 2013;14:627–37.

57. Ilson DH, Moughan J, Suntharalingam M, Dicker A, Kachnic LA, Konski AA, Chakravarthy B, Anker C, Thakrar HV, Horiba N, Kavadi V, Deutsch M, Raben A, Roof KS, Suh JH, Pollock J, Safran H, Crane CH. RTOG 0436: a phase III trial evaluating the addition of cetuximab to paclitaxel, cisplatin, and radiation for patients with esophageal cancer treated without surgery. J Clin Oncol. 2014;32:–4007.

58. Macdonald JS, Smalley SR, Benedetti J, Hundahl SA, Estes NC, Stemmermann GN, Haller DG, Ajani JA, Gunderson LL, Jessup JM, Martenson JA. Chemoradiotherapy after surgery compared with surgery alone for adenocarcinoma of the stomach or gastroesophageal junction. N Engl J Med. 2001;345:725–30.

59. Fuchs CS, Niedzwiecki D, Mamon HJ, Tepper JE, Ye X, Swanson RS, Enzinger PC, Haller DG, Dragovich T, Alberts SR, Bjarnason GA, Willett CG, Gunderson LL, Goldberg RM, Venook

AP, Ilson D, O'Reilly E, Ciombor K, Berg DJ, Meyerhardt J, Mayer RJ. Adjuvant chemoradiotherapy with epirubicin, cisplatin, and fluorouracil compared with adjuvant chemoradiotherapy with fluorouracil and leucovorin after curative resection of gastric cancer: results from CALGB 80101 (alliance). J Clin Oncol. 2017;35:3671–7.

60. Sasako M, Sakuramoto S, Katai H, Kinoshita T, Furukawa H, Yamaguchi T, Nashimoto A, Fujii M, Nakajima T, Ohashi Y. Five-year outcomes of a randomized phase III trial comparing adjuvant chemotherapy with S-1 versus surgery alone in stage II or III gastric cancer. J Clin Oncol. 2011;29:4387–93.

61. Noh SH, Park SR, Yang HK, Chung HC, Chung IJ, Kim SW, Kim HH, Choi JH, Kim HK, Yu W, Lee JI, Shin DB, Ji J, Chen JS, Lim Y, Ha S, Bang YJ, investigators Ct. Adjuvant capecitabine plus oxaliplatin for gastric cancer after D2 gastrectomy (CLASSIC): 5-year follow-up of an open-label, randomised phase 3 trial. Lancet Oncol. 2014;15:1389–96.

62. Ando N, Iizuka T, Kakegawa T, Isono K, Watanabe H, Ide H, Tanaka O, Shinoda M, Takiyama W, Arimori M, Ishida K, Tsugane S. A randomized trial of surgery with and without chemotherapy for localized squamous carcinoma of the thoracic esophagus: the Japan Clinical Oncology Group Study. J Thorac Cardiovasc Surg. 1997;114:205–9.

63. Ando N, Iizuka T, Ide H, Ishida K, Shinoda M, Nishimaki T, Takiyama W, Watanabe H, Isono K, Aoyama N, Makuuchi H, Tanaka O, Yamana H, Ikeuchi S, Kabuto T, Nagai K, Shimada Y, Kinjo Y, Fukuda H, Japan Clinical Oncology G. Surgery plus chemotherapy compared with surgery alone for localized squamous cell carcinoma of the thoracic esophagus: a Japan Clinical Oncology Group Study--JCOG9204. J Clin Oncol. 2003;21:4592–6.

64. Ando N, Kato H, Igaki H, Shinoda M, Ozawa S, Shimizu H, Nakamura T, Yabusaki H, Aoyama N, Kurita A, Ikeda K, Kanda T, Tsujinaka T, Nakamura K, Fukuda H. A randomized trial comparing postoperative adjuvant chemotherapy with cisplatin and 5-fluorouracil versus preoperative chemotherapy for localized advanced squamous cell carcinoma of the thoracic esophagus (JCOG9907). Ann Surg Oncol. 2012;19:68–74.

65. The Cancer Genome Atlas Research N. Comprehensive molecular characterization of gastric adenocarcinoma. Nature. 2014;513:202.

66. The Cancer Genome Atlas Research N. Integrated genomic characterization of oesophageal carcinoma. Nature. 2017;541:169.

67. Dutton SJ, Ferry DR, Blazeby JM, Abbas H, Dahle-Smith A, Mansoor W, Thompson J, Harrison M, Chatterjee A, Falk S, Garcia-Alonso A, Fyfe DW, Hubner RA, Gamble T, Peachey L, Davoudianfar M, Pearson SR, Julier P, Jankowski J, Kerr R, Petty RD. Gefitinib for oesophageal cancer progressing after chemotherapy (COG): a phase 3, multicentre, double-blind, placebo-controlled randomised trial. Lancet Oncol. 2014;15:894–904.

68. Catenacci DVT, Tebbutt NC, Davidenko I, Murad AM, Al-Batran SE, Ilson DH, Tjulandin S, Gotovkin E, Karaszewska B, Bondarenko I, Tejani MA, Udrea AA, Tehfe M, De Vita F, Turkington C, Tang R, Ang A, Zhang Y, Hoang T, Sidhu R, Cunningham D. Rilotumumab plus epirubicin, cisplatin, and capecitabine as first-line therapy in advanced MET-positive gastric or gastro-oesophageal junction cancer (RILOMET-1): a randomised, double-blind, placebo-controlled, phase 3 trial. Lancet Oncol. 2017;18:1467–82.

69. Petty RD, Dahle-Smith A, Stevenson DAJ, Osborne A, Massie D, Clark C, Murray GI, Dutton SJ, Roberts C, Chong IY, Mansoor W, Thompson J, Harrison M, Chatterjee A, Falk SJ, Elyan S, Garcia-Alonso A, Fyfe DW, Wadsley J, Chau I, Ferry DR, Miedzybrodzka Z. Gefitinib and EGFR gene copy number aberrations in esophageal cancer. J Clin Oncol. 2017;35:2279–87.

70. Medical Research Council Oesophageal Cancer Working Group. Surgical resection with or without preoperative chemotherapy in oesophageal cancer: a randomised controlled trial. Lancet. 2002;359:1727–33.

Systemic Treatment for Metastatic or Recurrent Disease

14

Daniel H. Ahn and Tanios Bekaii-Saab

Despite the decreasing incidence and mortality rate, gastroesophageal (GE) cancers remain the third leading cause of cancer-related deaths worldwide [1]. This is in large part from the absence of symptoms in the early stages of disease, where 40% of patients present with advanced metastatic disease. Unfortunately, the prognosis in advanced gastroesophageal cancers is poor, where the 5-year overall survival is less than 5% [2]. During the past decade, therapeutic advances include the approval of several targeted therapies for patients with newly diagnosed and treatment-refractory metastatic gastroesophageal adenocarcinoma [3–5]. This progress, however, has only resulted in an incremental improvement in patient outcomes, highlighting the need to develop novel treatment strategies in this disease. In this chapter, we will review current therapies that are used and being investigated in ongoing clinical trials, which include targeted therapies and immunotherapeutic approaches in advanced esophageal cancers.

Targeting HER-2

The ErbB family consists of four plasma membrane-bound receptor tyrosine kinases including erB-2, also frequently called HER-2 (human epidermal growth factor receptor 2) protein or HER-2/neu. HER-2 plays a critical role in cancer cell biology by facilitating in cellular apoptosis, differentiation, and tumor proliferation. The activation of the HER-2 receptor occurs through hetero- or homo-dimerization with other ErbB family members, which result in the upregulation and aberrant activation of downstream signaling pathways. In gastric and gastroesophageal cancers (GE), HER-2 overexpression and/or amplification has been reported up to 34% and

D. H. Ahn · T. Bekaii-Saab (✉)
Division of Hematology/Medical Oncology, Mayo Clinic Arizona, Phoenix, AZ, USA
e-mail: Bekaii-saab.tanios@mayo.edu

© Springer Nature Switzerland AG 2020
N. F. Saba, B. F. El-Rayes (eds.), *Esophageal Cancer*,
https://doi.org/10.1007/978-3-030-29832-6_14

is associated with poor prognosis, where HER-2 overexpression was associated with poor survival and clinicopathological characteristics [6]. Thus, novel therapeutic agents that inhibit HER-2 are a rational treatment strategy for advanced GE cancers (Table 14.1).

Table 14.1 Phase 3 randomized clinical trials of targeted therapies

Study	Target	Regimen	Line of therapy	Primary EP	Results	Ref
TOGA	HER-2	XP chemotherapy +/− trastuzumab	1st	OS	Positive. HR 0.74; 95% CI 0.6–0.91; $p = 0.005$	[5]
JACOB	HER-2	XP chemotherapy, trastuzumab+/− pertuzumab	1st	OS	Negative. HR 0.84, 95% CI 0.71–100, $p = 0.0565$	[9]
TyTAN	HER-2	Paclitaxel +/− lapatinib	2nd	OS	Negative. HR 0.84; 95% CI 0.64–1.11; $p = 0.104$	[12]
LOGIC	HER-2	CapeOx +/− lapatinib	1st	OS	Negative. HR 0.91; 95% CI 0.73–1.12; $p = 0.350$	[11]
GATSBY	HER-2	T-DM1 vs. taxane	2nd	OS	Negative. HR 1.15; 95% CI 0.89–1.43; $p = 0.86$	[15]
AVAGAST	VEGFA	XP chemotherapy +/− bevacizumab	1st	OS	Negative. HR 0.87; 95% CI 0.73–1.03; $p = 0.100$	[20]
AVATAR	VEGFA	XP chemotherapy +/− bevacizumab	1st	OS	Negative. HR 1.11; 95% CI 0.79–1.56; $p = 0.557$	[21]
REGARD	VEGFR2	Ramucirumab vs. placebo	2nd	OS	Positive. HR 0.776; 95% CI 0.603–0.998; $p = 0.047$	[3]
RAINBOW	VEGFR2	Paclitaxel +/− ramucirumab	2nd	OS	Positive. HR 0.807; 95% CI 0.678–0.962; $p = 0.017$	[4]
RAINFALL	VEGFR2	XP chemotherapy +/− ramucirumab	1st	OS	Positive. HR 0.75; 95% CI 0.61–0.94; $p = 0.011$	[22]
Li et al.	VEGFR2	Apatinib vs. placebo	3rd	OS	Positive. HR 0.71; 95% CI 0.54-0.94; $p < 0.016$	[24]
ANGEL	VEGFR2	Apatinib vs. placebo	4th and beyond	OS	Ongoing (NCT03042611)	
INTEGRATE II	VEGFR2	Regorafenib vs. placebo	3rd	OS	Ongoing (NCT02773524)	

XP fluoropyrimidine/platinum, OS overall survival, EP endpoint, HR hazard ratio, HER-2 human epidermal growth factor receptor 2, VEGF vascular endothelial growth factor

Trastuzumab

In preclinical studies, trastuzumab, a monoclonal antibody (mAb) that targets the extracellular domain of the HER-2 protein, inhibited tumor growth in HER-2-overexpressing xenograft models of human gastric cancer cell lines and enhanced activity in combination with chemotherapy. These observations led to TOGA study, a randomized phase 3 clinical trial, where patients with treatment-naïve advanced or metastatic gastric or GE adenocarcinoma with overexpression of HER-2 received fluoropyrimidine/cisplatin chemotherapy alone or in combination with trastuzumab [5]. Patients were eligible if their tumor samples were scored as 3+ on immunohistochemistry or if they were FISH positive with a HER-2/CEP17 ratio $\geq$ 2. The primary endpoint of overall survival (OS) was met, where patients that received the combination experienced a median survival benefit of 2.7 months compared (13.8 months versus 11.1 months) to those that received chemotherapy alone (HR 0.74, 95% confidence interval (CI) 0.60–0.91, p = 0.0046) [5]. Treatment was well tolerated, where rates of grade 3 or higher adverse events did not differ between the two groups. The positive results from TOGA changed the treatment paradigm for patients with advanced HER-2+ disease, for whom treatment with platinum and fluoropyrimidine cytotoxic chemotherapy in combination with trastuzumab is now the standard of care.

Pertuzumab

Pertuzumab is a monoclonal antibody that inhibits HER-2 dimerization, where its mechanism of action differs and is complementary to trastuzumab. The combination of pertuzumab and trastuzumab significantly improved progression-free survival in patients with advanced HER-2+ breast cancer (CLEOPATRA trial), resulting in dual anti-HER-2-directed therapy the standard therapeutic approach [7]. Similar to the clinical activity observed in breast cancer, preclinical studies conducted in HER-2+ human gastric xenograft models showed significant anti-tumor activity from pertuzumab in combination with trastuzumab compared with each monotherapy [8]. Based on these results, JACOB, a randomized phase 3 trial, investigated whether pertuzumab in combination with trastuzumab, fluoropyrimidine, and cisplatin cytotoxic chemotherapy would improve overall survival in patients with HER-2+ advanced gastric or GE cancer [9]. Despite an observed median 3.3-month survival benefit in patients that received the combination, the results failed to achieve statistical significance (17.5 vs. 14.2 months, HR 0.84, 95% CI 0.71–100, p = 0.0565) [9]. From the negative results observed in JACOB, pertuzumab and specifically dual HER-2-targeted treatment strategies are not relevant in the treatment for advanced HER-2+ gastric or GE cancers.

Tyrosine Kinase Inhibitors (TKI) that Target HER-2

Lapatinib, an approved multi-target small molecular inhibitor in HER-2+ breast cancer [10], failed to demonstrate any significant clinical activity across two phase 3 trials. In the LOGIC study, patients with treatment-naïve metastatic HER-2+ GE cancer were randomized to receive CapeOx chemotherapy alone or in combination with lapatinib [11]. The addition of lapatinib to CapeOx chemotherapy failed to improve overall survival (12.2 vs. 10.5 months, HR 0.91, 95% CI 0.731–1.12, $p = 0.3492$). As part of their preplanned exploratory analysis, median overall survival among Asian patients was 16.5 months with lapatinib versus 10.9 months with placebo (HR 0.68, $p = 0.0261$) compared with 10.0 months (lapatinib arm) versus 9.1 months in patients from other parts of the world [11]. However, HER-2 status is not known to vary based on these patient characteristics, which are not reliable or predictive for patient outcomes in this setting. The lack of efficacy from lapatinib was consistent in the refractory setting where in the phase 3 TyTAN trial, patients who received the combination of lapatinib with paclitaxel chemotherapy failed to show a survival benefit compared to those that received chemotherapy alone (11.0 months with lapatinib versus 9.9 months with paclitaxel alone) [12].

Trastuzumab-Emtansine (T-DM1)

T-DM1 is an antibody drug conjugate that consists of the monoclonal antibody trastuzumab linked to the cytotoxic agent emtansine (DM-1) and functions by inducing tumor cell cytotoxicity and antibody-dependent cell-mediated cytotoxicity. Trastuzumab inhibits tumor cell growth by binding to the HER-2/neu receptor, whereas DM1 enters the cell and induces cytotoxicity by tubulin binding [13]. In gastric cancer cell xenograft models, enhanced tumoricidal activity was observed from T-DM1 compared to trastuzumab monotherapy [14]. This promising activity led to GATSBY, a phase 2/3 trial that investigated T-DM1 in patients with treatment-refractory advanced gastric or GE cancer [15]. In an open-label adaptive phase 2/3 trial, patients were randomized to receive either T-DM1 or taxane chemotherapy, with a primary endpoint of overall survival. T-DM1 failed to demonstrate a survival benefit over taxane chemotherapy arm (7.9 months vs. 8.6 months, respectively) [15].

Despite HER-2 overexpression/amplification being an established therapeutic target in breast and GE cancers, the discordance in clinical activity between the two diseases suggests that HER-2-positive tumors are not created equal. This is likely due to in part from the varying incidence in HER-2 positivity, pathologic concordance rates, and detection testing measures. The knowledge of HER-2 as a prognostic and predictive biomarker has been well established in breast cancer, which includes an understanding of mechanisms of de novo and acquired treatment resistance. While the information generated from breast cancer research does not directly apply to gastric or GE cancers, aspects can be utilized in the knowledge and future development of treatment strategies in HER-2+ GE cancers.

Targeting Angiogenesis

Vascular endothelial growth factors (VEGF) are integral in vasculature development and formation in adults. VEGF ligands (VEGFA, B, C, D, and E and placental growth factor) stimulate endothelial cell growth and induce angiogenesis [16]. Ligands mediate the angiogenic response by binding to their respective receptor tyrosine kinases (RTKs), VEGFR 1–3, and induce pro-angiogenic effects (increased angiogenesis, endothelial cell survival and migration, increased vascular permeability) through subsequent signal transduction. Angiogenesis is essential for tumor proliferation and without the necessary microenvironment, and its inhibition induces cessation of tumor growth. In GE cancers, VEGF overexpression was associated with known poor prognostic tumor markers and has been shown to be prognostic for patient outcomes in solid tumor malignancies [17–19]. As such, anti-angiogenic approaches represent a rational treatment strategy in GE cancers.

Bevacizumab

Bevacizumab is a monoclonal antibody that targets VEGF and has been approved for the treatment of several solid tumor malignancies, leading to its investigation in GE cancers. AVAGAST, a randomized phase 3 trial, investigated fluoropyrimidine/platinum chemotherapy with bevacizumab or placebo in treatment-naïve metastatic GE cancers [20]. Despite a 2.1 survival benefit that was observed in patients who received bevacizumab, the survival difference failed to reach statistical significance (12.1 vs. 10.1 months, HR 0.87, 95% CI 0.73–1.03, $p = 0.1002$). AVATAR, a similar randomized phase 3 trial conducted in China, also failed to demonstrate a significant survival benefit from bevacizumab in patients with treatment-naïve metastatic GE adenocarcinoma [21]. Despite the clinical activity seen in other gastrointestinal malignancies, the negative results observed in these two studies suggest bevacizumab should not be given as a potential treatment in advanced GE cancers.

Ramucirumab

Ramucirumab, a fully humanized IgG1 monoclonal antibody that targets VEGFR2, has been investigated and is approved for treatment-refractory advanced gastro-esophageal cancers. In the phase 3 REGARD trial, patients that previously failed platinum/fluoropyrimidine chemotherapy were randomized to receive ramucirumab versus placebo [3]. The study met its primary endpoint, where patients who received ramucirumab experienced a median 1.4-month survival benefit in comparison to the placebo arm (5.4 vs. 3.8 months, HR 0.77, 95% CI 0.603–0.998, $p = 0.047$) [3]. Adverse events were similar between the two groups, with the ramucirumab group experiencing higher rates of hypertension (16% vs. 8%) [3]. Based on these positive findings in conjunction with the results observed from COUGAR-02 which demonstrated a clinical benefit from taxane chemotherapy in treatment-refractory metastatic gastroesophageal cancer, the RAINBOW trial was conducted, where patients were randomized to receive weekly paclitaxel (80 mg/m^2 days 1, 8, and 15 every 28 days) with or without ramucirumab on days 1 and 15. The results showed a significant survival benefit favoring the ramucirumab arm, where patients experienced a 2.2-month survival benefit in comparison to the placebo arm (9.6 vs. 7.4 months, HR 0.807, 95% CI 0.678–0.962) [4]. In the ramucirumab arm, a higher proportion of patients experienced grade 3 or higher neutropenia (133 [41%] of 327 vs. 62 [19%] of 329), leucopenia (57 [17%] vs. 22 [7%]), hypertension (46 [14%] vs. 8 [2%]), fatigue (39 [12%] vs. 18 [5%]), anemia (30 [9%] vs. 34 [10%]), and abdominal pain (20 [6%] vs. 11 [3%]). The incidence of grade 3 or higher febrile neutropenia was low in both groups. Based on the positive results observed in REGARD and the RAINBOW trial, ramucirumab received FDA approval as a monotherapy or in combination with paclitaxel chemotherapy. Based on the degree of peripheral neuropathy, the ramucirumab in combination with paclitaxel is the preferred treatment choice. Based on the promising results observed in the refractory setting, the RAINFALL trial, a randomized phase 3 trial, was completed, which investigated ramucirumab in the first-line setting. Patients with treatment-naïve metastatic GE cancer received cisplatin/fluoropyrimidine (5-fluorouracil or capecitabine per investigator's choice) chemotherapy with or without ramucirumab. The primary endpoint of the study was PFS, with OS as its secondary endpoint. The study met its primary endpoint, which showed a statistically significant difference in PFS (HR 0.75, 95% CI 0.61–0.94, $p = 0.01$), favoring the ramucirumab arm [22]. However, the difference equated to a 0.3-month benefit in PFS (median PFS 5.7 versus 5.4 months) between the two treatment arms. No survival benefit was observed in patients that received ramucirumab. Thus, despite the study meeting its primary endpoint, the lack of a clinically meaningful improvement in PFS will likely not result in a significant change in practice, and ramucirumab should be reserved in the treatment-refractory setting, where there is a more pronounced benefit in patient outcomes.

Tyrosine Kinase Inhibitors that Target VEGF

Another strategy in targeting angiogenesis that has shown promise is with tyrosine kinase inhibitors that inhibit angiogenesis. Several agents have shown promise and are currently undergoing investigation in the treatment of GE cancers. Regorafenib, an oral multi-targeted tyrosine kinase inhibitor that inhibits several receptor tyrosine kinases including angiogenesis (through blocking VEGFR2 and endothelial-specific type 2), is approved in the treatment of metastatic colorectal cancer [23] and is under investigation in the treatment of advanced gastroesophageal cancers. INTEGRATE, an international randomized phase 2 trial, investigated the clinical efficacy of regorafenib versus best supportive care in patients with treatment-refractory advanced GE cancers. The study met its primary endpoint, where patients who received regorafenib demonstrated a significant improvement in PFS (2.6 vs. 0.9, HR 0.40, 95% CI 0.28–0.59, $p > 0.001$). A non-significant trend toward an improvement in OS was seen favoring the regorafenib arm (5.8 vs. 4.5 months, HR 0.74, 95% CI 4.4–6.8, p = 0.147). Toxicities related to regorafenib were similar to those in previous studies. To confirm the observed positive results, INTEGRATE II, an international randomized placebo controlled phase 3 trial, with a primary endpoint of overall survival is ongoing (ClinicalTrials.gov, NCT02773524) and, if positive, will offer another treatment option for patients with treatment-refractory disease. Apatinib, an oral tyrosine kinase inhibitor that selectively inhibits VEGFR2, showed a significant benefit in overall survival in a Chinese placebo controlled randomized phase 3 trial, where patients randomized to Apatinib experienced a 1.8-month survival benefit (6.5 vs. 4.7 months, HR 0.709, 95% CI 0.537–0.937, p = 0.0156) [24]. The most common grade 3 or 4 toxicities observed included neutropenia (37.5%), anemia (25%), thrombocytopenia (25%), palmar-plantar erythrodysesthesia (27.8%), proteinuria (47.7%), and hypertension (35.2%) [24]. To corroborate the clinical activity observed in the Chinese patient population, ANGEL, an internationally run placebo controlled phase 3 trial, is currently ongoing (ClinicalTrials.gov, NCT03042611).

Immunotherapy in the Treatment of Gastroesophageal (GE) Cancers

Over the past decade, immunotherapeutic approaches, most notably immune checkpoint inhibitors, epitomized by antibodies against T lymphocyte regulators CTLA-4 (cytotoxic T lymphocyte-associated protein 4) and programmed death-1 (PD-1), has emerged as a promising treatment option for many solid tumor malignancies and has garnered much enthusiasm as a potential treatment option in GE cancers [25–28].

In GE cancers, PD-1 and its ligands programmed death-ligand 1 (PD-L1) and programmed death-ligand 2 (PD-L2) have been shown to be overexpressed and play an integral role in regulating the immune response to cancer cells. In GE cancers, immunosuppressive PD-L1 protein expression has been shown to be associated with a poor prognosis [29]. Thus, targeting PD-1/PD-L1 with immune checkpoint inhibitors can potentially enhance the immune response to GE cancers and represent an innovative treatment strategy. Several PD-1, PD-L1, and CTLA-4 immune checkpoint inhibitors have been investigated in advanced GE cancers (Table 14.2).

ATTRACTION-02, a placebo controlled randomized phase 3 trial, was conducted in East Asia (Japan, South Korea, and Taiwan), where patients with treatment-refractory GE cancer were randomized to receive either nivolumab, a PD-1 inhibitor (3 mg/kg IV Q2 weeks), or placebo [30]. The primary endpoint of the study was OS, with secondary endpoints that included PFS, overall response rate (ORR), and disease control rate (DCR) [30]. The study met its primary endpoint, where patients who received nivolumab experienced a 1.12-month survival benefit compared to those randomized to the placebo arm (median OS 5.26 months vs. 4.14 months, HR 0.63, 95% CI 0.51–0.78, p < 0.0001). The survival benefit was observed regardless of PD-L1 expression status. Grade 3 or 4 treatment-related adverse events occurred

Table 14.2 Summary of data from early phase trials of checkpoint inhibitors in advanced GE cancers

Study	Agent	MoA	Phase	Outcomes	Comments	Ref
CHECKMATE-032	Nivolumab	PD-1 inhibitor	1, 2	ORR 8–24%	Up to 43% of pts experienced TRAEs	[37]
KEYNOTE-059	Pembrolizumab	PD-1 inhibitor	2	12%	16% (PD-L1+) vs. 6% (PD-L1-)	[38]
JAVELIN 300	Avelumab	PD-L1 inhibitor	3	Negative	Results pending	NCT02625623
CP1108	Durvalumab	PD-L1 inhibitor	1, 2	ORR 7%	2 PR; 12 weeks DCR 25%	NCT01693562
GO27831	Atezolizumab	PD-L1 inhibitor	1	Not reported	1 pt had TTP of 9.8 months	NCT01375842
Ralph et al.	Tremelimumab	CTLA-4 inhibitor	2	ORR 5%	1 pt with PR > 30 months, 4 pts with SD	[39]
KEYNOTE-012	Pembrolizumab	PD-1 inhibitor	1b	ORR 22%		[40]
KEYNOTE-061	Pembrolizumab	PD-1 inhibitor	3	Negative	Median OS 9.1 vs. 8.3 months (HR 0.82, 95% CI 0.66–1.03; $p = 0.0421$)	[32]

PD-1 programmed death-1, PD-L1 programmed death-ligand 1, CTLA-4 cytotoxic T lymphocyte-associated protein 4, ORR objective response rate, PR partial response, DCR disease control rate, TTP time to progression, pt patient, SD stable disease, TRAE treatment-related adverse events in 10% of the patients who received nivolumab compared to 4% in the placebo arm. No new safety signals were observed in the study. Similar results were observed in KEYNOTE-059, a global open-label single-arm multi-cohort phase 2 trial that investigated pembrolizumab, a PD-1 inhibitor, in patients with treatment-refractory GE cancers [31]. In Cohort 1, patients received pembrolizumab 200 mg Q3 weeks for up to 2 years or until disease progression or intolerable toxicity. The primary endpoint of the study was safety and ORR in all patients and in the subset of patients with PD-L1+ tumors. PD-L1 expression was evaluated by the PD-L1 IHC 22C3 pharmDx Kit (Dako), and PD-L1 positivity was based on a combined positive score (CPS) $\geq$ 1. CPS is determined by the number of PD-L1 staining cells (tumor cells, lymphocytes, macrophages) divided by the total number of tumor cells evaluated, multiplied by 100 [31]. Of the 259 patients enrolled in Cohort 1, an ORR of 11.6% was observed in all patients where patients with PD-L1+ had an ORR of 15.5% versus 6.4% in PD-L1- tumors [31]. Forty-six patients (17.8%) experienced one or more grade 3 to 5 treatment-related adverse events [31]. Based on these results, the FDA approved pembrolizumab for patients with locally advanced or metastatic GE adenocarcinoma whose tumors express PD-L1.

In contrast to the results observed in ATTRACTION-02 and KEYNOTE-059, several other randomized clinical trials that investigated PD-1 or PD-L1 inhibitors failed to demonstrate any meaningful clinical activity in GE cancers (Table 14.2). KEYNOTE-061, a randomized phase 3 trial, investigated pembrolizumab versus paclitaxel in patients with treatment-refractory GE cancers whose tumors expressed PD-L1 positivity [32]. The primary endpoints were overall survival and progression-free survival in patients with a programmed cell death-ligand 1 (PD-L1) combined positive score (CPS) of 1 or higher. Pembrolizumab did not significantly improve OS compared to paclitaxel, where patients treated with pembrolizumab had a median OS of 9.1 months versus 8.3 months in patients treated with paclitaxel (HR 0.82, 95% CI 0.66–1.03, p = 0.0421) [32]. There was no significant difference in PFS between the two treatment arms (1.5 months in patients treated with pembrolizumab versus 4.1 months with paclitaxel) (HR 1.27, 95% CI 1.03–1.57) [32]. JAVELIN Gastric 300 (NCT02625623), a global randomized phase 3 trial, investigated avelumab, a PD-L1 inhibitor, compared to physician's choice of chemotherapy (irinotecan or paclitaxel) in patients with advanced GE cancer that progressed or relapsed after two prior chemotherapy regimens. While the results have not been published, a press release stated that the study failed to demonstrate a survival benefit from avelumab therapy.

Thus, taking into consideration the positive and negative results observed across several phase 3 trials, it is evident that further work needs to be done to refine and identify patients with GE cancers that will benefit from immunotherapeutic approaches. In 2014, The Cancer Genome Atlas (TCGA) completed a comprehensive molecular assessment of GE cancers. The TCGA characterized four distinct molecular subtypes, Epstein-Barr virus (EBV), microsatellite instability (MSI), genomically stable (GS), and chromosomal instability (CIN), which were based on various alterations which included gene mutations, copy number alterations, gene expression, and DNA methylation [33]. Each of the molecular subtypes is characterized by distinct genomic characteristics, where tumors positive for EBV displayed *PIK3CA* mutations and PD-L1 amplification, in contrast to the CIN subtype, which was characterized by marked aneuploidy and focal amplification of receptor tyrosine kinases. Potentially, these findings will allow for improved patient selection for specified therapies, which includes identifying specific patient subgroups likely to benefit from immunotherapies. Given the prevalence for PD-L1 and PD-L2 expression in the EBV molecular subgroup, patients with EBV+ tumors may be preferred candidates for immunotherapies aimed at targeting the PD-1/PD-L1 axis [34]. In addition to the characterization of patients subgroups likely to benefit from immunotherapies, further work is needed in the identification of novel biomarkers predictive for immunotherapy response which include PD-L1 expression, gene expression signatures, serum-soluble factors, and tumor mutation burden [35]. While PD-L1 has been suggested to be a potential predictive biomarker, it appears to be prognostic, as clinical activity is observed in patients who tumors do not express PD-L1 [31]. However, given the association between MSI-H and response to checkpoint inhibitors, MSI positivity is predictive for response to PD-1 blockade and should be assessed in all patients with GE cancers [36]. While immune checkpoint inhibitors have demonstrated modest activity in patients that response to these agents, future strategies aimed at enhancing the anti-tumor immune response including the combination of various novel agents are needed. CHECKMATE-032 investigated nivolumab at varying doses in combination with ipilimumab, an anti-CTLA-4 antibody, in patients with treatment-refractory GE cancer, where the primary endpoint of the study was ORR. Despite including a relatively treatment-refractory cohort of patients, the combination of nivolumab (1 mg/kg Q3 weeks) and ipilimumab (3 mg/kg Q3 weeks) resulted in an ORR of 24%, where patients with PD-L1 positivity had a ORR of 40% (4 out of 10 patients) compared to 22% in the PD-L1 negative cohort (7 out of 32 patients) [37]. While the combination demonstrated promising clinical activity, 21% of patients treated with nivolumab (1 mg/kg Q3 weeks) and ipilimumab (3 mg/kg Q3 weeks) experienced serious treatment-related adverse events, of which 17% were grade 3 or 4 [37]. Thus, despite the encouraging clinical activity observed from the combination of PD-1 and CTLA-4 inhibitors, an improvement in the toxicity profile is needed prior to its application into clinical practice. Alternative strategies, aimed at targeting other suppressive immune checkpoint proteins including LAG-3 and IDO (tryptophan-catabolizing enzyme that contributes to an immunosuppressive tumor microenvironment), are ongoing in early phase trials.

Conclusions and Future Directions

Treatment of advanced GE cancers remains an unmet need, where standard treatment regimens provide modest improvement in patient outcomes. Recent advances, primarily in our understanding of the molecular subtypes present in GE cancers, are encouraging and have spurred further investigation in tailoring studies toward specific subgroups of patients. While early findings with immunotherapies are promising, further work is needed, primarily in the understanding of the immune system and the immunosuppressive tumor microenvironment, which will allow the development and investigation of novel alternate therapies aimed at stimulating the immune system.

References

1. Ferlay J, Soerjomataram I, Dikshit R, Eser S, Mathers C, Rebelo M, Parkin DM, Forman D, Bray F. Cancer incidence and mortality worldwide: sources, methods and major patterns in GLOBOCAN 2012. Int J Cancer. 2015;136:E359–86.
2. Howlader N, Noone AM, Krapcho M, Miller D, Bishop K, Kosary CL, Yu M, Ruhl J, Tatalovich Z, Mariotto A, Lewis DR, Chen HS, et al. SEER cancer statistics review, 1975-2014. Bethesda, MD: National Cancer Institute; 2018. https://seer.cancer.gov/statfacts/html/esoph.html, based on November 2016 SEER data submission, posted to the SEER web site, April 2018.
3. Fuchs CS, Tomasek J, Yong CJ, Dumitru F, Passalacqua R, Goswami C, Safran H, Dos Santos LV, Aprile G, Ferry DR, Melichar B, Tehfe M, et al. Ramucirumab monotherapy for previously treated advanced gastric or gastro-oesophageal junction adenocarcinoma (REGARD): an international, randomised, multicentre, placebo-controlled, phase 3 trial. Lancet. 2014;383:31–9.
4. Wilke H, Muro K, Van Cutsem E, Oh SC, Bodoky G, Shimada Y, Hironaka S, Sugimoto N, Lipatov O, Kim TY, Cunningham D, Rougier P, et al. Ramucirumab plus paclitaxel versus placebo plus paclitaxel in patients with previously treated advanced gastric or gastro-oesophageal junction adenocarcinoma (RAINBOW): a double-blind, randomised phase 3 trial. Lancet Oncol. 2014;15:1224–35.
5. Bang YJ, Van Cutsem E, Feyereislova A, Chung HC, Shen L, Sawaki A, Lordick F, Ohtsu A, Omuro Y, Satoh T, Aprile G, Kulikov E, et al. Trastuzumab in combination with chemotherapy versus chemotherapy alone for treatment of HER2-positive advanced gastric or gastro-oesophageal junction cancer (ToGA): a phase 3, open-label, randomised controlled trial. Lancet. 2010;376:687–97.
6. Jorgensen JT, Hersom M. HER2 as a prognostic marker in gastric cancer—a systematic analysis of data from the literature. J Cancer. 2012;3:137–44.
7. Baselga J, Cortes J, Kim SB, Im SA, Hegg R, Im YH, Roman L, Pedrini JL, Pienkowski T, Knott A, Clark E, Benyunes MC, et al. Pertuzumab plus trastuzumab plus docetaxel for metastatic breast cancer. N Engl J Med. 2012;366:109–19.
8. Yamashita-Kashima Y, Iijima S, Yorozu K, Furugaki K, Kurasawa M, Ohta M, Fujimoto-Ouchi K. Pertuzumab in combination with trastuzumab shows significantly enhanced antitumor activity in HER2-positive human gastric cancer xenograft models. Clin Cancer Res. 2011;17:5060–70.
9. Tabernero J, Hoff PM, Shen L, Ohtsu A, Shah MA, Cheng K, Song C, Wu H, Eng-Wong J, Kang YK. 616O Pertuzumab (P) + trastuzumab (H) + chemotherapy (CT) for HER2-positive metastatic gastric or gastro-oesophageal junction cancer (mGC/GEJC): final analysis of a Phase III study (JACOB). Ann Oncol. 2017;28:mdx369–mdx.
10. Geyer CE, Forster J, Lindquist D, Chan S, Romieu CG, Pienkowski T, Jagiello-Gruszfeld A, Crown J, Chan A, Kaufman B, Skarlos D, Campone M, et al. Lapatinib plus capecitabine for HER2-positive advanced breast cancer. N Engl J Med. 2006;355:2733–43.
11. Hecht JR, Bang YJ, Qin SK, Chung HC, Xu JM, Park JO, Jeziorski K, Shparyk Y, Hoff PM, Sobrero A, Salman P, Li J, et al. Lapatinib in combination with capecitabine plus oxaliplatin in human epidermal growth factor receptor 2-positive advanced or metastatic gastric, esophageal, or gastroesophageal adenocarcinoma: TRIO-013/LOGiC-a randomized phase III trial. J Clin Oncol. 2016;34:443–51.
12. Satoh T, Xu RH, Chung HC, Sun GP, Doi T, Xu JM, Tsuji A, Omuro Y, Li J, Wang JW, Miwa H, Qin SK, et al. Lapatinib plus paclitaxel versus paclitaxel alone in the second-line treatment

of HER2-amplified advanced gastric cancer in Asian populations: TyTAN--a randomized, phase III study. J Clin Oncol. 2014;32:2039–49.

13. LoRusso PM, Weiss D, Guardino E, Girish S, Sliwkowski MX. Trastuzumab emtansine: a unique antibody-drug conjugate in development for human epidermal growth factor receptor 2-positive cancer. Clin Cancer Res. 2011;17:6437–47.

14. Barok M, Tanner M, Koninki K, Isola J. Trastuzumab-DM1 is highly effective in preclinical models of HER2-positive gastric cancer. Cancer Lett. 2011;306:171–9.

15. Thuss-Patience PC, Shah MA, Ohtsu A, Van Cutsem E, Ajani JA, Castro H, Mansoor W, Chung HC, Bodoky G, Shitara K, Phillips GDL, van der Horst T, et al. Trastuzumab emtansine versus taxane use for previously treated HER2-positive locally advanced or metastatic gastric or gastro-oesophageal junction adenocarcinoma (GATSBY): an international randomised, open-label, adaptive, phase 2/3 study. Lancet Oncol. 2017;18:640–53.

16. Ferrara N, Gerber HP, LeCouter J. The biology of VEGF and its receptors. Nat Med. 2003;9:669–76.

17. Maeda K, Chung YS, Takatsuka S, Ogawa Y, Onoda N, Sawada T, Kato Y, Nitta A, Arimoto Y, Kondo Y, et al. Tumour angiogenesis and tumour cell proliferation as prognostic indicators in gastric carcinoma. Br J Cancer. 1995;72:319–23.

18. Hegde PS, Jubb AM, Chen D, Li NF, Meng YG, Bernaards C, Elliott R, Scherer SJ, Chen DS. Predictive impact of circulating vascular endothelial growth factor in four phase III trials evaluating bevacizumab. Clin Cancer Res. 2013;19:929–37.

19. Chen J, Zhou SJ, Zhang Y, Zhang GQ, Zha TZ, Feng YZ, Zhang K. Clinicopathological and prognostic significance of galectin-1 and vascular endothelial growth factor expression in gastric cancer. World J Gastroenterol. 2013;19:2073–9.

20. Ohtsu A, Shah MA, Van Cutsem E, Rha SY, Sawaki A, Park SR, Lim HY, Yamada Y, Wu J, Langer B, Starnawski M, Kang YK. Bevacizumab in combination with chemotherapy as first-line therapy in advanced gastric cancer: a randomized, double-blind, placebo-controlled phase III study. J Clin Oncol. 2011;29:3968–76.

21. Shen L, Li J, Xu J, Pan H, Dai G, Qin S, Wang L, Wang J, Yang Z, Shu Y, Xu R, Chen L, et al. Bevacizumab plus capecitabine and cisplatin in Chinese patients with inoperable locally advanced or metastatic gastric or gastroesophageal junction cancer: randomized, double-blind, phase III study (AVATAR study). Gastric Cancer. 2015;18:168–76.

22. Fuchs CS, Shitara K, Bartolomeo MD, Lonardi S, Al-Batran S-E, Cutsem EV, Ilson DH, Tabernero J, Chau I, Ducreux M, Mendez GA, Alavez AM, et al. RAINFALL: a randomized, double-blind, placebo-controlled phase III study of cisplatin (Cis) plus capecitabine (Cape) or 5FU with or without ramucirumab (RAM) as first-line therapy in patients with metastatic gastric or gastroesophageal junction (G-GEJ) adenocarcinoma. J Clin Oncol. 2018;36:5.

23. Grothey A, Van Cutsem E, Sobrero A, Siena S, Falcone A, Ychou M, Humblet Y, Bouche O, Mineur L, Barone C, Adenis A, Tabernero J, et al. Regorafenib monotherapy for previously treated metastatic colorectal cancer (CORRECT): an international, multicentre, randomised, placebo-controlled, phase 3 trial. Lancet. 2013;381:303–12.

24. Li J, Qin S, Xu J, Xiong J, Wu C, Bai Y, Liu W, Tong J, Liu Y, Xu R, Wang Z, Wang Q, et al. Randomized, double-blind, placebo-controlled phase III trial of apatinib in patients with chemotherapy-refractory advanced or metastatic adenocarcinoma of the stomach or gastro-esophageal junction. J Clin Oncol. 2016;34:1448–54.

25. Larkin J, Chiarion-Sileni V, Gonzalez R, Grob JJ, Cowey CL, Lao CD, Schadendorf D, Dummer R, Smylie M, Rutkowski P, Ferrucci PF, Hill A, et al. Combined nivolumab and ipilimumab or monotherapy in untreated melanoma. N Engl J Med. 2015;373:23–34.

26. Motzer RJ, Escudier B, McDermott DF, George S, Hammers HJ, Srinivas S, Tykodi SS, Sosman JA, Procopio G, Plimack ER, Castellano D, Choueiri TK, et al. Nivolumab versus everolimus in advanced renal-cell carcinoma. N Engl J Med. 2015;373:1803–13.

27. Nghiem PT, Bhatia S, Lipson EJ, Kudchadkar RR, Miller NJ, Annamalai L, Berry S, Chartash EK, Daud A, Fling SP, Friedlander PA, Kluger HM, et al. PD-1 blockade with pembrolizumab in advanced merkel-cell carcinoma. N Engl J Med. 2016;374:2542–52.

28. Reck M, Rodriguez-Abreu D, Robinson AG, Hui R, Csoszi T, Fulop A, Gottfried M, Peled N, Tafreshi A, Cuffe S, O'Brien M, Rao S, et al. Pembrolizumab versus chemotherapy for PD-L1-positive non-small-cell lung cancer. N Engl J Med. 2016;375:1823–33.
29. Tamura T, Ohira M, Tanaka H, Muguruma K, Toyokawa T, Kubo N, Sakurai K, Amano R, Kimura K, Shibutani M, Maeda K, Hirakawa K. Programmed death-1 ligand-1 (PDL1) expression is associated with the prognosis of patients with stage II/III gastric cancer. Anticancer Res. 2015;35:5369–76.
30. Kang YK, Boku N, Satoh T, Ryu MH, Chao Y, Kato K, Chung HC, Chen JS, Muro K, Kang WK, Yeh KH, Yoshikawa T, et al. Nivolumab in patients with advanced gastric or gastro-oesophageal junction cancer refractory to, or intolerant of, at least two previous chemotherapy regimens (ONO-4538-12, ATTRACTION-2): a randomised, double-blind, placebo-controlled, phase 3 trial. Lancet. 2017;390:2461–71.
31. Fuchs CS, Doi T, Jang RW, Muro K, Satoh T, Machado M, Sun W, Jalal SI, Shah MA, Metges JP, Garrido M, Golan T, et al. Safety and efficacy of pembrolizumab monotherapy in patients with previously treated advanced gastric and gastroesophageal junction cancer: phase 2 clinical KEYNOTE-059 trial. JAMA Oncol. 2018;4:e180013.
32. Shitara K, Ozguroglu M, Bang YJ, Bartolomeo MD, Mandala M, Ryu MH, Fornaro L, Olesinski T, Caglevic C, Chung HC, Muro K, Goekkurt E, et al. Pembrolizumab versus paclitaxel for previously treated, advanced gastric or gastro-oesophageal junction cancer (KEYNOTE-061): a randomised, open-label, controlled, phase 3 trial. Lancet. 2018;392:123–33.
33. Cancer Genome Atlas Research N. Comprehensive molecular characterization of gastric adenocarcinoma. Nature. 2014;513:202–9.
34. Saito R, Abe H, Kunita A, Yamashita H, Seto Y, Fukayama M. Overexpression and gene amplification of PD-L1 in cancer cells and PD-L1(+) immune cells in Epstein-Barr virus-associated gastric cancer: the prognostic implications. Mod Pathol. 2017;30:427–39.
35. Baniak N, Senger JL, Ahmed S, Kanthan SC, Kanthan R. Gastric biomarkers: a global review. World J Surg Oncol. 2016;14:212.
36. Le DT, Durham JN, Smith KN, Wang H, Bartlett BR, Aulakh LK, Lu S, Kemberling H, Wilt C, Luber BS, Wong F, Azad NS, et al. Mismatch repair deficiency predicts response of solid tumors to PD-1 blockade. Science. 2017;357:409–13.
37. Janjigian YY, Ott PA, Calvo E, Kim JW, Ascierto PA, Sharma P, Peltola KJ, Jaeger D, Evans TRJ, Braud FGD, Chau I, Tschaika M, et al. Nivolumab ± ipilimumab in pts with advanced (adv)/metastatic chemotherapy-refractory (CTx-R) gastric (G), esophageal (E), or gastroesophageal junction (GEJ) cancer: CheckMate 032 study. J Clin Oncol. 2017;35:4014.
38. Fuchs CS, Doi T, Jang RW-J, Muro K, Satoh T, Machado M, Sun W, Jalal SI, Shah MA, Metges J-P, Garrido M, Golan T, et al. KEYNOTE-059 cohort 1: efficacy and safety of pembrolizumab (pembro) monotherapy in patients with previously treated advanced gastric cancer. J Clin Oncol. 2017;35:4003.
39. Ralph C, Elkord E, Burt DJ, O'Dwyer JF, Austin EB, Stern PL, Hawkins RE, Thistlethwaite FC. Modulation of lymphocyte regulation for cancer therapy: a phase II trial of tremelimumab in advanced gastric and esophageal adenocarcinoma. Clin Cancer Res. 2010;16:1662–72.
40. Muro K, Chung HC, Shankaran V, Geva R, Catenacci D, Gupta S, Eder JP, Golan T, Le DT, Burtness B, McRee AJ, Lin CC, et al. Pembrolizumab for patients with PD-L1-positive advanced gastric cancer (KEYNOTE-012): a multicentre, open-label, phase 1b trial. Lancet Oncol. 2016;17:717–26.

Immunotherapy in Esophageal Cancer

15

Megan Greally and Geoffrey Y. Ku

Introduction

Esophageal cancer is a highly aggressive malignancy which accounted for approximately 17,290 cases and 15,850 deaths in the United States in 2018 [1]. Given that 50% of patients present with overt metastatic disease and the majority of patients initially treated for locoregional disease will develop recurrence, most patients will undergo systemic therapy during their disease course [2]. Chemotherapy remains the core treatment for metastatic disease and improves survival over best supportive care. However, the prognosis for patients with esophageal cancer remains poor as the majority of patients will develop chemotherapy resistance and treatment options beyond first- and second-line therapy are limited. With the exception of the addition of trastuzumab to first-line therapy for Her2-positive disease [3] and ramucirumab as monotherapy [4] or in combination with paclitaxel [5] as second-line treatment, clinical trials evaluating targeted therapies have been disappointing. Thus, there is a critical need to improve outcomes for those diagnosed with this virulent disease.

In recent years, immunotherapy has emerged as a novel treatment strategy that has transformed outcomes in several cancers with a historically poor prognosis such as melanoma and lung cancer. In 2011, ipilimumab, an anti-cytotoxic T lymphocyte antigen-4 (CTLA-4) antibody, became the first immune checkpoint inhibitor to be approved by the US Food and Drug Administration (FDA) for the treatment of advanced melanoma [6, 7]. More recently, antibodies that target the programmed death (PD-1) and PD-ligand-1 (PD-L1) pathways have undergone evaluation in multiple other solid tumors which has resulted in FDA approval of these agents in melanoma, non-small cell lung cancer, renal cell carcinoma, urothelial carcinoma,

M. Greally (✉) · G. Y. Ku
Gastrointestinal Oncology Service, Department of Medicine, Memorial Sloan Kettering Cancer Center, New York, NY, USA
e-mail: greallym@mskcc.org; kug@mskcc.org

© Springer Nature Switzerland AG 2020
N. F. Saba, B. F. El-Rayes (eds.), *Esophageal Cancer*,
https://doi.org/10.1007/978-3-030-29832-6_15

289

squamous cell carcinoma of the head and neck, classical Hodgkin's lymphoma, hepatocellular carcinoma, and microsatellite unstable (MSI) or mismatch repair protein-deficient (dMMR) cancers (irrespective of primary site, the first site-agnostic approval for any anti-cancer therapy).

There has been similarly strong interest in the evaluation of immune checkpoint inhibitors in esophageal cancer, and, in a landmark approval, the FDA approved pembrolizumab in September 2017 for patients with advanced gastric and gastro-esophageal (GE) junction adenocarcinoma whose tumors express PD-L1 and who have received two or more prior chemotherapy regimens.

This chapter will outline the biologic rationale for the use of immunotherapeutic strategies in the treatment of cancer and discuss the accumulating data regarding their use in esophageal cancer.

CTLA-4 and PD-1/PD-L1/PD-L 2 Pathways in Cancer

CTLA-4 is a protein receptor that was implicated as a negative regulator of T cell activation in the mid-1990s [8, 9]. When expressed on the cell surface of CD4+ and CD8+ T lymphocytes, it has higher affinity for the costimulatory receptors B7-1 and B7-2 present on antigen-presenting cells (APCs) than for the T cell costimulatory receptor CD28 [10]. Expression of CTLA-4 is upregulated by the degree of T cell receptor activation and cytokines such as interleukin-2 and interferon gamma, which form a feedback inhibition loop on activated T effector cells. Activation leads to downregulation of the immune response triggered by APCs. CTLA-4 was impli-cated in the immune surveillance of cancer in sarcoma and colon adenocarcinoma mouse models, in which inhibition of CTLA-4 led to tumor shrinkage [11]. Ipilimumab was subsequently the first immune checkpoint inhibitor approved, based on a phase III study demonstrating that it improved survival in patients with metastatic malignant melanoma [6].

PD-1 is a transmembrane protein expressed on T cells, B cells, and NK cells. Like CTLA-4, it is also an inhibitory immune checkpoint molecule [12]. It has two ligands, PD-L1 and PD-L2. PD-L1 is expressed on multiple tissue types, including tumor cells, while PD-L2 is mostly expressed on APCs. When PD-L1 expressed on tumor cells binds to PD-1 on activated T cells, an inhibitory signal is delivered to the T cell, which inhibits apoptosis of the tumor cell [13]. Unlike CTLA-4, which func-tions in T cell activation, the PD-1/PD-L1/PD-L2 pathway is thought to protect cells from attack by T cells [14].

CTLA-4 Inhibitors in Esophageal Cancer

By blocking the interaction between CTLA-4 and its ligands, CTLA-4 inhibition promotes antitumor responses through T cell activation and tumor infiltration. Two anti-CTLA-4 antibodies, ipilimumab and tremelimumab, have been evaluated in esophageal cancer. The results presented below suggest very modest single-agent activity for these drugs, and, indeed, further evaluation of this class of drug as monotherapy in esophageal cancer is not being undertaken.

Tremelimumab

Tremelimumab was the first immune checkpoint inhibitor to be evaluated in esophagogastric (EG) cancer when a phase II study investigated its role as second-line therapy in patients with metastatic gastric, GE junction, and esophageal adenocarcinomas [15]. Tremelimumab was administered every 3 months at a dose of 15 mg/kg. Of 18 patients who were enrolled, 15 had received 1 prior line of therapy, and 3 had received 2 lines of therapy. At the end of the first cycle of treatment, four patients (22%) had stable disease. One of these patients had incremental reduction in tumor burden and achieved a partial response (PR) after 8 cycles that was sustained after 33 months of follow-up. Median PFS was 2.83 months and median OS was 4.83 months. Encouragingly, however, 12-month OS was 33%. Of note, the dose of tremelimumab utilized in this study was lower than the 10 mg/kg every 4 weeks dose currently being evaluated in ongoing studies, although it is unclear if a dose-relationship curve exists for these drugs.

Ipilimumab

A phase II study subsequently evaluated ipilimumab monotherapy in patients with advanced gastric or GE junction adenocarcinoma [16]. Patients who had achieved at least stable disease after first-line fluoropyrimidine/platinum chemotherapy were randomized to ipilimumab, 10 mg/kg every 3 weeks for four doses followed by 10 mg/kg every 12 weeks for up to 3 years, or best supportive care (BSC), which mainly consisted of continuation of fluoropyrimidine maintenance. The primary endpoint of the study was immune-related progression-free survival (irPFS). In 114 patients accrued, there was disappointingly no improvement in irPFS (2.92 vs. 4.90 months) or median overall survival (OS; 12.7 vs. 12.1 months) with ipilimumab. Grade 3/4 treatment-related adverse events (TRAEs) occurred more frequently in the patients who received ipilimumab vs. those who received active BSC (23% vs. 9%) and included diarrhea, fatigue, and hypothyroidism.

PD-1 and PD-L1 Checkpoint Inhibitors in Esophageal Cancer

Based on prolonged overall survival (OS) in phase III trials and durable responses in phase II studies, antibodies inhibiting PD-1 (pembrolizumab and nivolumab) and PD-L1 (avelumab, durvalumab, and atezolizumab) have now been approved in several malignancies, and these drugs continue to be extensively evaluated in EG cancer. The following section provides a summary of the current data for PD-1 and PD-L1 blockade in this disease.

Pembrolizumab

The KEYNOTE-012 study was a phase Ib multicenter, open-label, multi-cohort study which evaluated the benefit of pembrolizumab (10 mg/kg every 2 weeks) in patients with PD-L1-positive recurrent or metastatic gastric and GE junction tumors [17]. PD-L1 positivity was defined as ≥1% membrane staining of tumor or contiguous mononuclear inflammatory cells. The PD-L1 positivity rate was 40% based on this criterion (65 of 162 tumors). Thirty-nine patients were enrolled on the study, 68% of whom had received ≥2 prior therapies for metastatic disease and 49% of whom were from Asia. Of 36 patients evaluable for response by central assessment, 8 (22%) had an objective response, all PRs. At the time of analysis, median duration of response (DOR) was 40 weeks, and four of the responders had ongoing response. Median PFS was 1.9 months, and median OS was 11.4 months, while the 6- and 12- month OS rates were 66% and 42%, respectively. Grade 3/4 TRAEs occurred in five patients (13%; six events), consisting of fatigue, pemphigoid, hypothyroidism, peripheral sensory neuropathy, and one case of grade 4 pneumonitis.

The similarly designed phase Ib KEYNOTE-028 trial enrolled a cohort of patients with advanced esophageal cancer [18, 19]. This study evaluated pembrolizumab (10 mg/kg every 2 weeks) in 23 patients with PD-L1-positive esophageal carcinoma, 17 with squamous cell carcinoma (SCC), 5 with adenocarcinoma, and 1 with mucoepidermoid carcinoma. Of the 90 patients screened, 41% had PD-L1-positive tumors. Most patients (87%) had received ≥2 prior therapies. The objective response rate (ORR) was 30%, all PRs, and two patients had stable disease. Five of seven responses were ongoing at the time of data analysis with a median DOR of 40 weeks. The 6- and 12-month PFS rates were 30.4% and 21.7%, respectively. Grade 3 TRAEs occurred in four patients including lymphopenia, anorexia, liver disorder, and generalized rash.

The promising activity of pembrolizumab in gastric/GE junction tumors led to the KEYNOTE-059 study, a large phase II study that enrolled such patients into several cohorts. Cohort 1 investigated pembrolizumab 200 mg every 3 weeks in patients who had received ≥2 prior therapies. Patients in cohort 2 received pembrolizumab 200 mg in addition to cisplatin 80 mg/m^2 and fluoropyrimidine (5-fluorouracil [5-FU] 800 mg/m^2 or capecitabine 1000 mg/m^2) in the first-line setting every 3 weeks for 6 cycles followed by pembrolizumab plus fluoropyrimidine maintenance for up to 2 years or until disease progression.

KEYNOTE-059 cohort 1 enrolled 259 patients, and data has been presented in abstract form [20]. In this heavily pretreated population (51.7% received 2 prior lines of therapy and 29% and 19.3% had received 3 or ≥4 prior lines of therapy, respectively), the ORR was 11.6% after a median follow-up of 5.8 months. The complete response (CR) rate was 2.3% and 9.3% of patients had a PR. The median DOR was 8.4 months. Patients treated in the third-line setting had an ORR of 16.4% vs. 6.4% in patients who had received ≥4 prior therapies. The median PFS and OS in the intention-to-treat population were 2.0 and 5.6 months, respectively, and the 12-month OS rate was 23.4%. ORRs were improved in the approximately 60% of patients with tumors that were PD-L1 positive (defined when the combined positive score or CPS [the sum of the percentage of PD-L1 staining tumor cells, lymphocytes, and macrophages divided by the percentage of PD-L1 staining tumor cells] is ≥1%) vs. PD-L1 negative (15.5% vs. 6.4%), and the median DOR was 16.3 months in the PD-L1-positive group vs. 6.9 months in the PD-L1-negative group. When patients who received pembrolizumab in the third-line setting were stratified by PD-L1 status, the ORR was 22.7% in those who had PD-L1-positive tumors vs. 8.6% in those with PD-L1-negative tumors. Treatment was well tolerated with 2.3% of patients experiencing a grade 3/4 TRAE and grade 3/3 immune-related AEs occurring in 4.6%.

These results suggest that pembrolizumab has promising, albeit modest, activity in pretreated advanced gastric and GE junction adenocarcinoma and led to US FDA approval of pembrolizumab in September 2017 for patients with advanced gastric/ GE junction adenocarcinoma whose tumors express PD-L1, as determined by the PD-L1 IHC 22C3 pharmDx Kit (Dako) companion test by CPS, and who have received ≥2 prior chemotherapy regimens. This accelerated approval is contingent on the results of a confirmatory trial.

Preliminary efficacy and safety data from cohort 2 of the KEYNOTE-059 study have also been presented in abstract form. This arm enrolled 25 patients to the combination of fluoropyrimidine/cisplatin and pembrolizumab as first-line therapy. The safety profile was encouraging. At a median follow-up of 14.7 months, grade 3/4 TRAEs occurred in 76% of patients, most commonly neutropenia and stomatitis. Three patients experienced grade 3 immune-related AEs (rash and nephritis). There were no treatment-related deaths. The ORR was 60% and 20% of patients had stable disease (for a disease control rate of 80%). The ORR was 69% in patients with PD-L1-positive tumor vs. 38% in patients with PD-L1-negative tumor. The median DOR was 4.6 months. Median PFS and OS were 6.6 and 20.8 months, respectively. While the small number of patients and relatively early follow-up preclude any specific conclusions, these early data suggest that combination pembrolizumab and cisplatin/fluoropyrimidine has a manageable toxicity profile and encouraging anti-tumor activity.

Nivolumab

The largest study to date evaluating nivolumab in EG adenocarcinoma is the ATTRACTION-2 trial [21]. This was a randomized phase III East Asian study of 493 patients who had received ≥2 prior chemotherapy regimens. Patients were randomized 2:1 to nivolumab vs. placebo. The study revealed a very modest improvement in PFS (1.61 vs. 1.45 months, hazard ratio or HR 0.60, $p < 0.0001$) and OS (5.26 vs. 4.14 months, HR 0.63, $p < 0.0001$) in patients who received nivolumab. The 12-month OS rate was a landmark 26.6% vs. 10.9% in favor of nivolumab in a chemorefractory population. The ORR was 11.2% (vs. 0% in the placebo group), with a median DOR to nivolumab of 9.53 months. An exploratory analysis retrospectively assessed PD-L1 expression status in approximately 40% of patients ($n = 192$); 13.5% ($n = 26$) of tumors were assessed to be PD-L1 positive using the

28-8 pharmDx assay (Dako) and by assessing PD-L1 staining only in tumor cells. Similar OS was observed (5.22 months vs. 6.05 months in patients with PD-L1-positive vs. PD-L1-negative tumors) irrespective of PD-L1 positivity (<1% vs. ≥1% of tumor cells). The HRs for OS favored nivolumab over placebo in both PD-L1-positive and PD-L1-negative groups, suggesting an OS benefit regardless of PD-L1 expression status. Based on this study, nivolumab received regulatory approval in Japan for use in all patients irrespective of PD-L1 status in October 2017.

When comparing outcomes from the nivolumab ATTRACTION-2 study with cohort 1 of the pembrolizumab KEYNOTE-059, we observe near identical results for OS, PFS, and ORR as outlined in Table 15.1. Taken together, both of these studies confirm activity for anti-PD-1 blockade in EG adenocarcinomas and would suggest no difference in activity between Asian and non-Asian patients.

As further evidence, CheckMate 032 was a phase I/II open-label study which demonstrated a comparable degree of benefit from nivolumab in a Western population of patients. This study evaluated the safety and activity of nivolumab alone or in combination with ipilimumab in advanced and metastatic solid tumors and enrolled 160 heavily pretreated patients (79% had received ≥2 regimens) with advanced chemotherapy-refractory gastric, esophageal, or GE junction cancer. Patients were enrolled sequentially to three different arms: 3 mg/kg of nivolumab every 2 weeks (N3), 1 mg/kg of nivolumab plus 3 mg/kg of ipilimumab (N1 plus I3), and 3 mg/kg of nivolumab plus 1 mg/kg of ipilimumab (N3 plus I1) every 3 weeks for 4 cycles followed by nivolumab 3 mg/kg every 2 weeks until disease progression or intolerable toxicity. Preliminary results have been presented in abstract form [22] now published - https://www.ncbi.nlm.nih.gov/pubmed/30110194.

Results from the 59 patients enrolled in the N3 cohort suggest similar activity to pembrolizumab and nivolumab in an Asian population, as outlined in Table 15.1. The ORR was 12%, with a median time to response of 1.6 months and DOR of 7.1 months in the responders. In this study, PD-L1 positivity was assessed using a cutoff of ≥1% tumor staining on immunohistochemistry (assessed by the Dako 28-8 pharmDx assay).

Finally, a Japanese open-label, single-arm, multicenter phase II study has evaluated nivolumab in patients with esophageal SCC [23]. This study enrolled 65 patients who had received a median of three prior therapies. Of 65 patients enrolled, 64 were evaluable for the primary endpoint of ORR, and all patients were assessable for safety. Eleven patients (17%) had an ORR. The median PFS and OS were 1.5 and 10.8 months, respectively. The toxicity profile was manageable, and there were no treatment-related deaths.

Avelumab

Avelumab is the anti-PD-L1 antibody that has undergone the most extensive evaluation to date.

The phase Ib JAVELIN study [24] enrolled patients with GE junction and gastric adenocarcinoma. This study enrolled patients to two cohorts. The first evaluated

Table 15.1 Published or completed trials in metastatic EG carcinoma current as of March 2018

		Phase	Line of therapy	Patients	ORR	Median PFS (months)	Median OS (months)	1-year OS
Pembrolizumab	KEYNOTE-012[13]	Ib	≥2	n = 39 PD-L1+ n = 39	22%	1.9	11.4	42%
	KEYNOTE-059[16] Cohort 1	II	≥2	n = 259 PD-L1+ n = 148 PD-L1− n = 109	11.6% 15.5% 6.4%	2.0	5.6	23.4%
	KEYNOTE-059[17] Cohort 2 (pembro + chemo)	II	1st	n = 25 PD-L1+ n = 16 PD-L1− n = 8	60% 68.8% 37.5%	6.6	20.8	NS
Nivolumab	CheckMate 032[19] N 3 mg	I/II	≥2	n = 59 PD-L1+ n = 16 PD-L1− n = 26	12% 19% 12%	1.4	6.2	39%
	ATTRACTION-2[22]	III	≥2	n = 493	11.2%	1.65	5.32	26.6%
Nivolumab + ipilimumab	CheckMate 032[19] N 1 mg + I3 mg	I/II	≥2	n = 49 PD-L1+ n = 10 PD-L1− n = 32	24% 40% 22%	1.4	6.9	35%
	CheckMate 032[19] N 3 mg + I1 mg	I/II	≥2	n = 52 PD-L1+ n = 13 PD-L1− n = 30	8% 23% 0%	1.6	4.8	24%
Avelumab	JAVELIN Solid Tumor[23]	Ib	≥2	N = 20 PD-L1+ n = NS PD-L1− n = NS	15% 20% 0%	11.6 weeks 36 weeks 11.6 weeks	NS	NS
Durvalumab[24]	N/A	I	≥2	n = 16	25%	NS	NS	NS

NS not stated, ORR overall response rate, mPFS median progression-free survival, mOS median overall survival, OS overall survival, N nivolumab, I ipilimumab patients who had progressed following first-line therapy ($n = 20$), and the second enrolled patients whose disease had not progressed on first-line therapy to maintenance therapy ($n = 55$). Both groups received avelumab 10 mg/kg every 2 weeks. In patients who received second-line avelumab, the ORR was 15% (3/20). PD-L1 expression ($\geq 1\%$ cutoff) was evaluable in 12/20 patients. Median PFS was 36 weeks (95% CI 6.0, 36.0) for patients with PD-L1-positive tumors and 11.6 weeks (2.1, 21.9) for those with PD-L1-negative tumors. In the cohort who received maintenance avelumab, the ORR was 7.3% (4/55, 1 complete response), and 47.3% had stable disease. The disease control rate was 54.5%. PD-L1 expression was evaluable in 43/55 patients, and median PFS for PD-L1-positive and PD-L1-negative status was 17.6 weeks (95% CI 5.9, 18.0) and 11.6 weeks (2.1, 21.9) respectively.

The small numbers here preclude a definitive conclusion. Activity appears to be generally comparable to anti-PD-1 antibodies and has paved the way for two phase III studies; the top-line results of one of which is discussed below.

Durvalumab

Durvalumab is a PD-L1 inhibitor also being evaluated in EG cancer. Data presented in abstract form reported an acceptable safety profile with early evidence of clinical activity in multiple tumor types. The ORR was 7% (2/28 patients) in the gastro-esophageal cohort with a disease control rate of 25% at 12 weeks [25].

A phase Ib/II study is currently enrolling patients with GE junction or gastric adenocarcinomas in the second- and third-line setting to single-agent durvalumab, single-agent tremelimumab, or the combination of both (NCT02340975).

Combination Immune Checkpoint Inhibition

Data for combination immune checkpoint blockade in EG carcinoma comes from the CheckMate 032 study [22] now published - https://www.ncbi.nlm.nih.gov/pubmed/30110194. As discussed above, this study enrolled patients into three cohorts, two of which evaluated combination ipilimumab and nivolumab. Forty-nine patients received N1 + I3, and 52 patients received N3 + I1. Almost half of patients in both cohorts had received ≥ 3 lines of therapy. The highest ORR of all three cohorts was 24%, reported in the N1 + I3 group. The ORR for the N3 + I1 group was 8%. Median OS was 6.9 months in the N1 + I3 and 4.8 months in the N3 + I1 group. In both groups, the ORR was higher in patients with PD-L1-positive tumors: 40% vs. 22% in the N1 + I3 group and 23% vs. 0% in the N3 + I1 group. Grade ≥ 3 toxicities were highest in patients who received N1 + I3 (35%). The most common G3/4 toxicities were diarrhea and elevated transaminases.

It is important that these results are interpreted with caution both because of the small numbers and also because patients were enrolled sequentially and not in a randomized fashion. Nevertheless, several hypothesis-generating observations arise. The ORR for the N3 + I1 arm (8%) was certainly not superior to that observed in the N3 arm

(12%)—and the KEYNOTE-059 and ATTRACTION-2 studies. In addition, despite a higher ORR (40%; the highest reported in any immunotherapy study in EG cancer) in the N1 + I3 arm than the N3 arm (12%), the 18-month OS rate was similar between the groups (28% vs. 25%). Of note, the 18-month OS was 13% in the N3 + I1 cohort. Based on the superior ORR (at the expense of significant additional toxicity, which is discussed below), the N1 + I3 dose was selected for study in the phase III CheckMate 649 trial.

Phase III Studies

Based on the results outlined in this chapter, numerous phase III studies are ongoing or planned, both in the metastatic and adjuvant settings, as noted in Table 15.2. Studies evaluating single-agent therapy include the KEYNOTE-061 study which is a randomized study investigating second-line therapy with pembrolizumab vs. paclitaxel in patients with advanced gastric or GE junction adenocarcinoma. In a recent press release, it was reported that the primary endpoints of OS and PFS were not met in patients whose tumors are PD-L1 positive [26]. We await presentation of the data. The KEYNOTE-063 study (NCT03019588) is a similarly designed study evaluating pembrolizumab vs. paclitaxel in an Asian population.

The KEYNOTE-181 trial (NCT02564263) is investigating pembrolizumab vs. physician's choice of paclitaxel, docetaxel, or irinotecan in metastatic adenocarcinoma or SCC of the esophagus and Siewert type I GE junction adenocarcinoma following progression of disease on first-line therapy. ONO-4538 is a phase III, randomized, open-label study (NCT02569242) evaluating nivolumab vs. paclitaxel or docetaxel in patients with advanced esophageal cancer who have progressed following standard therapies.

Finally, the JAVELIN 300 study also evaluated avelumab in the third-line setting in a phase III study which randomized patients to avelumab vs. physician's choice chemotherapy with paclitaxel or irinotecan (NCT02625623). In a recent press release, it was reported that the trial did not meet its pre-specified primary endpoint of improved OS for avelumab vs. chemotherapy, and again we await presentation of the data.

The KEYNOTE-062 study (NCT02494583) is investigating pembrolizumab monotherapy vs. 5-FU/cisplatin vs. 5-FU/cisplatin plus pembrolizumab as first-line therapy for patients with advanced PD-L1-positive, Her2-negative gastric or GE junction adenocarcinoma [27]. This trial has accrued, and results are anticipated. The CheckMate 649 trial (NCT02872116) is a phase III study which is currently enrolling patients with advanced gastric or GE junction tumor (irrespective of PD-L1 status) and randomizing them to ipilimumab/nivolumab vs. fluoropyrimidine/oxaliplatin plus nivolumab vs. fluoropyrimidine/oxaliplatin in the first-line setting [28]. The JAVELIN 100 (NCT02625610) study is evaluating an alternative strategy of avelumab administered as switch maintenance therapy compared with continuation of first-line chemotherapy after 12 weeks of induction 5-FU/oxaliplatin or capecitabine/oxaliplatin. This trial is a randomized, open-label, multicenter phase III study which will enroll 466 patients with GE junction and gastric carcinoma. Patients must have at least stable disease following 12 weeks of first-line therapy to be eligible for enrollment.

Table 15.2 Selected ongoing studies evaluating immune checkpoint inhibition +/− combinatorial strategies in EG adenocarcinoma current as of March 2018

Drug	Trial identifier	Phase	Neoadjuvant/adjuvant	1st line metastatic	2nd line metastatic	3rd line metastatic	Status
Pembrolizumab	KEYNOTE-062 (NCT02494583)	III		Pembro vs. pembro + cisplatin/5-FU vs. cisplatin/5-FU			Accrued
	KEYNOTE-061 (NCT02370498)	III			Pembro vs. paclitaxel in gastric or GE junction AC		Completed
	KEYNOTE-181 (NCT02564263)	III			Pembro vs. taxane or irinotecan in AC or SCC esophagus or Siewert I AC of GE junction		Recruiting
	KEYNOTE-180 (NCT02559687)	II				Pembro in AC or SCC esophagus or Siewert I AC of GE junction	Ongoing
	(NCT02918162)	II	Pembro + platinum/5-FU doublet or triplet for 3 cycles pre-op and 3 cycles post-op, followed by maintenance pembro X 1 year				Recruiting
	PROCEED (NCT03064490)	II	Pembro + carbo/taxol + radiation, followed by adjuvant pembro X 3 cycles				Recruiting
	(NCT02954536)	II		Pembro +trastuzumab + platinum/5-FU			Recruiting

Drug	Trial	Phase	Description	Comparison	Status
Nivolumab	CheckMate 649 (NCT02872116)	III		Nivo + Ipi vs. Nivo + FOLFOX vs. FOLFOX	Recruiting
	ONO-4538 (NCT02569242)	III		Nivo vs. taxane	Recruiting
	CheckMate 577 (NCT02743494)	III	Nivo vs. placebo as adjuvant therapy in pts with residual disease after multi-modal therapy		Recruiting
	FRACTION-GC NCT02935634	II Adaptive		Tx-naïve and Tx-experienced tracks Nivo + Ipi vs. Nivo + anti-LAG Other combinations will open Any line of therapy	Recruiting
	CheckMate 906 (NCT03044613)	Ib	Induction Nivo x2 cycles (arm A) vs. induction Nivo + Ipi x1 cycle (arm B) prior to CRT + Nivo followed by surgery in pts with stage II/III esophageal or GE junction cancer		Recruiting

(continued)

Table 15.2 (continued)

Drug	Trial identifier	Phase	Neoadjuvant/adjuvant	1st line metastatic	2nd line metastatic	3rd line metastatic	Status
Avelumab	JAVELIN 100 (NCT02625610)	III		Oxaliplatin/5-FU followed by maintenance avelumab vs. maintenance chemotherapy or BSC			Recruiting
	JAVELIN 300 (NCT02625623)	III				Avelumab + BSC vs. taxane or irinotecan +BSC or BSC alone	Ongoing
Durvalumab	(NCT02340975)	Ib/II			Durvalumab vs. tremelimumab vs. durvalumab + tremelimumab	Durvalumab + tremelimumab	Recruiting
	(NCT02658214)	Ib		Durvalumab + tremelimumab + oxaliplatin/5-FU			Recruiting
	NCT 02639065	II	Durvalumab every 4 weeks × 12 months in pts with residual disease after multi-modal therapy				Recruiting

5-FU indicates 5-fluorouracil; BSC best supportive care; carbo carboplatin; FOLFOX folinic acid, 5-fluorouracil, and oxaliplatin; Ipi ipilimumab; Nivo nivolumab; Pembro pembrolizumab; AC adenocarcinoma; SCC squamous cell carcinoma; GE gastroesophageal; pts patients; CRT chemoradiation; Tx treatment

Neoadjuvant and Adjuvant Therapy

Given the activity of immune checkpoint inhibitors in the advanced disease setting, the role of these agents in the perioperative setting in patients with stage II and III disease is now being investigated.

The CheckMate 577 is a global phase III study evaluating adjuvant nivolumab vs. placebo in patients with locally advanced esophageal or GE junction carcinoma who have persistent disease (defined as $ypT_{any}N+$ or $ypT1-4N_{any}$) following preoperative chemoradiation and surgery with clear margins [29]. The optimal treatment strategy for patients who do not achieve a pathologic complete response is unclear, and the current standard of care is surveillance following trimodality therapy. Thus, there is an unmet need in this patient population as the risk of disease relapse is high, particularly in patients with node-positive disease at surgery [30].

The KEYNOTE-585 study (NCT03221426) is a phase III study enrolling patients with $\geq T3$ and/or node-positive gastric and GE junction adenocarcinoma to perioperative chemotherapy (either a fluoropyrimidine/cisplatin doublet or the FLOT regimen of 5-FU/leucovorin/oxaliplatin/docetaxel) with or without pembrolizumab.

In Asian countries, postoperative adjuvant chemotherapy with tegafur-gimeracil-oteracil potassium (S-1) or oxaliplatin/capecitabine (CapeOx) is the standard of care in patients with pathologic stage II/III gastric and GE junction cancer. The ATTRACTION-05 study is a randomized phase III trial randomizing East Asian patients with stage II/III disease to adjuvant nivolumab or placebo in combination with physician's choice of S-1 or CapeOx [31].

Several phase I/II studies with various designs are assessing the safety and efficacy of nivolumab, pembrolizumab, durvalumab, and atezolizumab in the neoadjuvant setting, administered either sequentially or concurrently with neoadjuvant chemoradiation. See Table 15.2 for a list of selected adjuvant and neoadjuvant studies.

Ramucirumab and PD-1 or PD-L1 Inhibition

Targeted therapies against the vascular endothelial growth factor (VEGF) pathway elicit effects on tumor antigenicity and intratumoral T cell infiltration. These immunomodulating effects provide a rationale for combining anti-angiogenic therapies with immunotherapies [32–34]. Preclinical studies suggest that simultaneous blockade of the VEGFR-2 and PD-1/PD-L1 pathways induces synergistic antitumor effects by inhibiting tumor angiogenesis and promoting access of cytotoxic T cells to tumors while preventing exhaustion of T cells [35–37].

Ramucirumab is a monoclonal antibody against VEGFR2, which is approved as a single agent and in combination with paclitaxel for second-line therapy in EG adenocarcinoma. A multi-cohort phase Ia/b study was the first to evaluate the simultaneous targeting of both PD-1 and VEGFR2 in EG adenocarcinoma [38]. Forty-one patients with advanced gastric or GE junction adenocarcinomas were enrolled to three cohorts: previously treated with chemotherapy (cohorts A and B) or chemotherapy-naive (cohort A2). Ramucirumab was administered at 8 mg/kg on days 1 and 8 (cohorts A and A2) or 10 mg/kg on day 1 (cohort B) with pembro-lizumab 200 mg every 3 weeks. The response rate in cohorts A and B was 7%. PFS and OS rates at 6 months were 22.4% and 51.2%, respectively. Eighteen patients were enrolled to the A2 cohort with an ORR of 17%. Any grade toxicity was 80%, with a grade 3/4 toxicity rate of 24%, most commonly colitis (7%) and hypertension (7%).

Preliminary results from a phase Ib expansion of cohort A2 (treatment-naïve) reported an ORR of 25% (7/28 patients; 6 had PD-L1-positive tumors). An additional 12 patients (43%) had stable disease for a disease control rate (DCR) of 68%. The median PFS was 5.3 months and median OS was not reached. The most common grade 3 toxicity was hypertension [39].

Results from an ongoing multi-cohort phase I study evaluating ramucirumab plus durvalumab in patients with metastatic gastric or GE junction adenocarcinoma, who have progressed after one or two prior lines of therapy, reported an ORR of 17% (5/29 patients) and DCR of 55%. All responders had PD-L1 tumor expression ≥25%. The combination appears safe with hypertension the most common grade 3/4 TRAE reported [40].

While the safety profile in both studies is encouraging, the ORR observed with pembrolizumab/ramucirumab is modest when compared to that achieved with standard-of-care chemotherapy in the first-line setting. Furthermore, although the ORR of 17% achieved with durvalumab/ramucirumab compares relatively favorably to that observed with single-agent PD-1/PD-L1 therapy in the chemorefractory setting, the ORR seen with paclitaxel/ramucirumab in the second-line setting (28%) was substantially higher [5]. Ultimately, these likely represent sufficient data to justify further evaluation of this combinatorial strategy, although the increasingly crowded therapeutic environment and the awaited results of several potentially practice-changing phase III studies make the optimal setting for such evaluation unclear at this time.

Trastuzumab and PD-1 Inhibition

Trastuzumab has been shown to have immune-mediated mechanisms of action [41], and a preclinical study demonstrated that Her2-targeted therapy in combination with anti-PD-L1 therapy enhanced tumor growth inhibition, increasing the rates and durability of therapeutic response [42].

Our group at Memorial Sloan Kettering Cancer Center is currently evaluating pembrolizumab in combination with fluoropyrimidine/platinum and trastuzumab as first-line therapy in patients with metastatic Her2-positive EG adenocarcinoma with the rationale that dual Her2 and PD-1 blockade will result in enhanced antibody-dependent cell-mediated cytotoxicity (ADCC), NK cell degranulation, and synergistic activity in combination with fluoropyrimidine and platinum.

Immune-Related Toxicity from Checkpoint Inhibitors

In stimulating the immune system with immune checkpoint blockade, the goal is to achieve a hyper-activated T cell response directed toward tumor cells. However, this response can affect normal tissues and result in inflammatory side effects, termed immune-related adverse events (irAEs). The underlying mechanism has not been fully elucidated but is thought to relate to the role that immune checkpoints play in maintaining immunologic homeostasis [30]. IrAEs can affect any organ system but most commonly involve the skin, gastrointestinal tract, endocrine glands, and liver. Pulmonary, central nervous system, renal, ocular, pancreatic, cardiovascular, musculoskeletal, and hematologic immune-related toxicities occur less frequently [43, 44].

To date, the irAEs that have been observed in trials of checkpoint inhibitors in EG carcinoma have been similar to published data in other disease types with no new safety signals observed [45]. IrAEs are more likely to occur in patients treated with CTLA-4 blockade than those treated with PD-1 and PD-L1 blockade [45]. With respect to EG carcinoma, the highest rate of adverse events in any trial to date was observed in the CheckMate 032 study in patients who received the combination of nivolumab 1 mg/kg and ipilimumab 3 mg/kg [22]. Table 15.3 summarizes the grade 3–4 adverse events reported in studies of checkpoint inhibition in EGC to date.

Biomarkers of Response

The results of the discussed studies uniformly suggest that benefit from immune checkpoint inhibitors is modest in an unselected population. Most studies report a median PFS of less than 2 months, even in the setting of encouraging OS, suggesting that most patients develop rapid progression on these treatments. Therefore, the identification of biomarkers to select patients most likely to benefit from these expensive and potentially toxic agents is a priority.

Approximately 40–60% of gastric and GE junction cancers are PD-L1 positive [17, 20]. There has been significant effort to investigate if PD-L1 expression by IHC can be used as a biomarker to select patients for immune-directed therapy with PD-1/PD-L1 inhibition, and pembrolizumab is approved by the FDA only in patients with PD-L1-positive tumors, as determined by the PD-L1 IHC 22C3 pharmDx Kit (Dako) companion test, and who have received ≥2 prior chemotherapy regimens. However, PD-L1 has been demonstrated to be an imperfect biomarker in EG cancer and many other cancers. Although PD-L1-positive tumors appear more likely to respond to treatment with anti-PD-1 and anti-PD-L1 antibodies, many of the studies above report responses and disease control even in patients with PD-L1-negative tumors. There appear to be key differences between PD-L1 expression in EG carcinoma and lung cancer and melanoma, and its role as a biomarker does not appear to be generalizable between tumor types. In EG cancer, expression of PD-L1

Table 15.3 Grade 3–4 toxicity from checkpoint inhibitors in EGC clinical studies

		Fatigue	Rash	Pruritus	Diarrhea	Colitis	Elevated LFTs	Pneumonitis	Endocrinopathies	Nephritis	Myelotoxicity
Pembrolizumab	KEYNOTE-012	5%	3% (pemphigoid)	0%	0%	0%	0%	3%	3% (hypothyroidism)	0%	0%
	KEYNOTE-059 Cohort 1	2.3%	0.8%	0%	1.2%	1.2%	0%	0.8%	0.4% hypothyroidism 0.4% thyroiditis	0%	0%
	KEYNOTE-059 Cohort 2	8%	8%	0%	0%	0%	0%	0%	0%	4%	64% (low neutrophils) 8% (low platelets) 8% (anemia)
Nivolumab	CheckMate 032 N3 mg	2%	0%	0%	2%	0%	8%	0%	0%	0%	0%
	ATTRACTION-2	0.6%	0%	0%	0.6%	0%	0.9%	0%	0%	0%	0%
Nivolumab + Ipilimumab	CheckMate 032 N1 mg + I3 mg	6%	0%	2%	14%	0%	24%	0%	0%	0%	0%
	CheckMate 032 N3 mg + I1 mg	0%	0%	0%	2%	0%	6%	0%	0%	0%	0%
Avelumab	JAVELIN Solid Tumor	2.7%	0%	0%	0%	0%	0%	0%	0%	0%	2.7% (low platelets) 2.7% (anemia)
Tremelimumab	N/A	0%	0%	0%	0%	5.5%	5.5%	0%	0%	0%	0%

principally occurs on infiltrating myeloid cells at the invasive margin and much less frequently on cancer cells [46, 47]. One study reported only a 12% rate of tumor cell membranous expression, while 44% of immune stromal cells expressed PD-L1 [46]. It remains unclear if membranous versus stromal PD-L1 expression affects response in EG cancer. Of note, rates of PD-L1 staining on tumor cells and immune cells are higher in tumors that are Epstein-Barr virus (EBV) positive and MSI high [48].

Testing of PD-L1 status is also a complex issue as there are currently several antibodies available for PD-L1 testing which have not been directly compared against each other. In addition, expression is heterogeneous, and the optimal cutoff is uncertain, and concordance among pathologists is also more difficult to achieve when measuring PD-L1 positivity on immune cells. This is highlighted by the discrepancy in PD-L1 positivity rates reported between the KEYNOTE-012 and KEYNOTE-059 studies (40% and 60%, respectively) and the ATTRACTION-2 study which reported a 13.5% PD-L1 positivity rate. The lower PD-L1 positivity rate in the ATTRACTION-2 study is at least in part because only tumor cells were evaluated for PD-L1 staining (unlike the CPS used in the pembrolizumab studies, which includes both tumor cells and peri-tumoral mononuclear cells). Similarly, the difference in PD-L1 positivity rate between the KEYNOTE-012 and KEYNOTE-059 studies—despite the use of the same antibody and the CPS—can be explained because later studies have mandated rapid processing of cell blocks for central PD-L1 testing. In light of the current uncertainty regarding the utility of PD-L1 as a biomarker, ongoing studies are enrolling patients irrespective of PD-L1 status.

A mononuclear inflammatory cell density score (0–4) was assessed in the KEYNOTE-012 study as part of a clinical trial PD-L1 assay which scored expression separately in tumor cells and mononuclear inflammatory cells. Of 35 patients who had biopsies available to be assessed with this assay, 4 of 9 (44%) patients who had a mononuclear cell density score of 3 had a PR, compared with 4 of 26 (15%) of patients with a score of ≤ 2. While the number of patients whose tumors were analyzed is small, the data is provocative.

The KEYNOTE-012 also investigated the potential use of an interferon-γ signature that may correlate with an increased magnitude of benefit from immune checkpoint inhibitors. In the KEYNOTE-001 study a six-gene (*CXCL9, CXCL10, IDO1, IFNG, HLA-DRA*, and *STAT1*) signature of interferon-γ-related genes was associated with response to pembrolizumab in patients with melanoma [49]. In KEYNOTE-012, an interferon-γ composite score was calculated using gene expression profiling of RNA isolated from tumor samples. Only 30 tumor samples were evaluable. There was a trend toward treatment response in patients with a higher interferon-γ signature score (p = 0.070) [17]. An 18-gene T cell-inflamed gene expression signature, derived using pretreatment tissue samples from previous pembrolizumab studies across several cancer types, significantly predicted ORR and survival in patients treated with pembrolizumab [50, 51]. In the KEYNOTE-059 study, this gene expression signature was significantly associated with improved response to pembrolizumab (p = 0.014) in 144 patients who had pretreatment testing of tumor tissue [20]. These results suggest that this gene signature may be a meaningful predictor of treatment response. Further evaluation is attractive as it may be more reproducible and robust as a biomarker than PD-L1.

The Cancer Genome Atlas (TCGA) has characterized molecular subtypes of gastric and esophageal cancer, and an active area of investigation is correlation of response to immune checkpoint inhibition with the different subtypes identified. The four subtypes identified in gastric cancer are EBV positive, MSI, genomically stable (GS), and chromosomal instability (CIN) [52]. Esophageal adenocarcinomas strongly resemble the chromosomal instability variant of gastric adenocarcinoma. The EBV and MSI subtypes show elevated mutation rates. It is speculated that most patients who respond to single-agent checkpoint inhibitors may have these subtypes and patients with the genomically stable and chromosomally unstable subtypes may require combination immunotherapeutic strategies. Of note, MSI-high tumors occur very rarely in esophageal cancer, and squamous cell esophageal carcinomas show frequent genetic amplifications [53].

While the MSI subgroup accounted for 22% of gastric cancer patients in TCGA analysis, this subgroup is rarely seen in esophageal and GE junction cancers. In addition, this analysis was restricted to patients with operable tumors, and the incidence of MSI tumors in the metastatic setting appears to be much lower [54]. The presence of MSI is associated with an elevated mutation rate and has been identified as predictive of response to PD-1 inhibition.

Finally, it is now well recognized that PD-1 inhibitors are active in dMMR/MSI-high colorectal cancer, and Le et al. also reported significant activity in other mismatch repair-deficient gastrointestinal cancers, including gastric cancer [55]. In the first tissue site-agnostic approval, the FDA granted accelerated approval in May 2017 to pembrolizumab for adult and pediatric patients with unresectable or metastatic, MSI solid tumors that had progressed on one standard therapy. The approval was based on data from 149 patients with MSI cancers enrolled across 5 single-arm clinical trials [56], and 9 of these patients had EG carcinoma. In this group, ORR was 56% with five out of the nine patients achieving a PR. Given this approval, testing for MSI via PCR or MMR status by immunohistochemistry is now standard, along with Her2 and PD-L1 testing. In addition, the increasing use of next-generation sequencing assays will also identify patients with MSI tumors. Furthermore, high somatic mutational burden may be of value in predicting response to PD-1 inhibitors, and only melanoma, lung, and bladder cancers demonstrate a more mutated profile than esophagogastric cancers [57]. Elevated tumor mutation burden may occur independent of MSI disease and may be utilized in the future as a biomarker of response [54].

Future Directions

At the time of the writing of this manuscript, we are rapidly approaching the end of the era of evaluating single-agent immunotherapy or even single-agent PD-1 blockade combined with chemotherapy. The next decade of evaluation will involve combination immunotherapeutic strategies to try to increase the proportion of patients who benefit but also the magnitude of benefit obtained. Studies evaluating chemotherapy in combination with immune checkpoint inhibition are at an advanced stage, and selected studies are described in Table 15.2.

There are multiple ongoing or planned phase I/II studies investigating immune checkpoint inhibitors in combination with other immunotherapy drugs, targeted therapies, or locoregional approaches (such as radiation or ablative procedures).

An interesting combinatorial strategy that is being investigated in other cancers is the combination of immune checkpoint inhibition with locoregional therapy aiming to generate an abscopal effect which refers to response in gross tumor sites outside of a radiation field. The hypothesis is that lysis of tumor cells by a locoregional treatment results in the release of intracellular antigens which are then recognized by an activated immune system and resultant anti-cancer effect. This has previously been observed in patients with melanoma who were receiving ipilimumab and then received palliative radiation [58]. A number of studies are currently evaluating this strategy in microsatellite-stable/MMR-proficient colorectal cancer.

Other immunomodulators, vaccines, and targeted therapies are also being evaluated in combination with immune checkpoint inhibitors. Many of these studies are specifically enrolling patients with EG carcinoma but also include studies that are enrolling EG patients in dose-expansion cohorts.

Conclusions

The evaluation of immune checkpoint inhibitors both in solid tumors and more recently in EG cancer has occurred at a rapid pace. The ATTRACTION-2 (nivolumab) and KEYNOTE-059 (pembrolizumab) studies have now confirmed activity of single-agent anti-PD-1 antibodies in the chemorefractory setting, resulting in regulatory approval (pembrolizumab in the United States and nivolumab in Japan) for this indication. While this is positive progress in a disease that continues to have a dismal prognosis, benefit is modest with single-agent therapy. It is therefore important to harness the knowledge that we have gained to date in order to move forward with innovative immunotherapeutic strategies to further improve outcomes for patients with EG cancer. The results of the ongoing phase III studies are awaited with eager anticipation, and it is hoped that they will establish new treatment paradigms in this disease. Finally, these drugs are not without both clinical and financial toxicities, with responses rates observed in a small albeit significant population of patients. Therefore, it is imperative that we attempt to identify patients most likely to benefit from these therapies, through ongoing correlative efforts and the next generation of studies evaluating combinatorial strategies.

References

1. Siegel RL, Miller KD, Jemal A. Cancer statistics, 2018. CA Cancer J Clin. 2018;68(1):7–30.
2. Ku GY, Ilson DH. Management of gastric cancer. Curr Opin Gastroenterol. 2014;30(6):596–602.

 3. Bang YJ, Van Cutsem E, Feyereislova A, Chung HC, Shen L, Sawaki A, et al. Trastuzumab in combination with chemotherapy versus chemotherapy alone for treatment of HER2-positive advanced gastric or gastro-oesophageal junction cancer (ToGA): a phase 3, open-label, randomised controlled trial. Lancet. 2010;376(9742):687–97.
 4. Fuchs CS, Tomasek J, Yong CJ, Dumitru F, Passalacqua R, Goswami C, et al. Ramucirumab monotherapy for previously treated advanced gastric or gastro-oesophageal junction adenocarcinoma (REGARD): an international, randomised, multicentre, placebo-controlled, phase 3 trial. Lancet. 2014;383(9911):31–9.
 5. Wilke H, Muro K, Van Cutsem E, Oh SC, Bodoky G, Shimada Y, et al. Ramucirumab plus paclitaxel versus placebo plus paclitaxel in patients with previously treated advanced gastric or gastro-oesophageal junction adenocarcinoma (RAINBOW): a double-blind, randomised phase 3 trial. Lancet Oncol. 2014;15(11):1224–35.
 6. Hodi FS, O'Day SJ, McDermott DF, Weber RW, Sosman JA, Haanen JB, et al. Improved survival with ipilimumab in patients with metastatic melanoma. N Engl J Med. 2010;363(8):711–23.
 7. Robert C, Thomas L, Bondarenko I, O'Day S, Weber J, Garbe C, et al. Ipilimumab plus dacarbazine for previously untreated metastatic melanoma. N Engl J Med. 2011;364(26):2517–26.
 8. Chambers CA, Sullivan TJ, Allison JP. Lymphoproliferation in CTLA-4-deficient mice is mediated by costimulation-dependent activation of CD4+ T cells. Immunity. 1997;7(6):885–95.
 9. Tivol EA, Borriello F, Schweitzer AN, Lynch WP, Bluestone JA, Sharpe AH. Loss of CTLA-4 leads to massive lymphoproliferation and fatal multiorgan tissue destruction, revealing a critical negative regulatory role of CTLA-4. Immunity. 1995;3(5):541–7.
10. Walker LS, Sansom DM. The emerging role of CTLA4 as a cell-extrinsic regulator of T cell responses. Nat Rev Immunol. 2011;11(12):852–63.
11. Leach DR, Krummel MF, Allison JP. Enhancement of antitumor immunity by CTLA-4 blockade. Science. 1996;271(5256):1734–6.
12. Freeman GJ, Long AJ, Iwai Y, Bourque K, Chernova T, Nishimura H, et al. Engagement of the PD-1 immunoinhibitory receptor by a novel B7 family member leads to negative regulation of lymphocyte activation. J Exp Med. 2000;192(7):1027–34.
13. Zou W, Chen L. Inhibitory B7-family molecules in the tumour microenvironment. Nat Rev Immunol. 2008;8(6):467–77.
14. Sharma P, Allison JP. The future of immune checkpoint therapy. Science (New York, NY). 2015;348(6230):56–61.
15. Ralph C, Elkord E, Burt DJ, O'Dwyer JF, Austin EB, Stern PL, et al. Modulation of lymphocyte regulation for cancer therapy: a phase II trial of tremelimumab in advanced gastric and esophageal adenocarcinoma. Clin Cancer Res. 2010;16(5):1662–72.
16. Bang YJ, Cho JY, Kim YH, Kim JW, Di Bartolomeo M, Ajani JA, et al. Efficacy of sequential ipilimumab monotherapy versus best supportive care for unresectable locally advanced/metastatic gastric or gastroesophageal junction cancer. Clin Cancer Res. 2017;23(19):5671–8.
17. Muro K, Chung HC, Shankaran V, Geva R, Catenacci D, Gupta S, et al. Pembrolizumab for patients with PD-L1-positive advanced gastric cancer (KEYNOTE-012): a multicentre, open-label, phase 1b trial. Lancet Oncol. 2016;17(6):717–26.
18. Doi T, Piha-Paul SA, Jalal SI, Mai-Dang H, Yuan S, Koshiji M, et al. Pembrolizumab (MK-3475) for patients with advanced esophageal carcinoma: preliminary results from KEYNOTE-028. J Clin Oncol. 2015;33(15_suppl):4010.
19. Doi T, Piha-Paul SA, Jalal SI, Mai-Dang H, Saraf S, Koshiji M, et al. Updated results for the advanced esophageal carcinoma cohort of the phase Ib KEYNOTE-028 study of pembrolizumab (MK-3475). J Clin Oncol. 2016;34(4_suppl):7.
20. Fuchs CS, Doi T, Jang RW-J, Muro K, Satoh T, Machado M, et al. KEYNOTE-059 cohort 1: efficacy and safety of pembrolizumab (pembro) monotherapy in patients with previously treated advanced gastric cancer. J Clin Oncol. 2017;35(15_suppl):4003.
21. Kang YK, Boku N, Satoh T, Ryu MH, Chao Y, Kato K, et al. Nivolumab in patients with advanced gastric or gastro-oesophageal junction cancer refractory to, or intolerant of, at least two previous chemotherapy regimens (ONO-4538-12, ATTRACTION-2): a randomised, double-blind, placebo-controlled, phase 3 trial. Lancet. 2017;390(10111):2461–71.

22. Janjigian YY, Ott PA, Calvo E, Kim JW, Ascierto PA, Sharma P, et al. Nivolumab ± ipilimumab in pts with advanced (adv)/metastatic chemotherapy-refractory (CTx-R) gastric (G), esophageal (E), or gastroesophageal junction (GEJ) cancer: CheckMate 032 study. J Clin Oncol. 2017;35(15_suppl):4014.
23. Kudo T, Hamamoto Y, Kato K, Ura T, Kojima T, Tsushima T, et al. Nivolumab treatment for oesophageal squamous-cell carcinoma: an open-label, multicentre, phase 2 trial. Lancet Oncol. 2017;18(5):631–9.
24. Chung HC, Arkenau H-T, Wyrwicz L, et al. Safety, PD-L1 expression, and clinical activity of avelumab (MSB0010718C), an anti-PD-L1 antibody, in patients with advanced gastric or gastroesophageal junction cancer. J Clin Oncol. 2016;34:167.
25. Segal N, Hamid O, Hwu W, Massard C, Butler M, Antonia S, et al. 1058PD—A phase I multi-arm dose-expansion study of the anti-programmed cell death-ligand-1 (PD-L1) antibody MEDI4736: Preliminary data. Ann Oncol. 2014;25(4):361–72.
26. http://www.mrknewsroom.com/news-release/corporate-news/merck-provides-update-keynote-061-phase-3-study-keytruda-pembrolizumab-p 2017.
27. Tabernero J, Bang Y-J, Fuchs CS, Ohtsu A, Kher U, Lam B, et al. KEYNOTE-062: phase III study of pembrolizumab (MK-3475) alone or in combination with chemotherapy versus chemotherapy alone as first-line therapy for advanced gastric or gastroesophageal junction (GEJ) adenocarcinoma. J Clin Oncol. 2016;34(4_suppl). TPS185-TPS.
28. Janjigian YY, Adenis A, Aucoin J-S, Barone C, Boku N, Chau I, et al. Checkmate 649: a randomized, multicenter, open-label, phase 3 study of nivolumab (Nivo) plus ipilimumab (Ipi) versus oxaliplatin plus fluoropyrimidine in patients (Pts) with previously untreated advanced or metastatic gastric (G) or gastroesophageal junction (GEJ) cancer. J Clin Oncol. 2017;35(4_suppl). TPS213-TPS.
29. Kelly RJ, Lockhart AC, Jonker DJ, Melichar B, Andre T, Chau I, et al. CheckMate 577: a randomized, double-blind, phase 3 study of nivolumab (Nivo) or placebo in patients (Pts) with resected lower esophageal (E) or gastroesophageal junction (GEJ) cancer. J Clin Oncol. 2017;35(4_suppl). TPS212-TPS.
30. Postow MA, Sidlow R, Hellmann MD. Immune-related adverse events associated with immune checkpoint blockade. N Engl J Med. 2018;378(2):158–68.
31. Terashima M, Kim YW, Yeh TS, Chung HC, Chen JS, Boku N, et al. 778TiPATTRACTION-05 (ONO-4538-38/BMS CA209844): a randomized, multicenter, double-blind, placebo- controlled Phase 3 study of Nivolumab (Nivo) in combination with adjuvant chemotherapy in pStage III gastric and esophagogastric junction (G/EGJ) cancer. Ann Oncol. 2017;28(suppl_5). mdx369.160-mdx369.160.
32. Hughes PE, Caenepeel S, Wu LC. Targeted therapy and checkpoint immunotherapy combinations for the treatment of cancer. Trends Immunol. 2016;37(7):462–76.
33. Motz GT, Coukos G. The parallel lives of angiogenesis and immunosuppression: cancer and other tales. Nat Rev Immunol. 2011;11(10):702–11.
34. Huang Y, Chen X, Dikov MM, Novitskiy SV, Mosse CA, Yang L, et al. Distinct roles of VEGFR-1 and VEGFR-2 in the aberrant hematopoiesis associated with elevated levels of VEGF. Blood. 2007;110(2):624–31.
35. Yasuda S, Sho M, Yamato I, Yoshiji H, Wakatsuki K, Nishiwada S, et al. Simultaneous blockade of programmed death 1 and vascular endothelial growth factor receptor 2 (VEGFR2) induces synergistic anti-tumour effect in vivo. Clin Exp Immunol. 2013;172(3):500–6.
36. Zou W, Wolchok JD, Chen L. PD-L1 (B7-H1) and PD-1 pathway blockade for cancer therapy: mechanisms, response biomarkers, and combinations. Sci Transl Med. 2016;8(328):328rv4.
37. Allen E, Jabouille A, Rivera LB, Lodewijckx I, Missiaen R, Steri V, et al. Combined antiangiogenic and anti-PD-L1 therapy stimulates tumor immunity through HEV formation. Sci Transl Med. 2017;9(385):eaak9679.
38. Chau IBJ, Calvo E, et al. Ramucirumab (R) plus pembrolizumab (P) in treatment naive and previously treated advanced gastric or gastroesophageal junction (G/GEJ) adenocarcinoma: a multi-disease phase I study. J Clin Oncol. 2017;35(15_suppl):4046.

39. Chau I, Penel N, Arkenau H-T, et al. Safety and antitumor activity of ramucirumab plus pembrolizumab in treatment naïve advanced gastric or gastroesophageal junction (G/GEJ) adenocarcinoma: Preliminary results from a multi-disease phase I study (JVDF). J Clin Oncol. 2018;36:101.
40. Bang Y-J, Golan T, Lin C-C, et al. Interim safety and clinical activity in patients (pts) with locally advanced and unresectable or metastatic gastric or gastroesophageal junction (G/GEJ) adenocarcinoma from a multicohort phase I study of ramucirumab (R) plus durvalumab (D). J Clin Oncol. 2018; 36:92.
41. Park S, Jiang Z, Mortenson ED, Deng L, Radkevich-Brown O, Yang X, et al. The therapeutic effect of anti-HER2/neu antibody depends on both innate and adaptive immunity. Cancer Cell. 2010;18(2):160–70.
42. Junttila TT, Li J, Johnston J, Hristopoulos M, Clark R, Ellerman D, et al. Antitumor efficacy of a bispecific antibody that targets HER2 and activates T cells. Cancer Res. 2014;74(19):5561–71.
43. Weber JS, Hodi FS, Wolchok JD, Topalian SL, Schadendorf D, Larkin J, et al. Safety profile of nivolumab monotherapy: a pooled analysis of patients with advanced melanoma. J Clin Oncol. 2017;35(7):785–92.
44. Naidoo J, Page DB, Li BT, Connell LC, Schindler K, Lacouture ME, et al. Toxicities of the anti-PD-1 and anti-PD-L1 immune checkpoint antibodies. Ann Oncol. 2015;26(12):2375–91.
45. El Osta B, Hu F, Sadek R, Chintalapally R, Tang SC. Not all immune-checkpoint inhibitors are created equal: meta-analysis and systematic review of immune-related adverse events in cancer trials. Crit Rev Oncol Hematol. 2017;119:1–12.
46. Thompson ED, Zahurak M, Murphy A, Cornish T, Cuka N, Abdelfatah E, et al. Patterns of PD-L1 expression and CD8 T cell infiltration in gastric adenocarcinomas and associated immune stroma. Gut. 2017;66(5):794–801.
47. Derks S, Nason KS, Liao X, Stachler MD, Liu KX, Liu JB, et al. Epithelial PD-L2 expression Marks Barrett's esophagus and esophageal adenocarcinoma. Cancer Immunol Res. 2015;3(10):1123–9.
48. Derks S, Liao X, Chiaravalli AM, Xu X, Camargo MC, Solcia E, et al. Abundant PD-L1 expression in Epstein-Barr Virus-infected gastric cancers. Oncotarget. 2016;7(22):32925–32.
49. Ribas A, Robert C, Hodi FS, Wolchok JD, Joshua AM, Hwu W-J, et al. Association of response to programmed death receptor 1 (PD-1) blockade with pembrolizumab (MK-3475) with an interferon-inflammatory immune gene signature. J Clin Oncol. 2015;33(15_suppl):3001.
50. Piha-Paul SA, Bennouna J, Albright A, Nebozhyn M, McClanahan T, Ayers M, et al. T-cell inflamed phenotype gene expression signatures to predict clinical benefit from pembrolizumab across multiple tumor types. J Clin Oncol. 2016;34(15_suppl):1536.
51. Ayers M, Lunceford J, Nebozhyn M, Murphy E, Loboda A, Kaufman DR, et al. IFN-gamma-related mRNA profile predicts clinical response to PD-1 blockade. J Clin Invest. 2017;127(8):2930–40.
52. The Cancer Genome Atlas Research N. Comprehensive molecular characterization of gastric adenocarcinoma. Nature. 2014;513(7517):202–9.
53. The Cancer Genome Atlas Research N. Integrated genomic characterization of oesophageal carcinoma. Nature. 2017;541:169.
54. Janjigian YY, Sanchez-Vega F, Jonsson P, Chatila WK, Hechtman JF, Ku GY, et al. Genetic predictors of response to systemic therapy in esophagogastric cancer. Cancer Discov. 2018;8(1):49–58.
55. Le D, Uram J, Wang H, Kemberling H, Eyring A, Bartlett B, et al. PD-1 blockade in mismatch repair deficient non-colorectal gastrointestinal cancers. J Clin Oncol. 2016;34:195.
56. https://www.accessdata.fda.gov/drugsatfda_docs/label/2017/125514s014lbl.pdf. 2017.
57. Alexandrov LB, Nik-Zainal S, Wedge DC, Aparicio SA, Behjati S, Biankin AV, et al. Signatures of mutational processes in human cancer. Nature. 2013;500(7463):415–21.
58. Postow MA, Callahan MK, Barker CA, Yamada Y, Yuan J, Kitano S, et al. Immunologic correlates of the abscopal effect in a patient with melanoma. N Engl J Med. 2012;366(10):925–31.

Palliative Approaches in Esophageal Cancer

16

Baiwen Li, Shanshan Shen, Cicily T. Vachaparambil, Vladimir Lamm, Qunye Guan, Jie Tao, Hui Luo, Huimin Chen, and Qiang Cai

Esophageal cancer is a lethal malignant disease and its incidence is still increasing. Despite progress in diagnosis and therapy that has been achieved in recent years, esophageal cancer remains a devastating disease and is one of the most frequent causes of cancer-related death in the world [1–3]. Esophageal cancer is usually clinically obscure until it has reached advanced stage. Substantially more than 50% of patients with esophageal cancer present at an incurable stage. Prolonged progression-free survival is possible only in a few of them. Thus, palliation rather than cure is the treatment goal for the majority of patients [4, 5]. The primary goals of palliative treatment are relieving dysphagia, managing pain, and improving quality of life. Caring for these patients requires a multidisciplinary approach including external beam radiation therapy (EBRT), chemotherapy, endoscopic dilatation and/ or stenting, photodynamic therapy, laser therapy, and palliative surgery. Dysphagia is the most common presenting symptom, often occurring secondary to intraluminal tumor growth and later secondary to treatment-induced fibrosis, postoperative

B. Li · H. Luo · H. Chen
Department of Gastroenterology, Shanghai General Hospital, Shanghai Jiaotong University, Shanghai, China

S. Shen
Department of Gastroenterology, Nanjing Drum TOwer Hospital, Nanjing University, Nanjing, China

C. T. Vachaparambil · V. Lamm · Q. Cai (✉)
Department of Medicine, Emory University, Atlanta, GA, USA
e-mail: qcai@emory.edu

Q. Guan
Department of Gastroenterology, Weihai Municipal Hospital, Weihai, China

J. Tao
Department of Hepatobiliary Surgery, The First Affiliated Hospital of Xi'an Jiaotong University, Xi'an, China

© Springer Nature Switzerland AG 2020
N. F. Saba, B. F. El-Rayes (eds.), *Esophageal Cancer*,
https://doi.org/10.1007/978-3-030-29832-6_16

Table 16.1 Current palliative modalities for dysphagia associated with esophageal cancer

Endoscopic techniques	Stent placement
	Photodynamic therapy (PDT)
	Nd:YAG
	Cryotherapy
	Ablation
	Argon plasma coagulation (APC)
	Chemical injection therapy
	Dilation
	Nasoenteric feeding tube
	Percutaneous endoscopic gastrostomy (PEG)
Non-endoscopic techniques	Radiation therapy
	Brachytherapy
	External beam radiotherapy
	Chemotherapy

anastomotic stricture, or pseudo-achalasia secondary to cancer infiltration of the myenteric plexus [6]. Dysphagia often progresses rapidly to the stage when patients lose their ability to swallow liquids and even saliva, which leads to sialorrhea, aspiration, and malnutrition [7, 8].

Since most patients with incurable esophageal cancer live no longer than 6 months, the aims of palliative treatment are to relieve dysphagia promptly, maintain swallowing function, improve nutrition, and avoid serious complications. It is important to realize that treatment of incurable esophageal cancer should be individualized and based on tumor stage, medical condition, performance status, and personal willingness of the patient. In addition, both the available expertise and results of prospective, randomized studies should be taken into consideration [9, 10]. A wide range of recently developed palliative treatment modalities are available (Table 16.1).

The main options can be divided into endoscopic and non-endoscopic approaches. The current available palliative treatment techniques are equally effective for esophageal adenocarcinoma (including adenocarcinoma located in the gastrointestinal junction, the GE junction) and esophageal squamous cell carcinoma [10]. We will mainly discuss the endoscopic palliative modalities in this chapter. Non-endoscopic procedures will be mentioned in other chapters.

In recent years, the advancement of endoscopy has offered physicians a variety of nonsurgical means to palliate malignant obstruction of the esophagus. Although there are many therapeutic options, they all have some limitations. Not all methods described here can be performed at every institution. Both physician and institutional experiences often influence the selection of treatment.

Stents and Stent Placement

In the 1990s, esophageal stenting was performed using plastic stents. Stent placement at that time required extensive esophageal dilation because the stent had a diameter of 15–20 mm which couldn't pass the stricture without dilation. Although

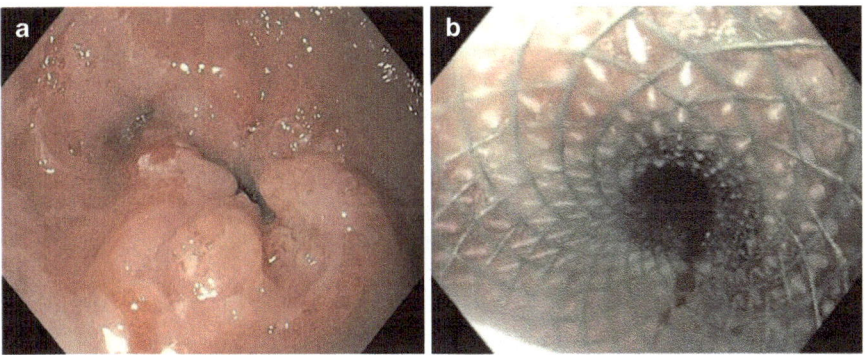

Fig. 16.1 (**a**) Middle esophageal adenocarcinoma with esophageal stricture; (**b**) partially covered metal esophageal stent placed (23 mm × 12 cm)

the plastic stents were inexpensive and relatively effective at palliation of malignant esophagobronchial fistulas, the thick and stiff walls of the stent caused chest pain and poor relief from dysphagia. In addition, old plastic stents were associated with a high incidence of complications, including perforation, migration, and high procedure-related mortality [6, 11]. During the past decade or so, self-expanding metal stents (SEMS) have become available for the treatment of malignant dysphagia and have almost replaced plastic stents. SEMS can be used to treat intrinsic and extrinsic tumors that cause malignant dysphagia. They are assembled in a tightly bound unit on a delivery catheter, greatly reducing the diameter of the delivery system. After endoscopic placement of the delivery system across the stricture, SEMS are deployed under endoscopic and fluoroscopic guidance, frequently without the need for pre-dilation [7, 8]. Once in proper position, SEMS is deployed by releasing the stent from the delivery system and allowing it to expand to its maximal diameter in a few hours. They can relieve dysphagia promptly (Fig. 16.1). Placement of SEMS is a minimally invasive procedure, with a significantly smaller risk of perforation compared with placement of plastic stents [12, 13].

Currently Available Covered Metal Stents

In light of the disadvantage of re-obstruction of the original uncovered metal stents due to tumor ingrowth [14–18], the new-generation stents are covered or partially covered [19]. Generally, an ideal metal stent should have the following characteristics: an internal diameter big enough for the passage of normal diet, flexible to avoid trauma during placement, resist to migrate, and removable if necessary [10]. Although this ideal stent does not exist at this time, all available covered stents do meet some of these criteria. The frequently used covered metal stents are as follows:

The Ultraflex stent (Boston Scientific, Natick, MA, USA) consists of a knitted nitinol wire tube, and the covered version has a polyurethane layer which covers the midsection of the stent extending to within 1.5 cm of either end of the stent. The stent has a proximal flare with two sizes: 28 mm (distal diameter 23 mm) and 23 mm (distal diameter 18 mm). It is important to remember that all these stents become 30–40% shorter after placement. The radial force of the Ultraflex stent is the lowest among the currently available metal stents. Partial obstruction of the stent can occur in stents that are sharply angled beyond the GE junction. The Wallstent (Boston Scientific) is made from a cobalt-based alloy and is formed into a tubular mesh. It is available in two designs: the Wallstent II and the Flamingo Wallstent. Stents of both designs are easy to place. The Wallstent can be repositioned during the procedure because recapture remains possible, while less than 50% of the stent is deployed. The degree of shortening after placement is about 20–30%. Both designs have a high radial force. The Wallstent II flares to 28 mm at both ends, with a diameter of 20 mm at its midsection. It is covered with a silicone polymer layer, with 2 cm left exposed at the proximal and distal ends. The Flamingo Wallstent is designed specifically for use in the distal esophagus/gastric cardia. However, it can be used in the proximal esophagus as well. The conical shape of this stent is designed to apply a variable radial force throughout the length of the stent to address anatomical differences in the distal esophagus and cardia. The stent is covered by a polyurethane layer, which is applied from the inside, extending to within 2 cm of either end of the stent. Both a large-diameter stent (proximal and distal diameters 30 and 20 mm) and a small-diameter stent (proximal and distal diameters 24 and 16 mm) are available. The Wallstent II and the Flamingo Wallstent are both very pliable, with the diameter of the stent unaffected even when angled. The Z-stent (Wilson-Cook Medical, Winston-Salem, NC, USA) with a Korean modification, the Choo stent (MI Tech, Seoul, Korea), consists of a wide "Z"-mesh of stainless steel covered over its entire length by a polyethylene layer. The Z-stent is available with or without fixing barbs in the central segment. The introduction system is more complex than that of the Wallstent and the Ultraflex stent. The stent does not shorten on release and is the least flexible of the currently available metal stents. The Z-stent flares to 25 mm at both ends with a diameter at its midsection of either 18 mm or 22 mm. Partial obstruction can also occur with Z-stents if they are sharply angled after passing across the GE junction [10].

Comparison of Different Types of Metal Stents

With the wide availability of different metal stents on the market, it is important to investigate which stent offers the most optimal palliation for malignant dysphagia. Several retrospective or prospective studies compared the outcome of different types of metal stents.

One retrospective study compared the uncovered Ultraflex, the covered and uncovered versions of the Wallstent, and the covered Z-stent on 96 patients. There were no differences in the outcome and complication rate among the different stent types [20]. Covered versions of the Wallstent and the Ultraflex stent were compared in another retrospective trial, showing a higher early complication rate with the

Wallstent but a higher re-intervention rate with the Ultraflex stent [9, 21]. In a prospective study, 100 patients were randomized into 1 of 3 types of covered metal stents, Ultraflex stent, Flamingo Wallstent, and Z-stent. No significant differences were found in dysphagia improvement, the occurrence of complications, or recurrent dysphagia, although there was a trend toward more complications with Z-stent (Ultraflex stent 8/34 (24%) and Flamingo Wallstent 6/33 (18%) than Z-stent 12/33 (36%); $P = 0.23$) [22]. In another prospective trial, the Ultraflex stent and the Flamingo Wallstent were compared in patients with distal esophageal cancer. The two types of stents were equally effective in the palliation of dysphagia in this patient group, and the complication rate associated with their use was also comparable (Ultraflex stent 7/31 (23%) and Flamingo Wallstent 5/22 (23%)) [9, 23].

We can conclude that there are only slight differences between the most frequently used types of stents. The choice of stent should therefore depend on the location and anatomy of the malignant stricture as well as the specific characteristics of the stent.

The Efficacy and Complications of Self-Expanding Mental Stent

Generally, the technical success rate for placement of metal stents is close to 100%. Almost all patients experience rapid improvement of dysphagia within a few days. The dysphagia grade usually improves from a median of 3 (able to drink liquids only) to a median of 1 (able to eat most solid foods). Limitations to successful placement include severe pain during procedure; extensive tumor growth in the stomach; failure of the stent to release from the introduction system, as can occur with Ultraflex stents; and immediate stent migration when the stent has been placed too distally. Procedure-related complications after metal stent placement mainly consist of perforation, aspiration pneumonia, fever, bleeding, and severe chest pain and occur in 5–15% of patients. Minor complications are mild retrosternal pain and gastroesophageal reflux, which are reported in 10–20% of patients. Delayed complications and recurrent dysphagia following stent placement are an important problem and occur in 30–45% of patients. This includes hemorrhage, fistula formation, stent migration, tumor over- or ingrowth, and food bolus obstruction. Treatment of fistula formation, stent migration, and tumor overgrowth or ingrowth mostly consists of placement of a second stent. This is an effective treatment and improves dysphagia scores [9, 24].

Stent Placement for Esophagorespiratory Fistulas

Esophagorespiratory fistula is a dreaded complication of esophageal cancer, which can lead to aspiration and respiratory failure, and occurs in 5% of all cases. It may also arise secondary to lung cancer and trachea and larynx cancer and have high morbidity and mortality rates because of comorbid conditions such as aspiration pneumonia [6, 25]. Placement of a covered metal stent is the choice of treatment for esophagorespiratory fistula. Complete sealing of a fistula is established in more than 90% of patients with no significant difference between the currently available covered metal stents. Moreover, dysphagia scores improve significantly as well. The complication rate (early and late complications) varies between 10% and 30% [26–30].

New Stent Designs

New stent designs focus on two aspects, changing of configuration and optimization of materials. For example, metal stents with an anti-reflux mechanism have been developed to prevent gastroesophageal reflux of distal esophageal cancer. The design of completely covered stents, like the Polyflex stent and the Niti-S stent, might be able to overcome ingrowth of tumoral tissue. Further, the Niti-S stent with a double-layer configuration, consisting of an inner polyurethane layer to prevent tumor ingrowth and an outer uncovered nitinol wire tube to allow the mesh to embed itself in the esophageal wall, has been designed to reduce stent migration.

A recently reported cause of recurrent dysphagia is the ingrowth and overgrowth of non-tumoral, inflammatory tissue, over and through the uncovered meshes at the ends of partially covered stents [31]. So, in addition to progressive tumor growth, benign tissue is also able to cause stent obstruction. Therefore, stents made with biodegradable materials, such as magnesium alloy or polymerid, may relieve obstruction and degrade after a period of time [32]. Relative studies are still on the way and further comparative studies are needed [33].

Laser Therapy: Nd:YAG Laser

Treatment of obstructing esophageal cancer with the high-power neodymium-yttrium-aluminum-garnet (Nd:YAG) laser is another relatively safe but often temporary palliation for dysphagia. Nd:YAG laser therapy delivers an intense beam of light that heats and vaporizes tumor tissue, thereby restoring patency to the esophageal lumen. Dysphagia relief occurs often immediately, and successful tumor recanalization can be achieved in more than 90% of appropriately selected patients. Tumors that are relatively short in length (<6 cm), exophytic, and located in the mid esophagus are most amenable to laser ablation. It is not recommended for tumors in submucosa, tumors causing extrinsic compression, and tumors with angulation. It is less effective for cancer of the proximal esophagus or gastroesophageal junction. However, many patients (70–95%) require multiple treatment sessions and are usually reassessed at 4–6 weekly intervals [34, 35].

Laser therapy offers similar dysphagia relief to esophageal stents. An early study suggested that laser therapy was associated with fewer complications than esophageal stenting [36]. A limitation of this retrospective study was that many of the patients in the stenting group received a plastic endoprosthesis rather than SEMS. A prospective randomized study subsequently concluded that laser therapy carried a higher risk of fistula formation, bleeding, and need for repeating intervention when compared to esophageal stents [19]. Therefore, this therapy is not widely utilized.

Photodynamic Therapy (PDT)

PDT, a non-thermal tissue ablative technique, involves intravenous injection of a photosensitizing agent that is preferentially taken up by neoplastic cells, followed by endoscopic application of laser therapy to the malignant stricture. Porphyrin compounds, such as porfimer sodium, have been the most commonly used photosensitizers for the palliation of malignant dysphagia. PDT with porfimer, a hematoporphyrin derivative, is thought to have a direct toxic effect on malignant cell via the production of singlet oxygen, which damages the microvasculature of the tumor and renders it ischemic [37]. Porfimer preferentially accumulates in malignant tissue after intravenous injection. The area is then exposed to an endoscopically placed low-powered laser diffuser with monochrome light (630 nm), which initiates a photochemical reaction resulting in tumor necrosis. The malignant tissue can be treated repeatedly to provide optimal tissue ablation [6].

PDT appears to be effective at palliating dysphagia, but its widespread acceptance is limited by the high cost of the photosensitizing agent and the requirement for patients to avoid sunlight for several weeks to avoid skin phototoxicity [38, 39]. Furthermore, patients require repeating intervention within a mean interval of 2 months. Major complications, including perforation, fistula formation, and strictures, have been reported in up to 30% of patients [38].

Cryotherapy

During cryoablation, liquid nitrogen or carbon dioxide at super cold temperatures (−76 to −158 °C) is sprayed directly on the tumor for 20–40 s. The tissue is then allowed to thaw before spraying again for 20–40 s. Typically, 2–4 freeze-thaw cycles of liquid nitrogen or 4–8 freeze-thaw cycles of carbon dioxide are administered. These freeze-thaw cycles cause intracellular disruption and ischemia, which leads to ablation of tumor tissue (thermal ablation) (Fig. 16.2). High-quality data has demonstrated the safety and effectiveness of this

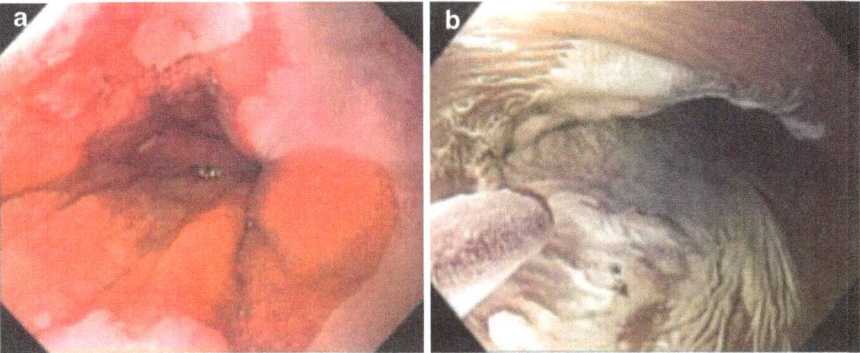

Fig. 16.2 Cryotherapy of esophageal cancer and Barrett's esophagus. (**a**) Before cryotherapy. (**b**) Immediately after therapy

technology in Barrett's esophagus and early esophageal cancer. The published literature on the efficacy of this modality for esophageal cancer palliation is primarily from smaller case series [40], and long-term survival has been reported [41]. Further research is necessary to clarify the role of cryoablation in esophageal cancer palliation.

Argon Plasma Coagulation

Argon plasma coagulation (APC) is an ablative endoscopic technique. A type of monopolar electrocautery, APC causes tissue coagulation, desiccation, and destruction via the transfer of energy from the APC probe to the malignant tissue in the form of ionized, electrically conductive argon gas ("plasma"). The APC probe produces a plasma arc that destroys tissue to a depth of approximately 2–3 mm and is most useful in superficial lesions [42].

Several studies have assessed its effectiveness in the palliation of malignant dysphagia. In one retrospective study of 32 patients, recanalization was achieved in 89% of patients [43]. A separate report of 83 patients found a similar recanalization rate of 86% [44]. Most of these patients required multiple sessions to maintain patency, averaging five to six sessions per patient, usually at an interval of 3–4 weeks. Perforation was seen in 1–1.8% of procedures, a rate comparable to that seen in other modalities [45, 46]. Argon plasma coagulation seems to be a safe and easy alternative to laser treatment. Further prospective trials are needed for comparison [42].

Radiofrequency Ablation (RFA)

With the advent of radiofrequency (RF), radiofrequency ablation (RFA) has been reported widely in recent decades. The energy of the radiofrequency current can radiate off solid tumors by electromagnetic waves [47, 48]. Due to its precise orientation, smaller trauma, and less pain, RFA has become increasingly recommended as a new option for esophageal tumors, which in part averts both pain and poor life quality in advanced patients [49]. In clinical practice, the endoscopic RFA can not only ablate tumors in the esophagus directly but also can further offer space for the stent extension by ablating ingrowth tumor, therefore keeping the stent patent for a longer time [50] (Fig. 16.3).

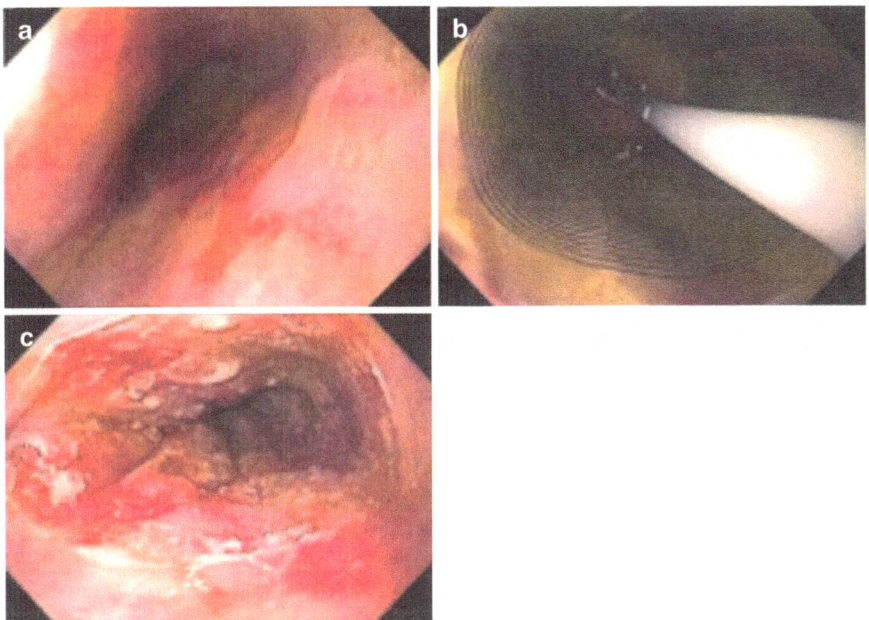

Fig. 16.3 Radiofrequency ablation of esophageal cancer and Barrett's esophagus. (**a**) Before therapy, (**b**) during therapy, (**c**) immediately after therapy

Dilatation

The normal functional lumen diameter of the esophagus in adults is 25 mm. If it decreases to 13 mm, symptoms of dysphagia to solid and regular diet appear. Esophageal dilation is generally used for benign or postoperative strictures and not recommended for malignant stricture. But in some special situations, dilatation might provide temporary relief. Endoscopically directed balloon dilatation or wire-guided polyvinyl bougies can bring temporary relief of dysphagia until more definitive treatment is given. Several sessions with balloon, Savary, and Maloney dilators can safely dilate most malignant strictures up to 17 mm. The relief duration obtained from dilatation is short; repeated dilatation is required in 1–2 weeks. Dilatation of malignant stricture should only be used as a preliminary modality before endoscopic tumor ablation or placement of an enteral feeding tube prior to chemoradiation therapy [6, 51–53].

Alcohol Injection

Direct injection of pure ethanol into malignant tissue is the simplest and least expensive technique that can recanalize an obstructed esophagus. Alcohol injected under endoscopic visualization can cause tissue fixation, tumor ulceration, and necrosis. It has proved to be an effective modality in the relief of malignant dysphagia. Like laser therapy, alcohol injection is best suited for treating exophytic bulky lesions at all levels of the esophagus.

Significant relief of dysphagia was demonstrated in two uncontrolled trials [54]. In a randomized, controlled trial comparing neodymium-yttrium-aluminum-garnet (Nd:YAG) laser with ethanol injection, the dysphagia-free interval was 37 days and 30 days, respectively. An improvement in the dysphagia score of at least two points was noted in 88% of the laser group and 78% of the ethanol group, with no difference in median survival [34]. In one of the largest studies, 36 patients underwent alcohol injection therapy for palliation of dysphagia. The mean number of treatments required to "recanalize" the esophagus was 1.8, and the mean volume of alcohol injected per session was 7.8 milliliter (mL). All patients reported fever and chest pain for 12–24 h after the procedure. Dysphagia improved in 81% of patients. Seven of the 36 patients had no subjective improvement despite objective evidence of esophageal patency [7].

Despite this technique relying on readily available and inexpensive materials and capability by nearly all endoscopists, this procedure has not gained widespread use in the United States since it is performed simply by injection of ethanol in aliquots of 0.5–1.0 mL into protuberant portions of neoplastic tissue. Excessively firm or fibrotic tumors may lead to difficulties with injection. On the other hand, if tumors are too soft, without much resistance to alcohol injection, it may be difficult to estimate the amount of alcohol delivered. Thus, when using alcohol injection, dosimetry can be inaccurate [7].

In summary, there are a number of palliative modalities for advanced-stage esophageal cancer. Stent placement, RFA, APC, and cryotherapy are commonly used. Selection depends on patients' condition and expertise.

References

1. Jemal A, Siegel R, Xu J, et al. Cancer statistics. CA Cancer J Clin. 2011;61:69–90.
2. Krasna MJ. Surgical staging and surgical treatment in esophageal cancer. Semin Oncol. 1999;26:9–11.
3. Ponec RJ, Kimmey MB. Endoscopic therapy of esophageal cancer. Surg Clin N Am. 1997;77:1197–217.
4. Fan Z, Dai N, Chen L. Expandable thermal-shaped memory metal esophageal stent: experiences with a new nitinol stent in 129 patients. Gastrointest Endosc. 1997;46:352–7.
5. Fleischer D. Four things to recall about esophageal cancer. Endoscopy. 1998;30:311.
6. Javle M, Ailawadhi S, Yang GY, et al. Palliation of malignant dysphagia in esophageal cancer: a literature-based review. J Support Oncol. 2006;4:365.
7. Adler DG, Baron TH. Endoscopic palliation of malignant dysphagia. Mayo Clin Proc. 2001;76:731–8.
8. Detsky AS. A controlled trial of an expansile metal stent for palliation of esophageal obstruction due to inoperable cancer. N Engl J Med. 1993;329:1302.
9. Homs MY, Kuipers EJ, Siersema PD. Palliative therapy. J Surg Oncol. 2005;92:246–56.
10. Siersema PD. New developments in palliative therapy. Best Pract Res Clin Gastroenterol. 2006;20:959–78.

11. Gasparri G, Casalegno PA, Camandona M, et al. Endoscopic insertion of 248 prostheses in inoperable carcinoma of the esophagus and cardia: short-term and long-term results. Gastrointest Endosc. 1987;33:354–6.

12. Segalin A, Bonavina L, Carazzone A, et al. Improving results of esophageal stenting: a study on 160 consecutive unselected patients. Endoscopy. 1997;29:701–9.

13. Bethge N, Sommer A, Gross U, et al. Human tissue responses to metal stents implanted in vivo for the palliation of malignant stenoses. Gastrointest Endosc. 1996;43:596–602.

14. Baron TH. Expandable metal stents for the treatment of cancerous obstruction of the gastrointestinal tract. N Engl J Med. 2001;344:1681.

15. Bartelsman JFW, Bruno MJ, Jensema AJ, et al. Palliation of patients with esophagogastric neoplasms by insertion of a covered expandable modified Gianturco-Z endoprosthesis: experiences in 153 patients. Gastrointest Endosc. 2000;51:134.

16. Siersema PD, Marcon N, Vakil N. Metal stents for tumors of the distal esophagus and gastric cardia. Endoscopy. 2003;35:79.

17. Raijman I, Siddique I, Ajani J, et al. Palliation of malignant dysphagia and fistulae with coated expandable metal stents: experience with 101 patients. Gastrointest Endosc. 1998;48:172.

18. Thompson AM, Rapson T, Gilbert FJ, et al. Endoscopic palliative treatment for esophageal and gastric cancer: techniques, complications, and survival in a population-based cohort of 948 patients. Surg Endosc. 2004;18:1257–62.

19. Vakil N, Morris AI, Marcon N, et al. A prospective, randomized, controlled trial of covered expandable metal stents in the palliation of malignant esophageal obstruction at the gastroesophageal junction. Am J Gastroenterol. 2001;96:1791–6.

20. May A, Hahn EG, Ell C. Self-expanding metal stents for palliation of malignant obstruction in the upper gastrointestinal tract. J Clin Gastroenterol. 1996;22:261.

21. Schmassmann A, Meyenberger C, Knuchel J, et al. Self-expanding metal stents in malignant esophageal obstruction: a comparison between two stent types. Am J Gastroenterol. 1997;92:400.

22. Siersema PD, Hop WC, Van BM, et al. A comparison of 3 types of covered metal stents for the palliation of patients with dysphagia caused by esophagogastric carcinoma: a prospective, randomized study. Gastrointest Endosc. 2001;54:145.

23. Sabharwal T, Hamady MS, Chui S, et al. A randomised prospective comparison of the Flamingo Wallstent and Ultraflex stent for palliation of dysphagia associated with lower third oesophageal carcinoma. Gut. 2003;52:922.

24. Homs MY, Steyerberg EW, Kuipers EJ, et al. Causes and treatment of recurrent dysphagia after self-expanding metal stent placement for palliation of esophageal carcinoma. Endoscopy. 2005;36:880.

25. Burt M, Diehl W, Martini N, et al. Malignant esophagorespiratory fistula: management options and survival. Ann Thorac Surg. 1991;52:1222.

26. Morgan RA, Ellul JP, Denton ER, et al. Malignant esophageal fistulas and perforations: management with plastic-covered metallic endoprostheses. Radiology. 1997;204:527–32.

27. Low DE, Kozarek RA. Comparison of conventional and wire mesh expandable prostheses and surgical bypass in patients with malignant esophagorespiratory fistulas. Ann Thorac Surg. 1998;65:919.

28. Dumonceau JM, Cremer M, Lalmand B, et al. Esophageal fistula sealing: choice of stent, practical management, and cost. Gastrointest Endosc. 1999;49:70.

29. May A, Ell C. Palliative treatment of malignant esophagorespiratory fistulas with Gianturco-Z stents. A prospective clinical trial and review of the literature on covered metal stents. Am J Gastroenterol. 1998;93:532–5.

30. Siersema PD, Schrauwen SL, Van BM, et al. Self-expanding metal stents for complicated and recurrent esophagogastric cancer. Gastrointest Endosc. 2001;54:579–86.

31. Mayoral W, Fleischer D, Salcedo J, et al. Nonmalignant obstruction is a common problem with metal stents in the treatment of esophageal cancer. Gastrointest Endosc. 2000;51:556–9.

32. Hirdes MM, van Hooft JE, Wijrdeman HK, et al. Combination of biodegradable stent placement and single-dose brachytherapy is associated with an unacceptably high complication rate in the treatment of dysphagia from esophageal cancer. Gastrointest Endosc. 2012;76:267–74.

33. Berg MWVD, Vries EMD, Walter D, et al. Su1522 Safety and Efficacy of a Biodegradable Stent During Neoadjuvant Therapy in Patients With Advanced Esophageal Cancer (Esnebio). Gastrointest Endosc. 2013;77:AB355.

34. Carazzone A, Bonavina L, Segalin A, et al. Endoscopic palliation of oesophageal cancer: results of a prospective comparison of Nd:YAG laser and ethanol injection. Eur J Surg. 1999;165:351.

35. Dallal HJ, Smith GD, Grieve DC, et al. A randomized trial of thermal ablative therapy versus expandable metal stents in the palliative treatment of patients with esophageal carcinoma. Gastrointest Endosc. 2001;54:549–57.

36. Gevers AM, Macken E, Hiele M, et al. A comparison of laser therapy, plastic stents, and expandable metal stents for palliation of malignant dysphagia in patients without a fistula. Gastrointest Endosc. 1998;48:383–8.

37. Marcon NE. Photodynamic therapy and cancer of the esophagus. Semin Oncol. 1994;21:20.

38. Moghissi K, Dixon K, Thorpe JA, et al. The role of photodynamic therapy (PDT) in inoperable oesophageal cancer. Eur J Cardiothorac Surg. 2000;17:95.

39. Litle VR, Luketich JD, Christie NA, et al. Photodynamic therapy as palliation for esophageal cancer: experience in 215 patients. Ann Thorac Surg. 2003;76:1687.

40. Vignesh S, Hoffe SE, Meredith KL, et al. Endoscopic therapy of neoplasia related to Barrett's esophagus and endoscopic palliation of esophageal cancer. Cancer Control. 2013;20:117.

41. Spiritos Z, Mekaroonkamol P, Elrayes BF, et al. Long -term survival in stage IV esophageal adenocarcinoma with chemoradiation and serial endoscopic cryoablation. Clin Endosc. 2017;50:491–4.

42. Adler DG, Merwat SN. Endoscopic approaches for palliation of luminal gastrointestinal obstruction. Gastroenterol Clin N Am. 2006;35:65–82. viii.

43. Eriksen JR. Palliation of non-resectable carcinoma of the cardia and oesophagus by argon beam coagulation. Dan Med Bull. 2002;49:346–9.

44. Heindorff H, Wojdemann M, Bisgaard T, et al. Endoscopic palliation of inoperable cancer of the oesophagus or cardia by argon electrocoagulation. Scand J Gastroenterol. 1998;33:21–3.

45. Jin M, Yang B, Zhang W, et al. Photodynamic therapy for upper gastrointestinal tumours over the past 10 years. Semin Surg Oncol. 1994;10:111.

46. Luketich JD, Christie NA, Buenaventura PO, et al. Endoscopic photodynamic therapy for obstructing esophageal cancer: 77 cases over a 2-year period. Surg Endosc. 2000;14:653–7.

47. Glazer ES, Massey KL, Zhu C, et al. Pancreatic carcinoma cells are susceptible to non-invasive radiofrequency fields after treatment with targeted gold nanoparticles. Surgery. 2010;148:319.

48. Zacharoulis D, Khorsandi SE, Vavra P, et al. Pilot study for a new bipolar radiofrequency ablation/aspirator device in the management of primary and secondary liver cancers. Liver Int. 2009;29:824–30.

49. Eisele RM, Neuhaus P, Schumacher G. Radiofrequency ablation of liver tumors using a novel bipolar device. J Laparoendosc Adv Surg Tech A. 2008;18:857–63.

50. Niu H, Zhang X, Wang B, et al. The clinical utility of RFA in esophageal and cardia cancer patients with severe malignant obstruction. Tumour Biol. 2016;37:1337–40.

51. Heit HA, Johnson LF, Siegel SR, et al. Palliative dilation for dysphagia in esophageal carcinoma. Ann Intern Med. 1978;89:629–31.

52. Hernandez LV, Jacobson JW, Harris MS, et al. Comparison among the perforation rates of Maloney, balloon, and savary dilation of esophageal strictures. Gastrointest Endosc. 2000;51:460.

53. Jr BH. Palliation of dysphagia of esophageal cancer by endoscopic lumen restoration techniques. Cancer Control. 1999;6:73.

54. Güitrón A, Adalid R, Huerta F, et al. Palliative treatment of esophageal cancer with transendoscopic injection of alcohol. Rev Gastroenterol Mex. 1996;61:208–11.

Nutritional Support in Esophageal Cancer

Tiffany Barrett

Malnutrition

Poor nutritional intake and weight loss due to cancer diagnosis or treatment can lead to malnutrition. Before diagnosis, 80% of all patients with esophageal cancer has over 10% of unintentional weight loss. Malnutrition is defined as "a state of nutrition in which a deficiency or excess or imbalance of energy, protein and other nutrients causes measurable adverse effects on tissue/body form and function and clinical outcome" [1]. Malnutrition leads to impaired immune response, reduced muscle strength, increased fatigue, impaired wound healing, impaired psycho-social function, reduced quality of life, reduced response, and tolerance to prescribed oncology treatment [2]. Malnutrition during cancer is a result of increased nutrient requirements, inadequate intake, decreased gastrointestinal absorption, and impaired digestion of nutrients. In 2009, the American Society for Parenteral and Enteral Nutrition (ASPEN) and the Academy of Nutrition and Dietetics developed a workgroup to standardize an approach to the diagnosis of malnutrition. Prior to this consensus, there was no universal approach to the diagnosis of adult malnutrition [3]. The identification of two or more of the six characteristics is recommended for diagnosis of either severe or nonsevere malnutrition (Table 17.1): weight loss, insufficient energy intake, loss of muscle mass, loss of body fat, fluid accumulation, and diminished functional status as measured by hand grip strength. Height and weight should be measured not estimated to determine body mass index.

T. Barrett (✉)
Winship Cancer Institute of Emory University, Nutritional Support in Esophageal Cancer, Atlanta, GA, USA
e-mail: Tiffany.barrett@emoryhealthcare.org

© Springer Nature Switzerland AG 2020
N. F. Saba, B. F. El-Rayes (eds.), *Esophageal Cancer*,
https://doi.org/10.1007/978-3-030-29832-6_17

Table 17.1 Clinical characteristics of malnutrition

Clinical characteristic	Malnutrition in the context of acute illness		Malnutrition in the context of chronic illness		Malnutrition in the context of social or environmental circumstances	
	Moderate	Severe	Moderate	Severe	Moderate	Severe
Weight loss	1–2% 1 week 5% 1 month 7.5% 3 months	>2% 1 week >5% 1 month >7.5% 3 months	5% 1 month 7.5% 3 months 10% 6 months 20% 1 year	>5%1 month >7.5% 3 months >10% 6 months >20% 1 year	5%/1 month 7.5%/3 months 10%/6 months 20%/1 year	>5%/1 month >7.5%/3 months >10%/6 months >20%/1 year
Energy intake	<75% of estimated energy requirement for >7 days	≤50% of estimated energy requirement for ≥5 days	<75% of estimated energy requirement for ≥1 month	≤75% of estimated energy requirement for ≥1 month	<75% of estimated energy requirement for ≥3 months	≤50% of estimated energy requirement for ≥1 month
Physical loss of subcutaneous fat	Mild	Moderate	Mild	Severe	Mild	Severe
Physical muscle loss	Mild	Moderate	Mild	Severe	Mild	Severe
Fluid accumulation generalized or localized evident on exam	Mild	Moderate to severe	Mild	Severe	Mild	Severe
Reduced grip strength	NA	Measurably reduced	NA	Measurably reduced	NA	Measurably reduced

Usual weight should be obtained in order to determine the percentage and to interpret the significance of weight loss. The National Center for Health Statistics defines "chronic" as a disease/condition lasting 3 months or longer. Serum proteins such as albumin and prealbumin are not included as defining characteristics of malnutrition because recent evidence analysis shows that serum levels of these proteins do not change in response to changes in nutrient intake

This table was developed by Annalynn Skipper, PhD, RD, FADA. The content was developed by an Academy workgroup composed of Jane White, PhD, RD, FADA, LDN, Chair; Maree Ferguson, MBA, PhD, RD; Sherri Jones, MS, MBA, RD, LDN; Ainsley Malone, MS, RD, LD, CNSD; Louise Merriman, MS, RD, CDN; Terese Scollard, MBA, RD; and Annalynn Skipper, PhD, RD, FADA and Academy staff member Pam Michael, MBA, RD. Content was approved by an ASPEN committee consisting of Gordon L. Jensen, MD, PhD, Co-Chair; Ainsley Malone, MS, RD, CNSD, Co-Chair; Rose Ann Dimaria, PhD, RN, CNSN; Christine M. Framson, RD, PhD, CSND; Nilesh Mehta, MD, DCH; Steve Plogsted, PharmD, RPh, BCNSP; Annalynn Skipper, PhD, RD, FADA; Jennifer Wooley, MS, RD, CNSD; and Jay Mirtallo, RPh, BCNSP Board Liaison and ASPEN staff member Peggi Guenter, PhD, CNSN. Subsequently, it was approved by the ASPEN Board of Directors. The information in the table is current as of February 1, 2012. Changes are anticipated as new research becomes available.

Adapted from: Skipper A. Malnutrition coding. In Skipper A (ed). *Nutrition Care Manual*. Chicago, IL: Academy of Nutrition and Dietetics; 2012 Edition

Nutrition Screening and Assessment

Early screening for malnutrition is important for improved outcomes. Nutrition screening identifies patients who may have a malnutrition diagnosis and benefit from an assessment by a registered dietitian. Several screening tools are available though there is not an agreement on the best way of screening the nutrition status for cancer patients. Validated tools in oncology patients include the malnutrition screening tool (MST), the malnutrition universal screening tool (MUST), patient-generated subjective global assessment (PG-SGA), and subjective global assessment. Evidence-based practice has recommended the use of scored patient-generated subjective global assessment (PG-SGA) within the oncology population [4]. Due to time constraints in a hospital or clinic setting, simplified screening methods can be beneficial. Development and research of patient-generated subjective global assessment short form (PG-SGA SF). Abbott et al. demonstrated an accurate and simple tool to detect risk of malnutrition when administered by a registered dietitian [4]. Malnutrition screening tool (MST) is a simple and quick tool consisting of two questions. It is a reliable tool for identifying malnutrition in adult oncology patients [5]. The MST has been shown to be validated and reliable. Decreased oral intake and weight loss should be addressed early in diagnosis. Early nutritional intervention assists with identifying the nutritional needs and can improve clinical outcomes.

Nutritional Needs of the Esophageal Cancer Patient

At cancer diagnosis, changes occur in carbohydrate, lipid, and protein metabolism. These abnormalities are the result of an inflammatory response of the tumor in addition to treatment side effects. This inflammation caused by the tumor has been defined as disease-related malnutrition [6]. Pro-inflammatory cytokines produced by the tumor disrupt metabolism in the body causing muscle wasting, fatigue, depression, and decreased physical activity [7].

Elevated resting energy expenditure (REE) has been found higher in esophageal, gastric, pancreatic, and lung cancer. Evaluating resting energy expenditure of newly diagnosed cancer, 46.7% were hypermetabolic, 43.5% were normometabolic, and 9.8% were hypometabolic [8]. Approximately 50% of cancer patients that lost weight were hypermetabolic compared to controls with similar weight loss [9]. Increased resting energy expenditure is due to hypermetabolism contributing to a negative nitrogen balance [10]. To maintain weight and prevent worsening malnutrition, the nutrition intake needs to meet energy requirements. The gold standard to determine resting energy needs is by indirect calorimetry. Indirect calorimetry calculates resting energy expenditure by measuring oxygen consumption and carbon dioxide production [11]. If calorimeters are not available, nutrient requirements are estimated by predictive equations. Commonly used equations include the Mifflin-St Jeor, the Harris-Benedict, Ireton-Jones, Penn State (critically ill), and kcal/kg equation [12]. There is limited research specific to esophageal cancer on estimating calories using predictive equations. Energy expenditure by indirect calorimetry using activity factors was compared to Harris-Benedict and pocket equation. Estimating calories using equation 30 kcal/kg was suitable in a small study of digestive tract cancers [11]. Newly diagnosed esophageal patients with weight loss have elevated energy expenditure and higher inflammation markers. Thirty-eight out of fifty-six patients were found to be hypermetabolic using both indirect calorimetry and predicted energy equation Harris-Benedict [13]. Other research has found Harris-Benedict to underestimate basal energy expenditure and overestimate when used with an injury factor. The results of basal energy needs for indirect calorimetry and Harris-Benedict (1.3 injury factor) equation were 1421.8 and 1703.8, respectively [14].

Protein is essential for building and repairing cells and maintaining muscle mass. Assuming normal renal function, protein needs range from 1.0 to 1.6 g/kg based on weight changes and lean body mass [15]. Fluid needs are based on nutrition assessment by using common equations:

- Body surface area = 1500 mL/m^2
- 1 mL fluid per 1 kcal of estimated energy needs
- Body weight 20–40 mL/kg/day

Vitamin and minerals should be supplied based on RDA recommendations unless tested deficiency. Estimating nutritional needs is based on physical assessment and current clinical data. Needs should be reassessed during intervals of treatment.

Sarcopenia

Sarcopenia is the loss of muscle mass and strength that commonly occurs in cancer patients. CT assessment is the gold standard method of analyzing muscle mass body composition in cancer patients, but is not always practical as a nutrition screening tool. Sarcopenia indicated poor prognosis in esophageal cancer patients without lymph node involvement status post-surgical resection or chemoradiation. Skeletal muscle mass was measured using standard computed tomography scans [16]. In a small study following participants from diagnosis to post-adjuvant therapy, both lean body and hand grip strength were reduced. Leading that nutrition support and exercise interventions should be recommended during preoperative therapy [17]. In another retrospective study, sarcopenia impacts long-term outcome following treatment for esophageal cancer. Sarcopenia was found in 61.5% of patients receiving neoadjuvant treatment with 28.5% having postoperative complications. Complications included pneumonia, anastomotic leakage, and conduit necrosis [18]. Loss of muscle and fat mass can often be disguised in overweight cancer patients who experience more weight loss when compared to underweight patients. Of the 72 studied esophageal patients, 43% was sarcopenic, and 14% had sarcopenic obesity, which is defined as sarcopenia with overweight and obesity based on body mass index (BMI). Dose-limiting toxicity during chemotherapy was high in both groups but higher in sarcopenic obesity [19]. Demonstrating the importance of nutrition intervention for all patients despite BMI, leading that sarcopenia can affect long-term outcome.

Nutrition During Treatment

As previously mentioned, weight loss, fatigue, and dysphagia are already present at the time of diagnosis. Treatments for esophageal cancer contribute to the development of malnutrition after diagnosis. Weight loss before the start of treatment has been shown to occur in up to 74% of patients and during treatment 40–57% [20]. Treatments are typically multimodal: surgery, chemotherapy, and radiation.

Adjuvant chemotherapy or chemoradiotherapy is common for the treatment of esophageal cancer. Chemotherapy-related toxicities include anemia, leukemia, fatigue, appetite changes, and stomatitis and taste aversions. Approaches to reduce the chemotherapy toxicities is needed for full benefit of treatment. Esophagitis is the main side effect during radiation, with nausea, vomiting, and anorexia common with chemotherapy. A complete nutrition assessment should not be ignored in this population. A retrospective study of esophageal patients treated with chemotherapy or radiation found a decline in weight loss of 3.5%. During treatment, 10% of curative patients did not meet with a dietitian despite prior weight loss. Patients that required a feeding tube completed treatment, with 72.2% completed treatment that required a stent [21]. This study concludes the importance of dietitian referral in a timely manner, with frequent follow-up during treatment. Including implementing a protocol of when to implement a feeding tube.

Limited data on the effectiveness of enteral nutrition reducing toxicities during chemotherapy is known. There is clinical evidence supporting enteral nutrition especially malnourished cancer patients. A randomized study revealed chemotherapy adverse effects leukopenia and neutropenia were reduced in patients supplemented with omega-3 containing enteral formula [22]. Omega-3 fatty acid support did not affect neutropenia, but did decrease stomatitis and diarrhea frequency [23]. Patients consumed ω-3 fatty acid-rich supplement orally or by nasogastric tube day 3 before chemo to day 12. Placing prophylactic feeding tubes prior to chemoradiotherapy can be controversial due to lack of evidence and complications from placement. Patients receiving induction chemotherapy and high-dose radiation therapy and experiencing greater weight loss (7.5% compared to 4.5%) were associated with feeding tube placement [24], concluding these patients should be followed closely and reevaluated to prevent nutrition decline during treatment.

Dysphagia and weight loss associated with diagnosis will continue to worsen during neoadjuvant therapy (chemotherapy alone or concurrent with radiation). Self-expanding stents have been used to allow increased oral intake and maintain nutrition status during neoadjuvant therapy. In patients hospitalized with dysphagia, placement of feeding tubes is the most common intervention [25]. Nutrition therapy prior to initiation of neoadjuvant therapy restores normal swallowing, maintains weight, and may prevent feeding tube placement. Patients were provided an individualized regimen as determined by a dedicated upper gastrointestinal cancer nutritionist. Follow-up meetings continued during neoadjuvant chemotherapy to maximize macronutrient intake. Of the 130 patients treated, 78 reported dysphagia at baseline. Weight did not significantly change after one cycle of chemotherapy. Intense nutrition support prior and during treatment assisted with resuming oral intake [26].

Surgical Resection

After concurrent chemotherapy and radiation, patient's immune system can be comprised with esophagectomy further causing immune suppression. Side effects of surgery include early satiety, reflux, nausea, vomiting, dumping syndrome, dysphagia, anastomotic leak, and pain. Literature reports prevalence of postoperative symptoms dysphagia (35.7%), delayed gastric emptying (37%), reflux (39.4%), and dumping syndrome (21.4%) [27]. The normal gastrointestinal structure is altered causing intolerance to oral intake Importance should be paid to nutritional support preoperative and postoperatively. A worse overall 5-year survival in patients with preoperative weight loss ($\geq$10%) after esophagectomy was found in a 2014 cohort study [28]. This current study did not observe increase in post-op complications. In a review by Steenhagen et al., patients with preoperative weight loss was associated with worse outcomes and increasing post-surgical complications [29]. The preoperative prognostic nutritional index is a parameter for evaluating nutritional condition, immunology, and surgical risk: 10x serum albumin level (g/dl) + 0.005 x lymphocyte count in peripheral blood [30]. The PNI of salvage esophagectomy patients affects their overall survival [31]. Prior to esophagectomy, patients are likely immune suppressed due to chemotherapy and radiation, which leads to increased nutrition support and assessment. Parameters of pretreatment nutritional status were evaluated in a study of 101 esophageal patients eligible for neoadjuvant chemoradiation. Body weight, body mass index, handgrip strength, bioelectrical impedance analysis (measure fat-free mass), current energy, and protein intake were collected. Forty-nine percent of patients demonstrated deterioration of nutritional status, and 22% patients lose >5% weight. Malnutrition prevalence increased from pre-chemoradiation 8% to post-chemoradiation 17% [20]. Patients with higher risk for deterioration had higher fat-free mass. It is recommended to carefully evaluate all patients both well-nourished and malnourished.

Perioperative Nutrition

Perioperative nutrition support for patients at high risk for malnutrition has been studied including carbohydrate treatment, vitamin D supplementation, and immunonutrition. Vitamin D deficiency is thought to worsen postoperative lung injury. There is limited data on Vitamin D deficiency and supplementation perioperative for esophagectomy. Immunonutrition refers to supplementation of nutrients including arginine, omega-3 fatty acids, and glutamine. These nutrients enhance the immune system, are anti-inflammatory, and stimulate protein syntheses. Immunonutrition has been reviewed in major surgery, burns, trauma, and critical illness. The timing, delivery method, quantity, and combinations of nutrients have all been studied. In a systematic review of 19 trials, reduced wound infection following gastrointestinal surgery was found. Gastrointestinal surgeries are included in the review: total and subtotal gastrectomy, pancreatectomy, and esophagectomy. Shorter hospital length of stay and reduced risk of wound infection are found with the enteral immunonutrition group, though inconsistencies were found due to study size and population. Also immunonutrition could be beneficial for specific patients (e.g., diabetics and malnourished) [32].

Omega-3 fatty acids (ω-3 fatty acids) are polyunsaturated fatty acids that have a number of functions in the body including reducing inflammation. The three types of omega-3 fatty acids are α-linolenic acid (ALA), eicosapentaenoic acid (EPA), and docosahexaenoic acid (DHA) [33]. Postoperatively following esophagectomy, patients supplemented with enteral immunonutrition formula improved oxygenation and maintained body composition. The formula contained eicosapentaenoic acid, γ-linolenic acid, and antioxidants, and control group received standard formula. All participants were initiated on continuous feedings 48 h post-op and continued for 2 weeks by jejunostomy tube. Subjects did not receive formula preoperatively [34]. The anti-inflammatory properties of immunonutrition formula were thought to improve the oxygenation.

Enhanced recovery after surgery (ERAS) protocol was developed and implemented in colorectal surgery and reduced length of stay without increase in complications. The goal of the protocol is to improve postoperative recovery. ERAS has expanded to include other surgical sites and also involing the multidisciplinary team including dietitians. Benton et al. found patients on ERAS protocol initiated oral intake earlier and upgraded to solids when compared to control group. Patients undergoing esophagectomy were assessed by registered dietitian preoperatively, jejunostomy tube was placed during surgery, and enteral nutrition was initiated day 1 following surgery (Table 17.2) [35]. Overnight fasting prior to surgery depletes glycogen stores and increased catabolism. There is now evidence that clear liquids 2 h prior to surgery and solids 6 h are safe [36]. To reduce the loss of skeletal muscle, carbohydrate loading had gained popularity. Studies on fasting and carbohydrate loading are limited with esophagectomy but have been performed in other

Table 17.2 Diet advancement after esophagectomy

Surgical time frame	Usual care	ERAS
−7	Food diary	Food diary
0	Surgery	Surgery
+1	J tube feeding starts	J tube feeding starts
+3		Clear fluids + J tube
+6	Clear fluids and J tube	Oral fluids + overnight 50% J tube feeds
+7	Oral fluids and J tube feeds	Oral soft diet+ overnight J tube feeds
+8		Discharge
+12	Discharge	

surgeries. Carbohydrate loading 2–3 h prior to surgery shows reduced postoperative insulin resistance and protein loss [29].

Oral intake after esophagectomy is delayed due to risk of aspiration pneumonia and anastomotic leakage. Evidence to evaluate safety is needed. Following immediate oral intake of clear liquids, 28% developed pneumonia compared to 40% of the delayed intake. Tube feeding was required in 38% of patients as oral intake was not tolerated. Advancing oral intake only without enteral may result in insufficient energy and protein intake, worsening malnutrition. Complications should be monitored closely [37].

Early enteral feeding is a consideration to reduce complications after esophagectomy. Early feeding definition has changed over the years and been controversial after an esophagectomy. Subjects that received enteral nutrition within 48 h of surgery had the earliest fecal passage and lowest length of stay and hospitalization expenses. The present study included enteral nutrition initiated within 48 h, 48–72 h, or after 72 h. The longer the length of time to initiate enteral nutrition, the higher the incidence of pneumonia and worse nutrition status [38].

Postoperative

Weight loss following esophagectomy is highest within the first 6 months due to inadequate energy and protein intake and most likely due to long-term gastrointestinal symptoms. Postoperatively patients lost 5–12% of weight at 6 months and >10% at 12 months (Table 17.3) [39]. Other studies have reported 6 months postoperatively weight loss of >10% of body weight in 60% of patients and >20% loss of weight in 20% of studied patients [40]. Enteral nutrition support varied among studies within time frame and percentage of meeting nutrient needs. Demonstrating the importance on long-term nutrition support and management of symptoms.

Home Tube Feeding Postoperatively

Postoperative home jejunostomy feeding varies from centers and is selective based on patients' nutrition at discharge. Indications include post-op complications, poor oral intake tolerance, or increased weight loss. After surgery, enteral nutrition can assist the transition to oral intake while preventing nutrition decline. At 6 weeks patients not using jejunostomy tube lost 3.9 kg more than intervention group receiving enteral feedings. These differences continued at 3–6-month follow-up. Home feeding was re-started in the control group at 33% due to loss of fat and muscle [41]. At discharge oral intake is poor, meeting only 9% for calorie and 6% protein needs. After 3 months, intake improves 61% calorie and 55% for protein needs. In this study, home jejunostomy feedings contributed to calorie and protein needs to supplement poor oral intake. This was an advantage in preventing weight loss and preserving strength. Twenty-six percent of participants not receiving home enteral support required rescue feedings, with overall 76% of participants receiving

Table 17.3 Nutrition symptoms after esophagectomy

Author	Data collection time	Assessment tool	Patient reported symptoms
Ginex et al.	6 m, 12 m	MSAS-SF	Dysphagia 30% (6 m), 22% (12 m) Anorexia 33% (6 m), 27% (12 m) Feeling bloated 40% (6 m), 42% (12 m) Reflux 38% (6 m), 44% (12 m)
Greene et al.	Single point (10–19 yr)	GIQLIMOS SF-36	Dysphagia 12% Postprandial dumping 33% Early satiety 50% Reflux 19%
Haverkort et al.	1 wk, 1 m, 3 m, 6 m, 12 m	Non-validated institutional questionnaire	Dysphagia 53–63% (all time points) Postprandial dumping 74–78% (all time points) Anorexia 51–76% (all time points) Early satiety 87–90% (all time points) Reflux 54–65% (all time points)
McLarty et al.	Single point (5 yr)	Non-validated institutional questionnaire MOS SF-36	Dysphagia 25% Odynophagia 9% Dumping 50% Reflux 60%

jejunostomy feeding [42]. In a result from a prospective cohort study, home enteral nutrition was tolerated with compliance and patient satisfaction. One hundred forty-nine patients were studied, and overnight enteral nutrition by jejunostomy tube continued 4 weeks after discharge. Tube was removed if weight was maintained within 5 kg of discharge weight. At 6 months, 39% of patients lost >10% of weight compared preoperatively. The type of neoadjuvant treatment did not affect weight loss results. Responses from patient satisfaction included enhanced recovery, reduced worry about weight loss, allowed earlier discharge, and reassurance about adequate intake [43], which continues with the question on how much weight loss is acceptable and percentage of supplemental nutrition should be recommended during recovery. Zeng et al. found 12 weeks after esophagectomy incidence of malnutrition was less in patient receiving home enteral nutrition. Patients had resumed fully oral intake within 24 weeks post-surgery. Quality-of-life scores were higher in the enteral group at 12 weeks, but similar to control at 24 weeks. Increased diarrhea was found in the home enteral group which could be related to pump rate and formula selection [44]. Patients decided by themselves when to decrease enteral feedings based on oral intake without recommendations of a trained nutrition professional. To support the benefit of home enteral nutrition, another study found malnutrition was reduced with improved quality of life 3 months after esophageal surgery. BMI, albumin, and hemoglobin were higher in the home enteral nutrition group after

3 months. And patients reported nausea, vomiting, fatigue, and pain [45]. Patients were able to manage feeding tube pump independently after education and guidelines to decrease rate based on improvement in oral intake. Tube feeding placement does have complications including clogging, dislodgement, skin irritation, and leakage. Jejunostomy tube complications were increased in gastrectomy than esophagogastrectomy [46]. The majority of complications were easily resolved by telephone or clinic follow-up. Extended jejunostomy feedings meeting macronutrient and micronutrient needs play an important role in body status and malnutrition.

Long-Term Nutrition

As the survival rate in patients following esophagectomy increases, quality of life is important. Symptoms of dysphagia, reflux, diarrhea, dumping syndrome, and nausea persisted at 12 months. Weight loss greater than 10% at 6 months was found in 41% of patients investigated and 33% at 12 months [47]. Weight loss, persistent eating difficulties, and reduced quality of life have been found to persist up to 10 years in a small cohort study [48], which demonstrate the need for continuous nutrition support for these patients long term. Dietitian-directed nutrition support has been shown to reduce postoperative complications. Twenty-eight patients post-esophagectomy received diet counseling from surgical oncology dietitians. Patients were provided diet recommendations and tube feeding if unable to meet set goals. Patients also received follow-up until a year after surgery. Patients in the nutrition therapy group have increased weight, less postoperative complications, and reduced length of hospital stay [49].

Managing Side Effects

When esophageal patients need to relearn how to eat again nutrition support and education should be provided. Patients can be assisted with making a timetable dividing intake into 5–6 meals daily. Smaller volumes are better tolerated foods with high nutritional content rec. Modify the consistency of food, and give smaller quantities to ease swallowing and prevent fatigue. Food with soft moist texture if solid, creamy if liquids. Foods at room temp, oral hygiene, avoid irritants. For patients who are not able to meet nutritional feedings orally should be.

Side effect	Nutrition intervention
Poor appetite/early satiety	Frequent small meals of calorie-dense foods
	Protein-rich small meals
	Eat by time not by hunger cues/view eating as treatment
	Easy to prepare meals/snacks
	Consume liquids between meals instead of with meals
Nausea/vomiting	Limit exposure to food odors
	Avoid high-fat, greasy foods
	Liquids between meals
	Foods at room temperature

Side effect	Nutrition intervention
Diarrhea/dumping	Multiple small meals
	Avoid fluids with meals
	Avoid intake of simple sugars
	Protein-rich foods
	Increase soluble fiber
Mucositis/esophagitis	Soft foods: add sauce, gravy, and oils
	Oral hygiene
	Limit acidic, citrus-based foods
	Foods at room temperature

Recommendations from patients for improving nutrition care [50]:

- Provide consistent nutrition messaging and practice
- Provide detailed instruction on home tube feeding
- Specialized dietitian assessment with specific goals
- Emphasize real food over oral nutrition supplements
- Educate family members throughout the treatment process
- Discuss rehabilitation at the beginning of treatment and continue after all treatments are completed

Summary

Esophageal cancer patients have many barriers to maintain adequate nutrition status. Increased incidence of malnutrition is associated with reduced treatment efficacy, increased morbidity, and hospital admissions. Nutrition support can be accomplished by increasing oral intake with counseling from RD or supplementing with enteral nutrition. Early nutrition education and support provided earlier in diagnosis and throughout the stages of treatment assist with limiting malnutrition and weight loss. A multidisciplinary approach should be developed to coordinate decisions and improve patient outcomes.

References

1. Straton RJ, Hackston A, Longmore D, Dixon R, Price S, Stroud M, King C, Marinos E. Malnutrition in hospital outpatients and inpatients: prevalence, concurrent validity and ease of use of the 'malnutrition universal screening tool' ('MUST') for adults. Br J Nutr. 2004;92:799–808.
2. Barker LA, Gout BS, Crowe TC. Hospital malnutrition: prevalence, identification and impact on patients and the healthcare system. Int J Environ Res Public Health. 2011;8:514–27.
3. White JV, Guenter P, Jensen G, Malone A, Schofield M, the Academy Malnutrition Work Group, A.S.P.E.N. Malnutrition Task Force and the A.S.P.E.N. Board of Directors. Consensus statement: Academy of Nutrition and Dietetics and American Society for Parenteral and Enteral Nutrition: characteristics recommended for the identification and documentation of adult malnutrition (undernutrition). JPEN J Parenter Enteral Nutr. 2012;36:275–83.
4. Abbott J, Teleni L, McKavanagh D, Watson J, McCarthy A, Isenring E. Patient-generated subjective global assessment short form (PG-SGA SF) is a valid screening tool in chemotherapy outpatients. Support Care Cancer. 2016;24:3883–7.

5. Academy's Oncology Expert Work Group, E. A. (2012).
6. Cederholm T, Barazzoni R, Austin P, Ballmer P, Biolo G, Bischoff S, et al. ESPEN guidelines on definitions and terminology of clinical nutrition. Clin Nutr. 2017;36:49–64.
7. Arends J, Baracos V, Bertz H, Bozzetti F, Calder P, Deutz N, et al. ESPEN expert group recommendations for action against cancer-related malnutrition. Clin Nutr. 2017;36:1187–96.
8. Cao D, Wu G, Zhang B, Quan Y, Wei J, Jin H, et al. Resting energy expenditure and body composition in patients with newly detected cancer. Clin Nutr. 2010;29:72–7.
9. Bosaeus I, Daneryd P, Svanberg E, Lundholm K. Dietary intake, resting energy expenditure in relation to weight loss in unselected cancer patients. Int J Cancer. 2001;93:380–3.
10. Gangadharan A, Choi SE, Hassan A, Ayoub NM, Durante G, Balwani S, et al. Protein calorie malnutrition, nutritional intervention and personalized cancer care. Oncotarget. 2017;8:24009–30.
11. Alves A, Zucnoi CP, Correia MI. Energy expenditure in patients with esophageal, gastric, and colorectal cancer. JPEN J Parenter Enteral Nutr. 2016;40:499–506.
12. Academy EAL. (n.d.).
13. Wu J, Huang C, Xiao H, Tang Q, Cai W. Weight loss and resting energy expenditure in male patients with newly diagnosed esophageal cancer. Nutrition. 2013;29:1310–4.
14. Veronese CB, Guerra LT, Grigolleti SS, Vargas J, Pereira da Rosa AR, Kruel CD. Basal energy expenditure measured by indirect calorimetry in patients with squamous cell carcinoma of the esophagus. Nutr Hosp. 2013;28:142–7.
15. Hamilton KK. Oncology nutrition for clinical practice: nutritional needs of the adult oncology patient. Oncology nutrition dietetic practice group of the academy of nutrition and dietetics. 2013.
16. Harada K, Ida S, Baba Y, Ishimoto T, Kosumi K, Izumi D, et al. Prognostic and clinical impact of sarcopenia in esophageal squamous cell carcinoma. Dis Esophagus. 2016;29:627–33.
17. Guinan E, Doyle S, Bennett A, O'Neill L, Gannon J, Elliott J, et al. Sarcopenia during neoadjuvant therapy for oesophageal cancer: characterising the impact on muscle strength and physical performance. Support Care Cancer. 2018;26:1569–76.
18. Paireder M, Asari R, Kristo I, Rieder E, Tamandl D, Ba-Ssalamah A, Schoppmann S. Impact of sarcopenia on outcome in patients with esophageal resection following neoadjuvant chemotherapy for esophageal cancer. Eur J Surg Oncol. 2017;43:478–84.
19. Anandavadivelan P, Brismar TB, Nilsson M, Johar AM, Martin L. Sarcopenic obesity: a probable risk factor for dose limiting toxicity during neo-adjuvant chemotherapy in oesophageal cancer patients. Clin Nutr. 2016;35:724–30.
20. Rietveld SC, Witvliet-van Nierop J, Ottens-Oussoren K, van der Peet DL, de van der Schueren MA. The prediction of deterioration of nutritional status during chemoradiation therapy in patients with esophageal cancer. Nutr Cancer. 2018;70:1–7.
21. Mak M, Bell K, Ng W, Lee M. Nutritional status, management and clinical outcomes in patients with esophageal and gastro-oesophageal cancers: a descriptive study. Nutr Diet. 2017;74:229–35.
22. Miyata H, Yano M, Yasuda T, Hamano R, Yamasaki M, Hou E, et al. Randomized study of clinical effect of enteral nutrition support during neoadjuvant chemotherapy on chemotherapy-related toxicity in patients with esophageal cancer. Clin Nutr. 2012;31:330–6.
23. Miyata H, Yano M, Yasuda T, Yamasaki M, Murakami K, Makino T, et al. Randomized study of the clinical effects of ω–3 fatty acid-containing enteral formula nutrition support during neoadjuvant chemotherapy on chemotherapy related toxicity in patients with esophageal cancer. Nutrition. 2017;33:204–10.
24. Verma V, Allen PK, Lin SH. Evaluating factors for prophylactic feeding tube placement in gastroesophageal cancer patient undergoing chemoradiotherapy. Font Oncol. 2017;7:235.
25. Modi RM, Mikhail S, Ciombor K, Perry KA, Hinton A, Stanich PP, et al. Outcomes of nutritional interventions to treat dysphagia in esophageal cancer: a population based study. Dis Esophagus. 2017;30:1–8.
26. Cools-Lartigue J, Jones D, Spicer J, Zourikian T, Rousseau M, Eckert E, et al. Management of dysphagia in esophageal adenocarcinoma patients undergoing neoadjuvant chemotherapy: can invasive tube feeding be avoided? Ann Surg Oncol. 2015;22:1858–65.

27. Deldycke A, Daele EV, Ceelen W, Nieuwenhove YV, Pattyn P. Functional outcome after Ivor Lewis Esophagectomy for cancer. J Surg Oncol. 2015;113:24–8.
28. Van Der Schaaf M, Tilanus H, Van Lanschot J, Johar A, Lagergren P, Wijnhoven BP. The influence of preoperative weight loss on the postoperative course after esophageal cancer resection. J Thorac Cardiovasc Surg. 2014;147:490–5.
29. Steenhagen E, van Vulpen JK, Hillegersberg R v, May AM, Siersema PD. Nutrition in perioperative esophageal cancer management. Expert Rev Gastroenterol Hepatol. 2017;11:663–72.
30. Sun J, Wang D, Mei Y, Jin H. Value of the prognostic nutritional index in advanced gastric cancer treated with preoperative chemotherapy. J Surg Res. 2017;209:37–44.
31. Sakai M, Sohda M, Miyazaki T, Yoshida T, Kumakura Y, Honjo H, et al. Association of preoperative nutritional status with prognosis in patients with esophageal cancer undergoing salvage esophagectomy. Anticancer Res. 2018;38:933–8.
32. Wong CS, Aly EH. The effects of enteral immunonutrition in upper gastrointestinal surgery: a systemic review and meta-analysis. Int J Surg. 2016;29:137–50.
33. Omega 3 Supplements: In Depth. (2015, August). Retrieved from National Center for Complementary and Integrative Health: https://nccih.nih.gov/health/omega3/introduction.htm
34. Matsuda Y, Habu D, Lee S, Kishida S, Osugi H. Enteral diet enriched with omega 3 fatty acid improves oxygenation after thoracic esophagectomy for cancer: a randomized controlled trial. World J Surg. 2017;41:1584–94.
35. Benton K, Thomson I, Isenring E, Smithers BM, Agarwal E. An investigation into the nutritional status of patients receiving an enhanced recovery after surgery (ERAS) protocol versus standard care following Oesophagectomy. Support Care Cancer. 2018;26:2057–62.
36. Ljungqvist O. ERAS—enhanced recovery after surgery: moving. JPEN J Parenter Enteral Nutr. 2014;38:559–66.
37. Weijs TJ, Berkelmans GH, Nieuwenhuijzen GA, Dolmans AC, Kouwenhoven EA, Rosman C, et al. Immediate postoperative oral nutrition following esophagectomy: a multicenter clinical trial. Ann Thorac Surg. 2016;102:1141–8.
38. Wang G, Chen H, Liu J, Ma Y, Jin H. A comparison of postoperative early enteral nutrition with delayed enteral nutrition in patients with esophageal cancer. Nutrients. 2015;7:4308–17.
39. Baker ML, Halliday V, Robinson P, Smith K, Bowrey DJ. Nutrient intake and contribution of home enteral nutrition to meeting nutritional requirements after oesophagectomy and total gastrectomy. Eur J Clin Nutr. 2017;71:1121–8.
40. Martin L, Lagergren P. Long-term weight change after esophageal cancer surgery. Br J Surg. 2009;96:1308–14.
41. Bowrey D, Baker M, Halliday V, Thomas AL, Pulikottil-Jacob R, Smith K, et al. A randomised controlled trial of six weeks of home enteral nutrition versus standard care after oesophagectomy or total gastrectomy for cancer: a report on a pilot and feasibility study. Trials. 2015;16:531.
42. Baker M, Halliday V, Williams RN, Bowrey DJ. A systematic review of the nutritional consequences of esophagectomy. Clin Nutr. 2016;35:987–94.
43. Donohoe C, Healy L, Fanning M, Doyle S, Mc Hugh A, Moore J, et al. Impact of supplemental home enteral feeding postesophagectomy on nutrition, body composition, quality of life and patient satisfaction. Dis Esopagus. 2017;30:1–9.
44. Zeng J, Hu J, Chen Q, Feng J. Home enteral nutrition' effect on nutritional status and quality of life after esophagectomy. Asia Pac J Clin Nutr. 2017;26:804–10.
45. Wu Z, Wu M, Wang Q, Zhan T, Wang L, Pan S, Chen G. Home enteral nutrition after minimally invasive esophagectomy can improve quality of life and reduce the risk of malnutrition. Asia Pac J Clin Nutr. 2018;27:129–36.
46. Choi AH, O'Leary MP, Merchant SJ, Sun V, Chao J, Raz DJ, et al. Complications of feeding jejunostomy tubes in patients with gastroesophageal cancer. J Gastrointest Surg. 2017;21:259–65.
47. Soriano T, Eslick G, Vanniasinkam T. Long-term nutritional outcome and health related quality of life of patients following esophageal cancer surgery: a meta analysis. Nutr Cancer. 2018;70:192–203.

48. Anandavadivelan P, Wikman A, Johar A, Lagergren P. Impact of weight loss and eating difficulties in health related quality of life up to 10 years after oesophagectomy for cancer. Br J Surg. 2017;105:410–8.

49. Ligthart-Melis G, Weijs P, te Boveldt N, Buskermolen S, Earthman C, Verheul H, et al. Dietician-delivered intensive nutritional support is associated with a decreased in severe postoperative complications after surgery in patients with esophageal cancer. Dis Esophagus. 2013;26:587–93.

50. Alberda C, Korenic-Alvadj T, Mayan M, Gramlich L. Peer support nutrition care in patients with head and neck or esophageal cancer: the patient perspective. Nutr Clin Pract. 2017;32:664–74.

Printed by Printforce, the Netherlands